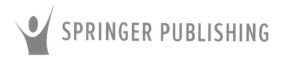 SPRINGER PUBLISHING

GET THE MOST FROM YOUR BOOK

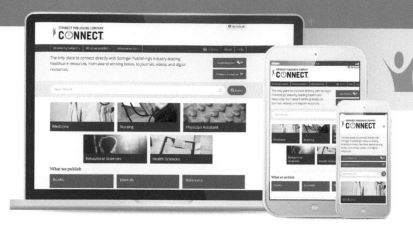

 SPRINGER PUBLISHING
CONNECT™

VOUCHER CODE:

TS3F5WLS

Online Access

Your print purchase of *Delivering Culturally Competent Nursing Care: Working With Diverse and Vulnerable Populations,* Third Edition, includes **online access via Springer Publishing Connect**™ to increase accessibility, portability, and searchability.

Insert the code at http://connect.springerpub.com/content/book/978-0-8261-8302-6 or scan the QR code and insert the voucher code today!

Having trouble? Contact our customer service department at **cs@springerpub.com**

Instructor Resource Access for Adopters

Let us do some of the heavy lifting to create an engaging classroom experience with a variety of instructor resources included in most textbooks SUCH AS:

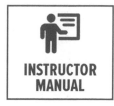

INSTRUCTOR MANUAL

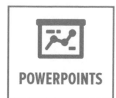

POWERPOINTS

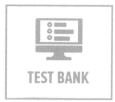

TEST BANK

Visit **https://connect.springerpub.com/** and look for the **"Show Supplementary"** button on your **book homepage** to see what is available to instructors! First time using Springer Publishing Connect?

Email **textbook@springerpub.com** to create an account and start unlocking valuable resources.

DELIVERING CULTURALLY COMPETENT NURSING CARE

Gloria Kersey-Matusiak, PhD, RN, is professor emerita and former coordinator for diversity at Holy Family University. She is an RN educator who has taught both undergraduate and graduate courses in nursing. Dr. Kersey-Matusiak was the 2016 recipient of the Christian R. and Mary F. Lindback Award for Teaching Excellence at Holy Family.

Currently, Dr. Kersey-Matusiak serves as an adjunct in the Health Science Program at St. Joseph's University, teaching Medical Terminology, Health and the School-Aged Child, and Leadership and Diversity in Healthcare.

Dr. Kersey-Matusiak holds a PhD in Psycho-Educational Processes from Temple University; a certificate in Culturally Competent Human Services from the former Multicultural Training and Research Institute, Temple University; an MSN in Nursing from Villanova University; and a BSN from Gwynedd-Mercy University.

As a diversity trainer, Dr. Kersey-Matusiak has led numerous workshops and conferences for various businesses, colleges, and medical institutions on issues of diversity and cultural competence throughout the United States.

Besides teaching heath science and nursing students, Dr Kersey-Matusiak enjoys writing and teaching language skills to people for whom English is a second language (ESL). In 2022, she earned a certificate of program completion at Villanova's Interdisciplinary Studies Training for Immigrant Accompaniment (VIISTA), Advocacy, and Trial Training.

DELIVERING CULTURALLY COMPETENT NURSING CARE

Working With Diverse and Vulnerable Populations

THIRD EDITION

Gloria Kersey-Matusiak, PhD, RN

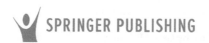 SPRINGER PUBLISHING

First Springer Publishing edition 978-0-8261-9381-0 (2013); subsequent edition 2019

Springer Publishing Company, LLC
902 Carnegie Center/Suite 140, Princeton, NJ 08540
www.springerpub.com
connect.springerpub.com

Acquisitions Editor: Joseph Morita
Compositor: Thomson Digital
Senior Production Manager: Kris Parrish

ISBN: 978-0-8261-8301-9
e-book ISBN: 978-0-8261-8302-6
DOI: 10.1891/9780826183026

SUPPLEMENTS:

 A robust set of instructor resources designed to supplement this text is located at http://connect.springerpub.com/content/book/978-0-8261-8302-6. Qualifying instructors may request access by emailing textbook@springerpub.com.

Instructor Materials:
LMS Common Cartridge (All Instructor Resources) ISBN: 978-0-8261-8305-7
Instructor PowerPoints ISBN: 978-0-8261-8304-0
Mapping to AACN Essentials ISBN: 978-0-8261-8311-8
Transition Guide for the Third Edition ISBN: 978-0-8261-8303-3

24 25 26 27 / 5 4 3 2 1

This book is dedicated to my children, Robbie, Troy, and Brian, and to all my students, past and present, who have inspired and motivated me to write this book.

Contents

Contributors

Claire L. Dente, PhD, MSW, LCSW
Professor of Social Work, West Chester University of Pennsylvania, West Chester, Pennsylvania

Catherine McGeehin Heilferty, PhD, RN
Associate Professor, University of Delaware, Newark, Delaware

Gloria Kersey-Matusiak, PhD, RN
Adjunct Professor, Saint Joseph's University, Professor Emerita, Holy Family University, Philadelphia, Pennsylvania

Janet Roman, DNP, APRN, ACNP-BC, CHFN, ACHPN
Special Advisor of Diversity, Equity, and Inclusion, University of South Florida, Tampa, Florida

Preface

So much has happened since the publication of the last edition of this text just 4 years ago that has forever changed our understanding of what it means to be a nurse. For the first time in my nearly half-century-long career in nursing, two national, unrelated major events and the world's response to them have made a tremendous impact on the profession of nursing: the COVID-19 pandemic and the death of George Floyd. Despite the death and devastation those events left in their wake, there are invaluable lessons learned that give us all much hope for the future.

In the spring of 2020, I had the privilege of teaching a small group of young graduate nursing students at a university, off-campus site at a major trauma center in our city. Students took classes in the evening either before or after their shifts. Many of them worked in the ED or ICU, but had also committed to completing their final courses for the MSN program that term. Then, the COVID-19 pandemic happened, suddenly knocking our schedules, our classes, and us out of kilter. We adjusted class assignments to accommodate the students' rescheduling needs as they attempted to manage the growing numbers of critically ill patients with COVID-19 entering the hospital. Chaos ensued as national and local guidelines and protocols kept changing, having adequate personal protective equipment (PPE) was an issue, and the numbers of patients with COVID-19 accelerated. As COVID-19 raged on, what seemed manageable at first to my graduate nursing students became overwhelming, and the students' anxiety, fears, and frustration were palpable in the classroom. While I was not on the "front lines" with them, I was a first-hand witness to their dedication, perseverance, and resilience. I decided that my role as nursing instructor would include just listening, allowing my students to vent and providing a momentary pressure release before they went back to work in the trenches. At some point the city and the nation began acknowledging the phenomenal work that nurses and other healthcare professionals do while serving on the front lines, rising to whatever the crisis calls for in meeting the health needs of the public. However, this time, it was at great risk to the nurses' own health and the health of their families. As a former critical care nurse myself, I was never prouder to be a nurse than to hear people far and wide hail nurses as "heroes" for their long hours of dedicated service to patients.

Unfortunately, many nurses suffered acute stress disorder (ASD) or posttraumatic stress disorder (PTSD) because of fatigue and burnout, as well as the added psychologic and emotional stress of caring for so many patients dying with COVID-19. According to the National Council of State Boards of Nursing (NCSBN; 2023), approximately 100,000 RNs left the workforce during the COVID-19 pandemic in the last 2 years and 62% of the nurse respondents in the NCSBN study said that their workloads had increased. Some others have simply retired. The profession will need to attract many new nurses to offset the anticipated nursing shortage to meet the demands of an aging and increasingly diverse U.S. society. Nurses are needed now more than ever.

Within this social climate, the murder of a Black man, George Floyd, by a White police officer in Minnesota in May of 2020 was like a one–two punch for communities of color that was felt around the world. The outrage regarding the shooting was shared by Whites, Blacks, and other members of the Black, Indigenous, and People of Color (BIPOC) community. The good news was that irrespective of one's race, the horrific images of George Floyd finally drove home the significance of the moment. There was unprecedented solidarity around the acknowledgement of our common humanity that aroused international civil unrest, protests, and riots in response to the crime. While various past acts of discrimination and racism had often gone ignored, this single act has shone a brilliant light on the human cost of racism in our society.

Having weathered the great storm that was COVID-19 and the emotional aftermath of the George Floyd death, nurses are now armed with new knowledge gained from the invaluable lessons learned from those experiences. I can think of no better time to be a nurse. Therefore, we are excited to present *Delivering Culturally Competent Nursing Care: Working With Diverse and Vulnerable Populations*, Third Edition, to assist nurses on this journey. We have integrated some lessons learned into the content of this text and offer them as support to all nurses seeking to deliver patient-centered, culturally competent care.

LESSON 1: NURSES ARE VULNERABLE TOO

Never has the impact of nurses being frontline workers been clearer. The work of being a nurse already demands long hours and stamina born of good physical and mental health and a strong sense of one's own purpose and commitment to the profession. To serve increasing numbers of culturally diverse populations in a fast-paced, highly technological environment, without sacrificing their own well-being, nurses also need to commit to self-care that will facilitate that effort. We learned from COVID-19 that it is critical for nurses and nursing leaders in the workplace to be supportive of one another to minimize the potential for horizontal violence and burnout, especially during times of health crises. Chapter 3 of the text, Embracing the Diversity Among Our Ranks, focuses on building interpersonal relationships between culturally diverse coworkers, identifying communication and institutional barriers that threaten those relationships, and developing strategies for addressing them. This chapter also examines methods of eliminating the "isms" found in the workplace, such as ageism and racism, as well as horizontal and lateral violence.

LESSON 2: WE ARE ALL IN THIS TOGETHER

During the pandemic, as the reported numbers came in from the Centers for Disease Control and Prevention (CDC) regarding the impact of this devastating disease, it became clear that BIPOC populations were disproportionately represented among those who were sick and dying, especially among older adults with comorbidities. Nursing homes were hit hardest, and according to the CDC, the rate of deaths for Whites accounted for 51.3% of deaths from COVID-19. However, although Blacks and Hispanics represented only 12.5% and 18.5% of the U.S. population, they experienced death rates from COVID-19 of 18.7% and 24%, respectively (Gold et al., 2020). These startling statistics reinforced what we already knew about the power of the social determinants of health (such as inequities in housing, nutrition, physical activity, education, employment, transportation, health insurance, healthcare access, discrimination, and racism). These inequities placed members of BIPOC groups at higher risk of getting and dying from COVID-19, as well as many other diseases. In addition, members of these groups already had prevalence rates of comorbidities like diabetes, hypertension, asthma, and obesity that were higher than that of the general U.S. population. For many, Americans of all races, these comorbidities sealed their unfortunate fates.

LESSON 3: WE CAN DO THIS

In response to the outcry for redress to years of inequalities in healthcare, three important documents offer hope to nurses and other healthcare professionals for the road ahead: The National Academy of Medicine's *Future of Nursing 2020–2030*; the American Association of Colleges of Nursing's (AACN's) *Updated Essentials for Baccalaureate Education*; and the American Nurses Association's (ANA's) Racial Reckoning Statement offer effective strategies for managing the various roles in nursing in a manner that fosters positive interpersonal communication and collegiality between culturally diverse nurses and interdisciplinary partnerships in the workplace that will support all nurses while encouraging their support of one another. Each of these documents calls upon nurses to play an active role in the elimination of discrimination and racism; to reduce the harmful effects of social determinants of health; and to promote health equity and inclusion, as well as social justice in healthcare.

Delivering Culturally Competent Nursing Care: Working With Diverse and Vulnerable Populations, Third Edition, offers the reader an opportunity to focus their attention on groups whose voices are often unheard, those we consider among the vulnerable and less able to speak for themselves. Chapters include cultural considerations when caring for children of diverse groups, victims of human trafficking, veterans, migrants, the terminally ill, and the older adult, among others.

As a follow-up to the *Future of Nursing* report by the former Institute of Medicine in 2021, the National Academy of Medicine (Flaubert et al., 2021) acknowledged in its report, *The Future of Nursing 2020–2030: Charting a Path to Achieve Health Equity and Social Justice,* that nurses play a key role in the health of Americans. Further, the report reminds nurses of their responsibility to address issues of diversity, equity, and inclusion because of their Professional Code of Ethics and because nurses have the potential to be successful based on the long-standing trust society has placed in the profession. The report encourages nurses to promote health equity by addressing social determinants of health to ensure accessible care for all in clinical and community settings. Most importantly, today nurses are being called to use their individual and powerful collective voice (over 4 million strong) to advocate for policy changes to promote social justice.

The AACN has also provided leadership for nurses in this regard through its Cultural Competency Guidelines and Baccalaureate and Graduate Essentials. Since the writing of the first edition of this book, the authors have followed the AACN toolkit of resources written in 2008 for *Cultural Competency in Baccalaureate Nursing Education*. We have done so because each competency provides clear information about the attitudes, knowledge, and skills needed for baccalaureate graduates when working with culturally diverse populations. After reviewing the AACN's newest *Essentials for Undergraduates* that were written in 2021, we find that in writing this text we have adhered to the elements of AACN's domains and subdomains in the *Essentials for Baccalaureate Education* by applying principles of diversity, equity, and inclusion throughout the text; addressing the relationship between social determinants of health and healthcare disparities in each chapter; emphasizing patient-centered care; including current demographic information from reliable data sources in each chapter; providing readers with opportunities for self-assessment to determine their own attitudes and biases; by promoting respect for individual differences; and by maintaining safety and civility in the workplace, which is the focus of Chapter 3.

Readers are directed to use the Staircase Self-Assessment Model, written by the author, to assess their own attitudes and potential biases when caring for each of the selected patient populations. Use of this approach at the end of the chapters also facilitates students' self-analysis of their readiness to provide patient-centered care for the patient described in the case scenarios. Over the past several years, both undergraduates and graduate students have used this model in my classrooms to rate their placement on the Staircase, examine their own beliefs and attitudes, and determine ways to progress in their knowledge, attitudes, and skill development to move up the Staircase. A discussion about how best to utilize the model is found in Chapter 1 of the text.

In January 2021, the ANA, in collaboration with the National Black Nurses Association, National Coalition of Ethnic Minority Nurses Associations, and National Association of Hispanic Nurses, among others, formed the National Commission to Address Racism in Nursing with the goal of exploring racism within nursing nationwide; describe its impact on nurses, patients, communities, and healthcare systems; and to motivate all nurses to confront racism (ANA, 2023). Following a series of listening sessions, a national survey of 5,600 nurses, and a series of reports on how racism shows up in nursing practice and in education, the striking, historic ANA response was the Commission's development of the *Racial Reckoning Statement* in June 2022. The statement offers an apology to nurses of color, extends reconciliation, and makes a commitment to nurses and the profession to continue this work of examining the impact of racism on nursing. The Commission also invites all nurses to join in these efforts. As a member of the ANA and the Transcultural Nursing Society, I have read the document, and commend the Commission for its work and comprehensive review of nursing's history as it relates to racism. I concur with its belief that the change needed in nursing and healthcare will require everyone's contributions. Every nurse has a role to play in addressing the inequalities that have blemished our profession. Through our various roles in healthcare, all of us can make a positive difference.

My colleagues, Claire Dente, Catherine Heilferty, and Janet Roman, the three contributors to this book, and I have tried our best to do exactly that in writing this third edition of *Delivering Culturally Competent Nursing Care: Working With Diverse and Vulnerable Populations*. We believe the battle to overcome racism begins with a self-analysis of one's own implicit biases and the potential to discriminate against others.

As transcultural nurse educators, the co-authors and I wish to join the Academy of Medicine, the AACN, and the ANA in their effort to eliminate racism and to reduce the harmful impact of all the social determinants of health that have led to so many healthcare disparities. This text is our response to the call for all nurses to take action. In this edition, we have added three new chapters that we believe are pertinent to healthcare in the 21st century: Chapter 7, Culturally Competent Care to the Older Adult; Chapter 15, Cultural Considerations for Advanced Practice Registered Nurses (APRNs); and Chapter 16, Delivering Culturally Competent Care to Victims of Human Trafficking. Chapter 10, Cultural Considerations When Caring for the New Immigrant or Refugee, combines two chapters from previous editions, merging the chapter on geographically displaced individuals with a chapter on immigration. We have been intentional in providing activities in the text that afford students opportunities to practice care planning for culturally diverse patient situations before they must confront them in the real world. Many of these cases have been taken from previous clinical experiences of the authors. It is our hope that student nurses and practicing nurse readers will find guidance and support for the challenging situations they confront in the workplace on a regular basis. We have chosen to retain the terms *vulnerable* and *culturally competent* in the title of our text despite some controversy about their use. In our view, cultural competence is the more overarching term that best describes the development of knowledge, attitudes, and skills that one acquires through a lifelong process of self-development, making the term more comprehensive than cultural humility, cultural sensitivity, cultural congruence, or other related terms. In addition, we believe the term *vulnerable* best describes the populations in the text because the social determinants of health and the exposures to discrimination and/or racism have placed the selected populations in the chapters at greater risk for health disparities. Consequently, members of these populations are in fact more vulnerable to disease, illness, and premature death.

We welcome this opportunity to provide a useful tool once again for nurses at all levels to facilitate their personal journey in delivering culturally competent care to the most vulnerable patients of our society. The text is also an effort to raise nurses' spirits about the future of nursing and what is possible for them to achieve in the coming years. We invite our readers to join us in our efforts to combat discrimination, racism, and other barriers that threaten healthcare access to ensure health equity and social justice for all.

Gloria Kersey-Matusiak

REFERENCES

American Association of Colleges of Nursing. (2008). *Cultural competencies in baccalaureate education.* https://www.aacnnursing.org/Portals/42/AcademicNursing/CurriculumGuidelines/Cultural-Competency-Bacc-Edu.pdf

American Nurses Association. (2023). *Our racial reckoning statement.* https://www.nursingworld.org/practice-policy/workforce/racism-in-nursing/RacialReckoningStatement/

Flaubert, J. L., Le Menestrel, S., Williams, D. R., & Wakefield, M. K. (Eds.). (2021). *The Future of Nursing 2020-2030: Charting a Path to Achieve Health Equity.* National Academies Press. https://doi.org/10.17226/25982

Gold, J. A. W., Rossen, L. M., Ahmad, F. B., Sutton, P., Li, Z., Salvatore, P. P., Coyle, J. P., DeCuir, J., Baack, B. N., Durant, T. M., Dominguez, K. L., Henley, J., Annor, F. B., Fuld, J., Dee, D. L., Bhattarai, A., & Jackson, B. R. (2020). Race, ethnicity, and age trends in persons who died from COVID-19—From May to August 2020. *Morbidity and Mortality Report, 69*(42), 1517–1521. https://doi.org/10.15585/mmwr.mm6942e1

National Council of State Boards of Nursing. (2023). *NCSBN research projects significant nursing workforce shortages and crisis.* https://www.ncsbn.org/news/ncsbn-research-projects-significant-nursing-workforce-shortages-and-crisis

Acknowledgments

I remain forever grateful to the Divine and Holy Presence that guides my life and sustains my belief that all people matter and that we have a collective and individual responsibility to one another. With much humility and gratitude, I extend my sincere thanks to all the angels who were sent to support and encourage me during the writing of this edition: colleagues, family, and friends too numerous to name. Special thanks to my colleagues and friends Dr. Claire Dente and Dr. Catherine Heilferty, who once again said yes, despite their busy schedules and responsibilities, to helping me give voice to those who too often go unheard—the children of culturally diverse backgrounds and members of the LGBTQIA+ community. I extend my heartfelt appreciation for their invaluable contributions to this work. I also thank Dr. Janet Roman, who offered our readers a peek into the world of APRNs and their care of vulnerable populations. Thank you for sharing your wisdom and expertise and for inspiring and encouraging our readers to consider delivering culturally competent care throughout their careers. Thank you to Joe Morita, for his guidance, patience, understanding, and support throughout this project. without which this book would not be possible.

To all my personal angels, thank you for always being there. To my dear friend Connie, thank you for caring and sharing all these years, and for always encouraging me to keep going with this project. Love and much gratitude to my siblings Ernestine, Barbara, Ernest, and Evon for your love and support and for lifting me up during the physical challenges I faced during the writing of this edition. To my husband and fellow nurse, Bob, thank you for patiently traveling this journey with me again and for being the steady loving presence in my life. Finally, to my children, Robbie, Troy, and Brian, the light of my life and reason for being, I extend unwavering and unconditional love. To Rakeem, Lil' Troy, Brennen, Kahlil, Ariel, and Isaiah Franklin Kersey, thank you for the laughter and love that enriches my life, nourishes my spirit, and gives me great joy.

Gloria Kersey-Matusiak

Instructor Resources

 A robust set of instructor resources designed to supplement this text is located at http://connect.springerpub.com/content/book/978-0-8261-8302-6. Qualifying instructors may request access by emailing textbook@springerpub.com.

Instructor resources include:

- LMS Common Cartridge–All Instructor Resources

- Instructor PowerPoints

- Mapping to AACN Essentials: Core Competencies for Professional Nursing Education

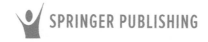

I

BUILDING CULTURAL COMPETENCY SKILLS

1

Defining Cultural Competency

Gloria Kersey-Matusiak

Faith is taking the first step, even when you don't see the whole staircase.
—MARTIN LUTHER KING JR.

LEARNING OBJECTIVES

After this chapter, the reader will be able to

1. Provide a rationale for a nurse to become culturally competent.
2. Define cultural competency as it relates to nursing practice.
3. Differentiate cultural competence from cultural humility.
4. Recall the American Association of Colleges of Nursing (AACN) cultural competencies for baccalaureate graduates.
5. Describe diversity in terms of healthcare populations and personnel in the 21st century.
6. Utilize the Staircase Self-Assessment Model as a means of determining one's level of cultural competency.
7. Determine strategies for strengthening culturally competent knowledge and skills.
8. Define related terms used in this chapter.
9. Identify relevant resources for further study of this topic.
10. Describe the impact of social determinants of health as they relate to healthcare disparities in the United States.

KEY TERMS

Acculturate	Culture
Assimilate	Diversity
CLAS standards	Healthcare disparities
Cultural competence	Reflective listening
Cultural humility	Social determinants of health
Cultural sensitivity	

WHY CULTURAL COMPETENCY?

Why Cultural Competence?

Because of the increasing global migration of refugees, asylum seekers, and other migrants, nurses often care for patients from cultural backgrounds that differ from their own (Kuwano & McMaster, 2020; Nolan et al., 2021). In addition, within the United States inequities exist between different cultural backgrounds regarding access to care, quality of care, and, consequently, healthcare outcomes. According to *Healthy People 2030*, "in the United States, 1 in 10 people live in poverty, and many people can't afford things like healthy foods, health care, and housing" (Office of Disease Prevention and Health Promotion, n.d.-a, para. 1). In a society where great wealth exists for some, those who are without health insurance or healthcare providers seek care only when they are very ill; at that point, healthcare is much more costly and sometimes too late to make a significant difference in health outcomes. Unfortunately, despite some efforts to address these issues over the past several years, limited healthcare access and disparities among members of marginalized and lower socioeconomic groups persist.

Social Determinants of Health

These disparities are attributed to the **social determinants of health**. In March 2005, the World Health Organization (WHO) created the Commission on the Social Determinants of Health (CSDH) with the goal of promoting global healthcare equity and an aim to foster health policy and social change between and within countries where major differences in health indicators existed. The CSDH wrote its final report in 2008. The group identified gross inequalities in health between countries such as differences in life expectancy at birth that ranged from 34 years in Sierra Leone to 81.9 years in Japan (Marmot, 2005). Even within countries like the United States, a 20-year gap in life expectancy existed between those "most and least advantaged" (Marmot, 2005, p. 1099). In another example of inequalities, child mortality rates varied between and within countries based on the socioeconomic level of the family. Thus, poorer health as evidenced by both communicable and noncommunicable disease and injury was linked to social conditions: poverty, education, living conditions, food security, access to safe drinking water, environmental conditions like clean unpolluted air, and access to medical care, among other prerequisites for optimal health. Further, the CSDH examined "causes of the causes" such as stress, social exclusion, unemployment, and one's early life and its impact on health.

In its recommendations, the CSDH stressed the need to address health disparities by identifying their social causes and recognizing that these disparities between and within countries are avoidable. Further, the members of the CSDH concluded that social inequalities in health are a matter of social justice. In addition, the goals of *Healthy People 2030* include the achievement of health equity, the elimination of health disparities, and the improvement of health for all. Because a primary goal of this text is to promote equity and social justice in healthcare for all, the concepts of **healthcare disparities** and the social determinants of health are integrated throughout the chapters where relevant. For example, the chapter on the poor and uninsured describes determinants socioeconomic status, poverty, and its impact on those who are medically uninsured.

Moreover, as people of all races and ethnicities age and suffer some of the chronic illnesses and cognitive, sensory, and functional losses that are common among older people, nurses will be expected to provide culturally sensitive care to older adults that addresses their specific cultural needs. Therefore, nurses in their day-to-day interactions with patients from culturally diverse groups are compelled to identify creative and effective ways of addressing these unfortunate dilemmas.

Madeleine Leininger, nurse, anthropologist, and founder of transcultural nursing, was visionary in her recognition of the need for nurses to provide care that was culturally congruent with their patients' "beliefs, values, and caring lifeways" (Nursing Theory, 2023). Leininger's theory, Culture Care Diversity and Universality, is also called Culture Care. Madeleine Leininger's Nursing Theory (nursing-theory.org) was developed in the 1950s, although it was published in 1991. Since that time, Leininger's seminal theory and lifelong work have served as guiding lights for nurses' clinical practice, education, and research.

Led by that work, later nurse theorists and other nurse leaders that followed Leininger have reminded nurses of her rich legacy and encouraged them to apply Culture Care Theory to their clinical practice. In support of those efforts, the American Nurses Association (ANA) in 2015 revised its Standards of Practice to include Standard 8: Culturally Congruent Care, and encouraged RNs to practice "in a manner that is congruent with cultural diversity and inclusion principles" (ANA, 2015, p. 69).

Additionally, to address the "[s]hifting U.S. population demographics, health workforce shortages, and persistent health inequities," (p. 5), the American Association of Colleges of Nursing (AACN), in outlining its undergraduate and graduate essentials for nursing education for the 21st century, stressed the need for diversity, equity, and inclusion as important values that support nursing workforce development and the preparation of nurses who can promote access to quality care for underserved populations. AACN also included among its 10 domains *person-centered care*, which is described in part as being care that "considers and includes the cultural context of the individual, family, and community" (AACN, 2022, p. 1).

Today, as the United States becomes increasingly more diverse, there seems to be a wide acceptance of the need for cultural competence among nurses. However, the controversy seems to be over what language or words best describe the goals and nurse behaviors that are appropriate to achieve it. Also, some nurses are concerned that cultural competence, while a lofty goal, is unlikely to be achieved in one's lifetime (Kersey-Matusiak, 2012). Rather, it is an ideal to aim for recognizing it as a lifetime endeavor. This caveat has always been true for those who are proponents of cultural competency (The Joint Commission, 2014).

So, Cultural Competency or Cultural Humility?

Others believe that perhaps nurses should strive for the attainment of **cultural humility** instead because it is action oriented and, as defined by many, "a lifetime commitment to self-evaluation and critique, to redressing power imbalances" (Nolan et al., 2021, p. 4). These authors believe that "cultural humility surpasses the knowledge-based notion of cultural competence" because it emphasizes actions that foster excellent patient care outcomes, heightens and redirects **cultural sensitivity**, shares power, and demands reverence for the patient perspectives in care when decision-making (Nolan et al., 2021; Zinan, 2021). Becze (2021) considered cultural humility as a clinical competency that may be used to overcome implicit and explicit bias among health professionals and achieve patient-centered care. Pierce-McDaniel (2021) touts the acceptance of cultural humility by many other disciplines "as an achievable guidance of patient centered care" (p. 12). Zinan (2021) proposed a Humility in Healthcare Model and identified the related behaviors that nurses can utilize to provide care. Using Zinan's model, the nurse begins incorporating humility in practice through self-reflection and self- critique, asking "internal questions" (p. 8) that examine potential sociocultural barriers to a therapeutic relationship. Active listening, flexibility in negotiation, and an openness to new paradigms of care are all aspects of this process of applying humility. Through this process, the nurse acknowledges their strengths and limitations as the care provider while elevating the patient's status to partner in this relationship, thereby establishing a relationship between patient and nurse that is born of mutual respect.

This writer believes that, while the evidence in support of cultural humility as a means of fostering a stronger and more egalitarian relationship between nurse and client is clear, demonstrating humility is still only one of the ways to ensure improved patient outcomes. The overarching goal for nurses remains gaining a level of cultural competence that includes building cultural knowledge. That knowledge is best gleaned from interacting with many patients from culturally diverse backgrounds. Developing the appropriate skills in listening and assessing each of them to determine what is best to do in their interests is a critical part of the process. Nurses need to use an arsenal of strategies to redress power imbalances and healthcare disparities. Yes, we must do these things with humility, acknowledging that neither the nurse, nor the physician for that matter, has all the answers. Nurses who demonstrate cultural humility also recognize that each member of the healthcare team can make mistakes, but each is willing to share in the decision-making with the patient. It is through the way we go about gaining cultural knowledge, listening actively, acknowledging the patient's role in care planning, and affirming the patient's dignity and value that we demonstrate cultural humility. In this way, the nurse embraces and acts on Leininger's message of providing care that is culturally congruent with the needs of the patient. Through an ongoing striving toward Leininger's vision, nurses become the best that they can be, always moving toward cultural competence, that distant star on the horizon, with cultural humility being the road they take to get there.

Culture, for purposes of this text, is defined as "the totality of socially transmitted behavioral patterns, arts, beliefs, customs, lifeways, and all other products of human work and thought characteristics of a population of people that guide their worldview and decision-making" (Purnell, 2013, p. 6). Culture is dynamic, because individuals' values, beliefs, and attitudes change or evolve with their life experiences. For example, many new immigrants bring with them certain values, attitudes, beliefs, languages, and talents. During an immigrant's stay in America, that individual may initially hold fast to their traditional beliefs and practices, but over time may adopt some of the cultural values and patterns of behavior held by the majority of Americans. The fact that culture is a determinant of one's healthcare decisions is well supported in the literature (Kersey-Matusiak, 2012; Purnell, 2019; Spector, 2017; U.S. Department of Health and Human Services [DHHS], 2016). Moreover, wide variations in access to healthcare and to specific treatment modalities have long been observed between members of culturally diverse groups. Linkages among culture, diversity, morbidity, response to treatment, and mortality are also well documented (ODPHP, n.d.-b). In some cases, these linkages among diseases, life expectancy, and cultural group membership seem inexplicable, suggesting a need for further medical and nursing research. The Centers for Disease Control and Prevention (CDC) National Prevention Information Network (2021) reports that such differences have led to healthcare disparities. These disparities include diseases and other illnesses that "disproportionately afflict individuals who are members of racial and ethnic minority groups" (Thomson et al., 2006, p. 185). High infant mortality rates, cancer mortality, and death from coronary heart disease and diabetes are some of the conditions that affect minority group members at higher rates than Whites in the United States. A vision held by the National Institute on Minority Health and Health Disparities is "an America in which all populations will have an equal opportunity to live long, healthy, and productive lives (2022, "Vision"). Many researchers emphasize the need for cultural competence in healthcare to address health disparities and to ensure equitable services for all (Jeffreys & Zoucha, 2018; Pierce McDaniel, 2021; Purnell, 2019).

Cultural competency frameworks and models are readily available to assist nurses in their journey toward cultural competency. For example, Giger et al. (2017) offered an early assessment model using six cultural phenomena. Some of these frameworks are presented in Chapter 2. While there are several models and frameworks available in the literature, this text will focus on the use of Purnell's Model for Culturally Competent Healthcare and the GKM Staircase Self-Assessment Model for nurses (Kersey-Matusiak, 2001). Limiting the focus of the discussion in the text to two models will afford readers an opportunity to concentrate their efforts on applying each of them during their clinical experiences. Colleges and universities, through their mission statements, policies, and recruitment efforts, are attempting to strengthen their diversity. These institutions recognize the need to provide a more diverse and culturally rich college experience for their students to better prepare them for citizenship in a multicultural society. All these efforts support the idea that nurses are called to become culturally competent if they are to be effective in delivering care in the 21st century and in helping to eliminate the healthcare disparities that exist.

For the purposes of this text, cultural competence is defined using the AACN's definition. This definition and the identified competencies are written as a framework for baccalaureate and masters level prepared nursing graduates (AACN, 2021). **Cultural competence** is defined as the attitudes, knowledge, and skills necessary for providing quality care to diverse populations. Although there are many other definitions found in nursing literature, most contain these three fundamental hallmarks of what it means for a nurse to be culturally competent. The attitudes one needs to be culturally competent include having an openness to an ongoing self-reflection about one's own values, beliefs, biases, and prejudices, and having a willingness to consider another individual's or group's perspective or worldview. This is not to say that culturally competent nurses adopt each patient's beliefs and attitudes; rather, the nurse accepts that differences exist between nurse and patient and is motivated to work toward transcending those differences for the sake of the nurse–patient relationship.

In addition to having attitudes that support positive interactions between nurses and culturally diverse patients, nurses must also be able to acquire cultural knowledge about themselves and the patient. The cultural assessment model that the nurse selects helps determine the kind of information needed to assess patients from diverse backgrounds. However, the nurse needs to know about the patient's history in the United States, geographical origin, the cultural or ethnic background, the context or situation, and the diversity within the group of reference. When nurses are able to obtain information about each of these areas, they are able to view the patient holistically and from the patient's cultural perspective.

The culturally competent nurse must also utilize various skills effectively to deliver care that is congruent with patients' cultural values. Primarily, these skills are communication skills that enhance the nurse–patient rapport and include active and **reflective listening**, speaking to patients using language they understand, interviewing the patient using a cultural assessment tool, and thinking critically to problem-solve cross-culturally. Reflective listening refers to a process of communication in which the nurse or other healthcare providers listen to the patient for understanding and intermittently seek clarification to be sure that they are accurately interpreting the patient's words. This style of communicating is especially important when the patient's verbal communication does not seem to reflect the nonverbal. Nurses must also keep in mind that medical jargon is a language all its own, and as such probably unfamiliar to most patients. Therefore, speaking to all patients in a language they understand means minimizing the use of medical jargon as much as possible and reserving it for use with colleagues and other healthcare providers. Communication is even more compromised when the patient and nurse speak different languages. When that is the case, a medically trained interpreter is the ideal person to translate for the nurse. The process of interpreting requires training and healthcare knowledge that family members and other laypeople who speak the language may not have. To maintain the patient's privacy, confidentiality, and comfort, clinicians should avoid using children to translate.

To obtain accurate cultural information about the patient, the nurse must *interview and assess* the patient and/or family using appropriate language and behaviors for the situation. Without some cultural knowledge of the patient's cultural norms and preferences, the chances of unintentionally making offensive remarks or demonstrating behaviors that the patient considers inappropriate increases. Therefore, nurses are encouraged to gain specific cultural knowledge about the populations they serve on a regular basis. It is impossible for nurses to know everything about all the various culturally diverse groups they may encounter; however, there are many current texts that nurses can reference to gain specific knowledge about a particular group. These include Purnell and Fenkl (2020), Spector (2017), and Giger and Haddad (2020). The more nurses experience individuals from the same group, the more they can strengthen their cultural knowledge. However, simply having knowledge about cultural groups is not enough, because nurses must also be able to apply what they know about themselves and their patients in various clinical situations. In addition, the nurse must be able to think critically about the information and to engage in cross-cultural problem-solving when it is needed.

In other words, nurses who can think critically about the patient's cultural needs will also be able to identify potential cultural conflicts among individuals, families, and/or institutions. These nurses identify cultural differences, determine their impact on care, and develop strategies for overcoming them. Nurses who function at this level of cultural competency can serve as mentors for others. Each of the previously described cultural competency skills takes patience and time for the nurse to develop. Most importantly, skill development takes practice.

The more knowledgeable nurses and other healthcare workers become about diversity as it impacts healthcare, the more likely they are to make a significant impact on healthcare disparities. The challenge, then, is for nurses and other healthcare providers to strive toward cultural competence and to begin implementing changes in care provision that respond to the needs of an increasingly diverse patient population.

DIVERSITY IN AMERICA

Throughout the history of the United States, diversity has always been a resilient and inter-woven thread that strengthens the fabric of our society. No longer considered a melting pot, America has more recently been likened to a beautiful mosaic or quilt, reflecting the diverse colors and attributes of the many people who have come to this country from different shores. Most often, Americans have benefited from the rich contributions of its culturally diverse people. At other times, however, differences in attitudes, beliefs, values, religion, language, and other characteristics threaten to undermine the ability of culturally diverse groups to coexist and to benefit equally from the nation's resources.

For the purposes of this text, **diversity** refers to all aspects of difference that may be found among healthcare populations as well as the intersectionality of those differences. Increasingly, both the nature and scope of our nation's diversity has changed to include a wide range of differences between and among members of diverse groups. Diversity in healthcare today includes, but is not limited to, age, culture, race, gender, ethnicity, language differences, sexual orientation, socioeconomic status, immigration status, military or veteran status, and any other group membership that may negatively influence one's access to culturally competent care. Moreover, intracultural or within-group differences may also have a significant influence on healthcare. Differences such as patterns or styles of communication, attitudes toward authority, and ways of knowing, addressing conflict, and making decisions may all differ even within the same ethnic or racial group based on one's age, gender, or personality. For example, today's political environment is one of polarization along partisan lines with party membership dictating some individuals' attitudes toward healthcare policies. However, research tells us that even within each sociopolitical group there are individuals who differ with one another. Therefore, one can never assume that one's beliefs are completely dictated by the party to which one belongs. The same applies to membership in racial, ethnic, or age groups. Therefore, the author warns nurses against adopting a "recipe" approach to assessing patients' specific healthcare needs based solely on commonalities attributed to the cultural group of reference. Cuellar (2017) reminded us that culturally competent care can only be delivered when patients values, beliefs and care needs are known. Recognizing the intragroup differences within patient populations will ensure that care is based on an accurate assessment of patients' specific care needs. Immigrants also differ in their desire to **assimilate** or **acculturate**, or not, based on their reasons for immigration. Acculturation refers to adapting or taking on some parts of another culture, whereas assimilation refers to being absorbed into another culture and relinquishing one's own (Im, 2015).

Among new immigrants, some, but not all, are able to communicate fluently in English. Those who cannot are much less able to negotiate the healthcare system. New immigrants with limited English skills must rely on hospitals and healthcare personnel to identify and respond to their specific health needs despite difficulties in communicating with them. Today, several institutions have accepted this challenge.

DIVERSITY AND HEALTHCARE

The DHHS Office of Minority Health, in its publication of the National Standards for Culturally and Linguistically Appropriate Services (CLAS) in healthcare, affirmed the need for nurses to become culturally competent (DHHS, 2001, 2004, 2016). These standards serve as a guide for all healthcare providers. Some serve as mandates to hospitals to conform to those standards deemed necessary in providing culturally competent healthcare. These 15 guidelines and mandates are intended to ensure equitable care for all patients. Since the inception of the **CLAS standards**, the response to them has been positive. Administrators of U.S. hospitals recognize the need for healthcare providers to understand the impact of language and culture on the quality of patient care. Patient safety is also impacted by the patient's and staff's ability to communicate effectively with one another. Therefore, qualified interpreters are needed to assist in improving health literacy and patient safety.

Having a diverse healthcare staff that is inclusive of age, culture, race, ethnicity, and religion is one way to better serve a diverse patient population. However, limited ethnic diversity within nursing's rank and file and society's general intolerance of difference are factors that hinder nurses' progress in becoming culturally competent. Although there has been a gradual increase in diversity within nursing, gender, ethnic, and racial diversity remains disproportionate to that of American society. For example, according to the National Council of State Boards of Nursing (NCSBN®) 2020 National Nursing Workforce Survey (2022), males accounted for 9.4% of the RN workforce in nursing, an increase of 0.3% since 2017. Black or African American nurses have also increased in number within the RN population and now more closely match their numbers (14%) in the U.S. population, growing from 6.0% in 2013 to 6.7% in 2020. However, both White RNs at 80.6% and Asian nurses at 7.2% are overrepresented, while Hispanic nurses are greatly underrepresented among the RN population at 5.6% as compared to their numbers (18.9%) in the U.S. population (NCSBN, 2022; U.S. Census Bureau, 2020). Data from the NCSBN survey reveal an aging nurse population with a median age of 52; 19% of nurses are 65 years and older, up from 14.6% in 2017 and 4.4% in 2013. This trend is expected to continue and is reflective of the aging U.S. population.

Curtin (2016) discussed the current multigenerational workforce and explained the challenges that it poses for the nursing leadership. Because nurses working today come from three different generations, there is the potential for intergenerational conflict based on their respective differences. The top causes of intergenerational conflict identified by the writer included "an aging workforce [with limited tolerance for certain behavior], continuation of historically embedded power inequities, lack of conflict-management training, [and] intolerance for the values and prejudices of older generations" (p. 48). In addition, this writer identified social changes like "increased incivility, pressures on families . . ., anxieties related to increased global tensions and diversity, vulnerabilities in a terror-filled world, and individuals' unmet expectations" (p. 48) as factors that make it even more difficult for diverse groups to work together. Curtin provided several strategies for minimizing the conflict that naturally results in such settings. She encouraged nurses to maintain an awareness of the nature of the diversity within the group; develop nonconfrontational strategies and behaviors; be careful of timing when raising an issue; be clear about the real issues; choose their words carefully; and, when someone complains, to listen.

In addition to the generational diversity of nurses, racial and ethnic diversity results from the migration of nurses from Asia, the Philippines, Africa, the Caribbean, and other places who are recruited to work alongside domestic nurses in the United States, Canada, United Kingdom, Australia, and Ireland. Tuttas (2015) discussed the perceptions of migrant or foreign-born minority nurses (MMN) of racial and ethnic prejudice and discrimination when working with domestic-born nurses. The writer identified various types of perceived discrimination, including isolate discrimination, small-group discrimination, direct institutional discrimination, and indirect institutional discrimination. At times, acts of discrimination were perceived to be perpetrated by patients and families toward the migrant nurses, while at other times these acts were behaviors exhibited by domestic nurses toward migrant nurses. This researcher found that the literature provides much evidence of "dominant group behavior aiming to protect a perceived domain that incorporates entitlements such as access to career advancement, placement in choice jobs, inclusion in social circles, recognition of competency, and acceptance as an equal team member" (p. 519). Further, Tuttas noted, while all of the nursing agencies and organizations encourage nurses to provide ethical and nondiscriminatory care to patients, there are no correlating statements or codes of conduct that advocate for nurses being nondiscriminatory to MMN. The author stated that research suggested a need for explicit position statements from the top nursing organizations on this behavior to foster policy development to address this problem. Tuttas also noted that recurrent training and monitoring were identified in the literature as a means of reducing nurse-to-nurse racial harassment. The literature also revealed that "perceptions of discrimination can be mitigated when the host country invests in measures to facilitate social networks and support for migrant nurses" (p. 519).

As Curtin (2016) reminded us, nurses usually manage to get along well despite our increasing diversity, because we all value the important work that we do. With these thoughts in mind, nurses should be encouraged to always strive toward maintaining a more nurturing and supportive work environment in which all nurses can thrive and deliver high-quality patient care (see Chapter 3).

PATIENT DIVERSITY

Efforts to deliver culturally competent care to patients from culturally diverse populations can be found throughout the healthcare literature (CDC NPN, 2021; Furness et al., 2020; Jeffreys & Zoucha, 2018; Rising, 2017; Substance Abuse and Mental Health Services Administration [SAMHSA], 2022; Tierney, 2017). For example, the ' SAMHSA website provides information regarding the care and treatment of military persons and veterans, especially those with limited English proficiency. The site emphasizes the need for providers to deliver patient-centered and culturally competent care that addresses the diversity within the military population. Toward that end, SAMHSA provides cultural competency training during orientation and at reasonable intervals for its care providers. In another study, Tierney (2017) explored nurses' attitudes toward patients with substance disorders in a review of the literature and identified intolerance, anger, distrust, powerlessness, anxiety, feelings of being manipulated, frustration, and disappointment among the many feelings expressed by nurses. Some nurses viewed substance abusers as irresponsible and treatment for them as hopeless. Further, the researcher noted, the literature revealed that "surveys from more recent years showed an improvement in nurses' attitudes, especially among younger nurses, although a significant minority continued to hold negative attitudes or biases toward substance abusers" (p. 7). These results have important implications for nurses caring for veterans and others experiencing problems with substance abuse. The researcher found that education on substance abuse and nursing support helped decrease bias in nurses toward substance abusers by reducing nurses' frustration and sense of powerlessness about caring for this population of patients, while improving their confidence and job satisfaction when caring for members of this group. Ashley and colleagues (2021) also identified special considerations for nurses working with veterans, especially during the pandemic, and suggested screening all patients for veteran status, recognizing their high risk for posttraumatic stress disorder (PTSD), depression, anxiety, and suicidal ideation. These writers reminded nurses of veterans' higher access to firearms, higher risk for suicide, and the need for nurses to build trust by creating a judgment-free setting. In such settings, a patient-centered relationship can be established and patients can be assisted in developing more appropriate and healthy coping strategies.

Furness and colleagues (2020) discussed the multiple disparities encountered by persons who are LGBT and the need to provide culturally affirming care for members of this population. Despite an increasing general acceptance of members of this group by society, many "continue to encounter stigma, bias, and discrimination in their daily lives" (p. 292). As the writers observe, chronic exposure to stressors and anti-LGBT stigma results in a myriad of problems that lead to decreased healthcare access and ultimately to disparities in health outcomes. Differences in sexual orientation are often overlooked in books that focus on cultural diversity and cultural competency; however, individuals who are gay, lesbian, bisexual, or transgender bring unique issues and concerns to the healthcare arena (see Chapter 9).

In 2015, at least 37 states and D.C. recognized same-sex marriage and all states had some court case pending on this topic (National Conference of State Legislatures [NCSL], 2015), but in June 2015, in a landmark decision by the Supreme Court, same-sex marriage became legal in all 50 states (Liptak, 2015). Yet, there are still many people in America who view the family as consisting solely of a married man and woman and their children. In many states, unmarried gay and lesbian partners in long-term relationships may be denied healthcare benefits for their partners and consequently worry about accessing healthcare, particularly as they age. This is because despite same-sex marriage being legalized, "growing numbers of employers have eliminated domestic partner health coverage... requiring couples to be married before an employee's partner can receive health care benefits" (Hannon, 2017, para. 2). Factors influencing these decisions include company culture and the desire to be inclusive and equitable, perceptions of fairness, and administrative costs to provide these benefits. The topic of caring for LGBTQIA will be explored more fully in Chapter 9.

Jeffreys and Zoucha (2018) explained the importance of promoting cultural congruence in the workplace, healthcare, and academic settings to accommodate the increasing number of multiracial and multiheritage individuals, those who identify with more than one race or ethnicity. In this article, the writers describe members of this population as "invisible and the fifth minority, because they are individuals whose cultural backgrounds and needs are often hidden and unmet" (p. 113). Using case scenarios, the writers demonstrate how outcome disparities may result from the use of culturally incongruent strategies and suggest using Leininger's Culture Care Theory and Jeffrey's Cultural Competence and Confidence model as a framework for assessment and decision-making to make a positive difference in outcomes.

Another area of difference that exists among healthcare recipients is socioeconomic status. The impact of poverty on health, irrespective of one's culture, race, or ethnicity; gender; or sexual orientation, is profound. Although minorities and some new immigrants represent a higher percentage of those who live below the poverty level, among all patients who are poor, many lack health insurance and are less able to access appropriate medical care. The topic of caring for the poor and uninsured is discussed in Chapter 11.

Despite differences among and between groups, as members of the human family every individual is in need of acceptance and understanding. Nurses are challenged to acknowledge the uniqueness of all individuals, families, and groups while recognizing their patients' ties to the rest of society. Nurses who acknowledge cultural differences while establishing collaborative partnerships with patients from diverse populations maximize their potential to provide culturally competent care. These nurses gain new insights by acting with cultural humility and relinquishing their power over patients to determine what the patient actually needs and wants. Differences between the patient and the nurse are considered, but the patient is always treated with dignity and respect despite those differences. The reader is encouraged to view "diversity" from an inclusive perspective and consider all the aspects of difference to have the potential to influence the quality of care a patient receives.

Today, the decision to develop cultural competency skills can no longer be viewed as optional for nurses. If nurses are ever to gain insight into the needs of their culturally diverse patients, they must view each patient's healthcare situation through that patient's own cultural lens. To gain the respect and trust of the culturally diverse groups they serve, nurses must be willing to provide care that is relevant and congruent with their patients' own healthcare values and beliefs, just as Leininger encouraged nurses to do many years ago (Leininger & McFarland, 2005).

Moreover, despite being the largest group of healthcare providers, nursing is but a microcosm of the society it represents. Consequently, the profession is plagued by the same societal ills, sexism, racism, homophobia, elitism, ageism, sizeism, and a host of other biases that exist in the larger society. Each of these characteristics can negatively influence the quality of care that some nurses provide and may prohibit them from being effective when working with individuals outside of their own reference groups. In becoming culturally competent, nurses learn to better address the specific needs of all patients and become much better prepared to work cooperatively as members of an increasingly diverse workforce. In settings where cultural competency is emphasized, nurses are encouraged to accept the differences and to treat colleagues with cultural sensitivity and respect. Interactions between members of diverse groups offer opportunities for professional growth in cultural knowledge and skill development. In such settings, nurses strive to provide one another with the same degree of cultural awareness and sensitivity that they are expected to provide their patients. Despite the many challenges, becoming culturally competent can be a rewarding experience that enhances both nurse–patient and nurse-to-nurse interactions.

UTILIZING THE STAIRCASE SELF-ASSESSMENT MODEL

The Cultural Competency Staircase Self-Assessment Model was developed in 1991 by the author as a self-assessment tool to assist student nurses and practicing nurses in assessing their personal level or degree of cultural competency. This model builds on ideas proposed by Cross (2012), who described a continuum of cultural competency with six stages: cultural destructiveness, cultural incapacity, cultural blindness, precompetency, basic cultural competency, and advanced cultural competency. As a nurse educator, the author over the past several years has observed both students and practicing nurses to be more easily grouped into the categories described by the Staircase Self-Assessment Model. Another purpose of the Staircase Self-Assessment Model is to provide nurses with a method of progressive movement through the various steps. This approach fosters the ongoing development of a nurse's cultural awareness, knowledge, skills, and expertise in cultural competency. Therefore, culturally competent behaviors must be adaptable to the changing or evolving needs of individuals within culturally diverse groups.

The Staircase Self-Assessment Model describes salient characteristics of the nurse at the various steps in becoming culturally competent; however, these characteristics may only be known to that individual. So, it is important that nurses honestly evaluate themselves during this self-assessment. The model also offers a possible rationale for the characteristics observed, identifies typical patient care–related behaviors, and suggests strategies for moving toward the next step. Therefore, a staircase to illustrate upward mobility seemed most appropriate. However, while the model is linear, the staircase moves toward infinity, illustrating a primary assumption that cultural competency is a lifelong process and aspiration, not a final goal to be achieved. Another assumption of this model is that nurses who reach Step 5 or 6 in encounters with certain groups may easily find themselves at a much lower level when encountering new groups with whom they have little experience. Therefore, nurses can ascend or descend the staircase based on the experience or encounters a nurse has had with members of a particular cultural group. Through multiple encounters with the same group, nurses gain more knowledge, skill, and facility in ascending the staircase. For example, a nurse may have much experience with Mexican patients through an emersion during which the nurse worked with migrant farm workers. That nurse might well be able to demonstrate cultural competency in situations with some Mexican patients at Step 5 or 6 of the staircase. At this level, the nurse can serve as mentor to other nurses who have not had such encounters. However, this same nurse may have little or no experience with Vietnamese clients and functions at Step 3 when caring for these patients. Nurses who perform a self-assessment on a regular basis when they encounter new groups will gain greater self-awareness, as well as new insights about cultural care. These nurses also recognize the need to seek appropriate resources to assist them and begin to develop a network of support.

Staircase Self-Assessment Model assumptions include the following. Culturally competent nurses:

- Increasingly develop self-awareness, cultural knowledge, and skills through encounters with culturally diverse patients.
- Strive to understand the patients or clients in their entire sociocultural context and with regard to all the dimensions of difference the patient represents, for example, a Black Muslim patient with multiple marriage partners; a new Vietnamese immigrant and single mother; a gay, Irish Catholic adolescent; a young, married female newly diagnosed with multiple sclerosis (MS); or the veteran returning from deployment or military service who may have experienced traumatic events and has become drug dependent. Each of these scenarios renders the patient unique and in need of very specific healthcare interventions.
- Consider the patient's geographical origins, history in the United States, cultural background, and within-group diversity.
- Make efforts to address healthcare disparities at the individual, institutional, or community levels through patient advocacy, mentoring, or educating other staff members, publications, or research.

FINDING YOUR PLACE ON THE STAIRCASE

Step 1. Nurses at Step 1 fail to recognize the significance of cultural influences when planning care. They may have grown up with limited exposure to people of culturally diverse backgrounds from their own upbringing and/or completed nursing school before cultural content was introduced and/or have limited exposure to culturally diverse patients in their social interactions.

Step 2. Nurses at Step 2 have a growing awareness of the influence that culture has on health but limited cultural self-awareness. They may be in denial about the role culture plays in their lives and have limited knowledge about other cultural groups.

Step 3. These nurses have begun to develop cultural self-awareness, acquire cultural knowledge about one or two culturally diverse groups, and attempt to include cultural information in care planning.

Step 4. Nurses in this category have a strong cultural self-awareness and an expanded social network from which to derive cultural information about diverse groups. These nurses consistently incorporate that knowledge into their care planning.

Step 5. Nurses at Step 5 are highly aware and readily apply cultural knowledge to care planning. They also anticipate potential culturally related patient problems or staff issues. They may serve as mentors and role models.

Step 6. Nurses at this level have a high level of self-awareness, a wide knowledge of another or multiple cultures that differ from their own, and an ability to problem-solve across cultural groups and to teach other nurses through mentoring, publication, and/or research.

See Table 1.1 to find strategies for progression.

TABLE 1.1 ■ CULTURAL COMPETENCY STAIRCASE SELF-ASSESSMENT MODEL

STEP	CHARACTERISTICS	RATIONALE	BEHAVIORS	STRATEGIES FOR PROGRESSION
Step 1	HC provider fails to recognize the significance of cultural influences, lacks motivation	• Has not accepted the influence of culture on own life, or • Has had negative experiences with members of diverse groups, or • Has had limited experiences with diversity, or • Completed nursing school before cultural content was presented	• May treat all patients the same • May care for patients based on own values and beliefs • May make assumptions that may be unfounded • May stereotype or demonstrate bias, prejudice, or discrimination	• Explore own cultural origins through interviews of family members and ethnographic study of one's cultural, ethnic heritage • Enhance internal motivation through encounters with members of culturally diverse groups; attend conferences and workshops • Seek culturally competent mentors, colleagues, and friends who are comfortable in cross-cultural situations
Step 2	HC provider is motivated and has growing awareness of culture's influence on health, but limited self-awareness or knowledge of other groups	• Is internally motivated to learn about own culture and culture of others • Is uncertain about how culture influences values	• May rely on texts for cultural information • Has limited experiences with diverse groups • May ignore intracultural differences • May make generalizations or stereotypes	• All of the previous strategies. Utilize a cultural assessment tool to determine intracultural differences • Broaden one's personal contacts beyond the comfort zone or usual social group in social and professional situations
Step 3	HC provider has developed a planned approach to developing cultural self-awareness and to acquire cultural knowledge about one or two culturally diverse groups	• Has developed a firm belief in the significance of culture and its impact on health and healthcare • Cultural competency is an identified value	• Attempts to include cultural information in care planning, but inconsistently • May overlook cultural competency behaviors when overwhelmed by other clinical roles and responsibilities	• All of the previous strategies. Seek professional workshops and conferences that focus on cultural competency development • Consider immersions in a cultural group of interest or professional engagement • Identify culturally competent role models in the workplace

(continued)

TABLE 1.1 ■ CULTURAL COMPETENCY STAIRCASE SELF-ASSESSMENT MODEL *(continued)*

STEP	CHARACTERISTICS	RATIONALE	BEHAVIORS	STRATEGIES FOR PROGRESSION
Step 4	Nurses have strong cultural self-awareness and an expanding social network. Consistently incorporates cultural knowledge into care planning	• Has observed cultural differences through interactions with family, close friends, and colleagues	• Consistently seeks to identify cultural information in plans of care	• All of the previous strategies • Continue to seek additional cultural resources through community, state, and federal organizations
Step 5	Nurses are highly self-aware, readily apply cultural knowledge in care planning, and anticipate potential cultural conflicts in patient care or staff issues	• Has ongoing experience and training in cultural diversity and/or transcultural nursing	• Serves as role model and coach in demonstrating cultural competency behaviors in patient-care settings	• All of the previous strategies • Seek cultural/diversity support networks as resources
Step 6	Nurses have attained a high level of self-awareness, a wide knowledge about a particular or multiple cultures, and an ability to problem-solve cross-culturally	• Has had multiple and ongoing transcultural formal and informal learning experiences and training	• Serves in a leadership capacity in area of diversity or transcultural situations • Problem-solves cross-culturally • Considered an expert in some areas of diversity • Has areas of diversity needing development	• All the previous strategies • Identify areas of diversity/transcultural nursing needing further development, e.g., language skills of interest (Spanish, Chinese) • Continue to attend workshops and conferences to strengthen knowledge • Utilize opportunities to immerse oneself in cultural learning experiences when possible

HC, healthcare.

Source: Kersey-Matusiak, G. (2001, April 2). An action plan for nurses: Building cultural competence. *Nursing Spectrum, 10*(7), 21–24. CE: 255; Reprinted with permission from *Nursing Spectrum.*

GENERAL STEP-CONSCIOUS QUESTIONS FOR NURSES TO ASK THEMSELVES TO DETERMINE THEIR LEVEL ON THE STAIRCASE

Step 1

• How much do I value becoming culturally competent?
• What actions have I taken recently or in the past when caring for culturally diverse patients that demonstrate my motivation? What can I do to become more skilled at caring for patients from backgrounds different from my own?

Step 2

• How much do I know about my own cultural heritage or racial identity and its relationship to my own healthcare beliefs and practices?

- Have I discussed these issues with my parents, grandparents, or other relatives?
- What cultural attitudes may be influencing the way I relate to members of diverse groups?

Step 3
- How much do I know about cultural groups that differ from my own?
- Am I aware of my own implicit or explicit biases and how might these impact the care that I give to patients (see Implicit Association Test [IAT])?

Step 4
- How culturally diverse is my social network?
- How many encounters with cultural group members outside my own social network do I have? Are these relationships superficial or do I have social contact beyond the workplace?
- Do I have resources within my social network from whom I might gain cultural knowledge or insight?

Step 5
- Am I able to independently identify the potential or actual problems that originate from cultural conflicts, or am I surprised by them?
- Do I serve as a culturally competent role model/mentor for others?

Step 6
- Have I developed problem-solving strategies to manage cultural conflicts?
- Am I able to manage or resolve cultural problems or issues that arise?
- Do I have personal and other resources to call on to assist when these conflicts occur?

STRATEGIES FOR STRENGTHENING CULTURAL COMPETENCY

Nurses can use seven strategies when practicing culturally competent care:

- **Strategy 1**

  Review a patient care scenario.
- **Strategy 2**

  Perform a self-assessment using the Staircase Self-Assessment Model.
- **Strategy 3**

  Select and apply a patient-centered cultural assessment to the scenario.
- **Strategy 4**

  Identify potential or actual barriers to culturally competent care.
- **Strategy 5**

  Establish patient-care goals based on barriers and patient needs.
- **Strategy 6**

  Develop a nursing action plan based on self-assessment, cultural assessment, barriers, and goals.
- **Strategy 7**

  Evaluate the effectiveness of culturally competent care planning and revise as needed. This strategy also allows the nurse to reflect on whether the interventions were effective.

IMPORTANT POINTS

1. The increasing global migration of refugees, asylum seekers, and other migrants challenges nurses to care for growing numbers of patients from culturally diverse backgrounds.
2. Within the United States there remain inequities in access to care, quality of care, and, consequently, healthcare outcomes.
3. According to *Healthy People 2030*, in the United States, 1 in 10 people live in poverty and do not have health insurance.
4. People living in poverty are less likely to have access to healthcare, healthy food, stable housing, and opportunities for physical activity and those without insurance are less likely to have a primary care provider.
5. As people of all races and ethnicities age and suffer some of the chronic illnesses and cognitive, sensory, and functional losses that are common among older people, nurses will be expected to provide culturally sensitive care to older adults that addresses their specific cultural needs.
6. The goals of *Healthy People 2030* include the achievement of health equity, the elimination of health disparities, and the improvement of health for all.
7. Madeleine Leininger, nurse, anthropologist, and founder of transcultural nursing, was visionary in her recognition of the need for nurses to provide care that was culturally congruent with their patients' "beliefs, values, and caring lifeways." Accessed at nursing-theory.org/theories-and-models/leininger-culture-care-theory.php
8. The American Nurses Association (ANA) in 2015 revised its Standards of Practice to include Standard 8: Culturally Congruent Care and encouraged registered nurses to "practice in a manner that is congruent with cultural diversity and inclusion principles" (p. 69).
9. The American Association of Colleges of Nursing (AACN), in outlining its undergraduate and graduate essentials for nursing education for the 21st century, stressed the need for diversity, equity, and inclusion as important values that support the nursing workforce.
10. Patient-centered care is emphasized under AACN's 10 domains, which is described in part as being care that considers and includes the cultural context of the individual, family, and community.
11. There is controversy over the use of cultural humility versus cultural competency in the literature.
12. Culture is defined as "the totality of socially transmitted behavioral patterns, arts, beliefs, customs, lifeways, and all other products of human work and thought characteristics of a population of people that guide their worldview and decision-making" (Purnell, 2013, p. 6).
13. Culture is dynamic because individuals' values, beliefs, and attitudes change or evolve with their life experiences.
14. There are several cultural competency frameworks and models readily available to assist nurses in their journey toward cultural competency.
15. Purnell's Model for Culturally Competent Healthcare is used to perform a patient cultural assessment.
16. The GKM Staircase Model is a means of assessing one's own level of cultural competence as a nurse or healthcare professional.
17. **Cultural competence** is defined by AACN as the attitudes, knowledge, and skills necessary for providing quality care to diverse populations.
18. The attitudes one needs to be culturally competent include having an openness to an ongoing self-reflection about one's own values, beliefs, biases, and prejudices.
19. The culturally competent nurse must also utilize various skills effectively to deliver care that is congruent with patients' cultural values. These skills include communication skills like reflexive listening.
20. Diversity refers to all aspects of difference that may be found among healthcare populations as well as the intersectionality of those differences.
21. The U.S. Department of Health and Human Services (DHHS) Office of Minority Health, in its publication of the National Standards for Culturally and Linguistically Appropriate Services (CLAS) in healthcare, affirmed the need for nurses to become culturally competent (DHHS, 2001).

Mrs. G, a 48-year-old, married, Spanish-speaking, recent immigrant from Colombia, is brought to the ED via ambulance. She was brought to the ED after her 18-year-old son, Roberto, discovered her in a chair in the living room with a cigarette in her hand that had fallen into her lap. Mrs. G's son began beating Mrs. G's clothing to extinguish the fire that was starting to ignite Mrs. G's dress. During the episode, Mrs. G remained silent and appeared confused. Mrs. G has a history of hypertension and type 2 diabetes mellitus (DM). She has smoked two packs of cigarettes a day for the past 40 years and has tried unsuccessfully to stop multiple times. Mrs. G is non-English speaking. Her son understands and speaks a little English, but has some difficulty communicating in English.

Roberto tells the nurse that his mother has been taking medication at home for DM and high blood pressure, but has not been to a doctor since coming to the United States 8 months ago.

The ER triage nurse becomes concerned when she realizes that the patient seems to be experiencing some neurologic changes. Communication with both the patient and son is difficult. Laboratory results reveal that the patient's blood sugar is 340 mg/dL.

STEPPING UP TO CULTURALLY COMPETENT CARE

Apply seven strategies to ensure culturally competent care.

Strategy 1

Perform a self-assessment using the Staircase Self-Assessment Model. The ED nurse in this situation has had many encounters with Spanish-speaking patients but has not cared for patients from Colombia. The nurse is able to speak enough Spanish to obtain and explain basic information to the patient. When speaking with Mrs. G, she learns that Mrs. G is a widow. During a recent self-assessment, the ED nurse rated herself between Steps 4 and 5 using the Staircase Self-Assessment Model. Today, she reflects on whether she needs the support of her colleague to assist her in this situation. The nurse knows a nurse practitioner (NP) who is fluent in Spanish and who she can call on to assist her in performing an assessment of the patient if necessary. Because of the complex nature of the patient's medical condition, which is likely to involve more than one diagnosis, the nurse decides to call on her friend, the NP, for assistance to expedite the assessment process.

Strategy 2

Review a patient-care scenario. The ED nurse considers this patient's entire cultural context and considers the following:

1. This patient and her son are both new immigrants and may be unfamiliar with the U.S. healthcare system.
2. The patient is unable to communicate in English. The son is not an appropriate translator or good historian, as he also has limited English skills.
3. The patient has been taking unknown medications at home. She may be using herbal medicine or folk medicine to treat health problems; these may be incompatible with medicine ordered by a physician in the hospital.

4. At age 48, is this patient employed? Does she have health insurance? What is the socio-economic status and education level of this patient? Have any of these issues impacted the patient's health in general, specifically blood pressure, or her understanding about her disease or its treatment?

Strategy 3

Select and apply a patient-centered cultural assessment to the scenario. The nurse selects from among Purnell's Twelve Domains of Culture (Purnell, 2013), selecting those attributes relevant to a cultural assessment of this case example. The attributes selected include the following:

- Inhabited locality
- Communication
- Family roles and organization
- Workforce issues
- Biocultural ecology
- High-risk behaviors
- Nutrition
- Spirituality
- Healthcare practices
- Healthcare practitioners

Strategy 4

Identify potential or actual barriers to culturally competent care.
Example: Language barrier

Strategy 5

Establish patient-care goals based on barriers and the patient's needs.
Example: The patient will understand health information and the plan of care.

Strategy 6

Develop a nursing action plan based on the previous strategies. A medically trained interpreter will assist with providing health information and the plan of care in the patient's own language.

Strategy 7

Evaluate the effectiveness of culturally competent care planning and revise as needed.

NCLEX®-TYPE QUESTIONS

1. What percentage of Americans speak a language other than English in the home?
   A. One in five
   B. One in 10
   C. One in 15
   D. One in 20

2. According to a report by the National Institutes of Health and the Centers for Disease Control and Prevention, health disparities are a result of
   A. Genetic predispositions
   B. Wide variations in healthcare access

C. Cultural diversity among various groups
D. Racial and ethnic characteristics

3. Which statement describes nurses' use of terms like *cultural humility, cultural awareness, cultural sensitivity,* and *cultural competency*? *Select all that apply.*
   A. The words all have the same meaning.
   B. The words convey different meanings and are often a source of confusion.
   C. Each term conveys some aspect of being culturally competent.

4. Which statement best illustrates what the nurse should consider when reflecting upon the patient's context?
   A. Social political, historical, and structural situations impacting the patient
   B. Folk and traditional health beliefs and attitudes
   C. Preferences for Western versus Eastern traditions
   D. Employment and economic status of the patient

5. Which statement best describes a culturally competent nurse?
   A. Having the motivation to provide quality care to assigned patients
   B. Having the desire to partner or collaborate with the patient
   C. Having the attitude, knowledge, and skills necessary to provide quality care to culturally diverse patients and groups
   D. Having the knowledge of multiple languages to address various patients' needs

ANSWERS TO NCLEX-TYPE QUESTIONS

1. A
2. B

3. B and C
4. A

5. C

AMERICAN ASSOCIATION OF COLLEGES OF NURSING END-OF-PROGRAM CULTURAL COMPETENCIES FOR BACCALAUREATE NURSING EDUCATION

1. Apply knowledge of social and cultural factors that affect nursing and healthcare across multiple contexts.
2. Use relevant data sources and best evidence in providing culturally competent care.
3. Promote achievement of safe and quality outcomes of care for diverse populations.
4. Advocate for social justice, including commitment to the health of vulnerable populations and the elimination of healthcare disparities.
5. Participate in continuous cultural competence development.

A robust set of instructor resources designed to supplement this text is located at http://connect.springerpub.com/content/book/978-0-8261-8302-6. Qualifying instructors may request access by emailing textbook@springerpub.com.

REFERENCES

American Association of Colleges of Nursing. (2021, April 6). *The Essentials: Competencies for professional nursing education.* https://www.aacnnursing.org/Portals/0/PDFs/Publications/Essentials-2021.pdf
American Association of Colleges of Nursing. (2022, October 4). *Domain 2: Person-centered care.* https://www.aacnnursing.org/Portals/42/AcademicNursing/Tool%20Kits/Essentials/Domain-2%20Person-Centered-Care-Toolkit.docx
American Nurses Association. (2015). *Nursing: Scope and standards of practice* (3rd ed.). Nursesbooks.org.
Ashley, M., Julaka, S., & Woodward, L. (2021, November). Nurses in action: Insights into providing care to veterans. *APNA News.* https://www.apna.org/news/providing-mental-health-care-for-veterans
Becze, E. (2021). Cultural humility is a nursing clinical competency. *ONSVOICE.* https://voice.ons.org/news-and-views/cultural-humility-is-a-nursing-clinical-competency
Centers for Disease Control and Prevention, National Prevention Information Network. (2021, September 10). *Cultural competence in health and human services.* https://npin.cdc.gov/pages/cultural-competence

Cross, T. (2012). Cultural competence continuum. *Journal of Child and Youth Care Work, 24,* 83–84. https://scholar.google.com/scholar?q=Cross+T.+1988+Cultural+Competence&hl=en&as_sdt=0&as_vis=1&oi=scholart

Cuellar, N. (2017). If you're not outraged, you're not paying attention. *Journal of Transcultural Nursing, 28*(6), 529. https://doi.org/10.1177/1043659617732850

Curtin, L. (2016). A kinder, gentler workplace, part 3: The generation gap. *American Nurse Today, 11*(11), 48. https://www.americannursetoday.com/wp-content/uploads/2016/11/ant11-Curtin-1021a-copy.pdf

Furness, B., Goldhammer, H., Montalvo, W., Gagnon, K., Bifulco, L., Lentine, D., & Anderson, D. (2020). Transforming primary care for lesbian, gay, bisexual, and transgender people: A collaborative quality improvement initiative. *Annals of Family Medicine, 18*(4), 292–302. https://doi.org/10.1370/afm.2542

Giger, J. E., Davidhizar, R. E., Purnell, L., Harden, J. T., Phillips, J., & Strickland O. (2017). American Academy of Nursing expert panel report: Developing cultural competence to eliminate health disparities in ethnic minorities and other vulnerable populations. *Journal of Transcultural Nursing, 18*(2), 95–102. https://doi.org/10.1177/1043659606298618

Giger, J. N., & Haddad, L. (2020). *Transcultural nursing: Assessment and intervention.* Elsevier.

Hannon, K. (2017, September 7). The health insurance surprise facing some same-sex couples. *Forbes.* https://www.forbes.com/sites/nextavenue/2017/09/07/the-health-insurance-surprise-facing-some-same-sex-couples

Im, E.-O. (2015). What makes an intervention culturally competent. *Journal of Transcultural Nursing, 26*(1), 5. https://doi.org/10.1177/1043659614545495

Jeffreys, M. R., & Zoucha, R. (2018). Cultural congruence in the workplace, healthcare, and academic settings for multiracial and multiheritage individuals. *Journal of Cultural Diversity, 25*(4), 113–126. https://www.proquest.com/docview/2190964216

Kersey-Matusiak, G. (2001). An action plan for nurses: Building cultural competence. *Nursing Spectrum, 10*(7), 21–24. http://search.ebscohost.com/login.aspx?direct=true&db=ccm&AN=106911179&site=ehost-live>

Kersey-Matusiak, G. (2012). Culturally competent care: Are we there yet? *Nursing Management, 43*(4), 34–39. https://doi.org/10.1097/01.NUMA.0000413093.39091.c6

Kuwano, N., & McMaster, R. (2020). Knowing ourselves: Self-awareness and culturally competent care. *Nursing & Health Sciences, 22*(4), 843–845. https;//doi.org/10.1111/nhs.12735

Leininger, M., & McFarland, M. R. (2005). *Culture care diversity and universality: A worldwide nursing theory.* Publication No. 15-2402. National League of Nursing Press.

Liptak, A. (2015, June 27). Supreme Court ruling makes same-sex marriage a right nationwide. *New York Times.* https://www.nytimes.com/2015/06/27/us/supreme-court-same-sex-marriage.html

Marmot, M. (2005). Social determinants of health inequalities. *Lancet, 365*(9464), 1099–1104. https://web-s-ebscohost-com.ezproxy.sju.edu/ehost/pdfviewer/pdfviewer?vid=27&sid=9296079f-8e77-4440-a3db-4e7d8511eda4%40redis

National Conference of State Legislatures. (2015). *Same sex marriage laws.* http://www.ncsl.org/research/human-services/same-sex-marriage-laws.aspx

National Institute on Minority Health and Health Disparities. (2022, February 21). *About NIMHD.* https://www.nimhd.nih.gov/about

Nolan, T., Alston, A., Choto, R., & Moss, K. (2021). Cultural humility: Retraining and retooling nurses to provide equitable cancer care. *Clinical Journal of Oncology Nursing, 25*(5), 3–9. https://doi.org/10.1188/21.CJON.S1.3-9

Nursing Theory. (2023). *Culture care theory.* Nursing-Theory.org. https://nursing-theory.org/theories-and-models/leininger-culture-care-theory.php

Office of Disease Prevention and Health Promotion. (n.d.-a). *Economic stability.* Retrieved October 3, 2023, from https://health.gov/healthypeople/objectives-and-data/browse-objectives/economic-stability

Office of Disease Prevention and Health Promotion. (n.d.-b)., *Healthy people 2030, ND.* https://health.gov/healthypeople/priority-areas/social-determinants-health

Pierce McDaniel, V. (2021). Cultural humility in nursing building the bridge to best practices. *Virginia Nurses Today, 29*(2), 12–14. https://www.proquest.com/docview/2532701904

Purnell, L. D. (2013). *Transcultural health care: A culturally competent approach* (4th ed.). F. A. Davis Company.

Purnell, L. (2019). Update: The Purnell Theory and Model for culturally competent health care *Journal of Transcultural Nursing, 30*(2), 98–105. https://doi.org/10.1177/1043659618817587

Purnell, L., & Fenkl, E. A. (Eds.). (2020). *Textbook of healthcare: A population approach: Cultural competence concepts in nursing care* (5th ed.). Springer Publications. https://doi.org/10.1177/1043659616632046

Rising, M. L. (2017). Truth Telling as an element of culturally competent care at end of life. *Journal of Transcultural Nursing: Official Journal of the Transcultural Nursing Society, 28*(1), 48–55. https://doi.org/10.1177/1043659615606203

Spector, R. (2017). *Cultural diversity in health and illness* (9th ed.). Pearson.

Substance Abuse and Mental Health Services Administration. (2022). *Cultural competency for serving the military and veterans.* https://www.samhsa.gov/certified-community-behavioral-health-clinics/section-223/cultural-competency/military-veterans

The Joint Commission. (2014). *Advancing effective communication, cultural competence, and patient and family centered care: A roadmap for hospitals* (Vol. 26, No. 1, p. 5). Author. Retrieved from https://www.jointcommission.org/roadmap_for_hospitals/

Thomson, G. E., Mitchell, F., & Williams, M. B. (Eds). (2006). *Examining the health disparities research plan of the National Institutes of Health: Unfinished business*. National Academies Press. https://www.ncbi.nlm.nih.gov/books/NBK57031

Tierney, M. (2017, April 12). Improving nurses' attitudes toward patients with substance use disorders. *American Nurse Today, 11*(11), 6–9. https://www.americannursetoday.com/improving-nurses-attitudes-toward-patients-substance-use-disorders

Tuttas, C. A. (2015). Perceived racial and ethnic prejudice and discrimination experiences of minority migrant nurses: A literature review. *Journal of Transcultural Nursing, 26*(5), 514–520. https://doi.org/10.1177/1043659614526757

U.S. Census Bureau. (2020). *2020 Census results*. https://www.census.gov/programs-surveys/decennial-census/decade/2020/2020-census-results.html

U.S. Department of Health and Human Services. (2000). *Healthy People 2010: Understanding and improving health* (2nd ed.). U.S. Government Printing Office.

U.S. Department of Health and Human Services. (2001). *National standards for culturally linguistically appropriate services in health care*. Author.

U.S. Department of Health and Human Services. (2016). *The national CLAS standards*. https://minorityhealth.hhs.gov/omh/browse.aspx?lvl=2&lvlid=53

U.S. Department of Health and Human Services, Office of Minority Health. (2004). *Setting the agenda*. Author.

Walden University. (2022). *Standard 8: What every nurse should know about culturally congruent practice*. https://www.waldenu.edu/online-masters-programs/master-of-science-in-nursing/resource/standard-eight-what-every-nurse-should-know-about-culturally-congruent-practice

Zinan, N. (2021). Humility in health care: A model. *Nursing Philosophy, 22*(3), e12354. https://doi.org/10.1111/nup.12354

IMPORTANT WEBSITES

American Association of Colleges of Nursing. Retrieved from www.aacnnursing.org/Education-Resources/Tool-Kits/Cultural-Competency-in-Nursing-Education

American Nurses Association Standard 8: Culturally Congruent Practice. Retrieved from www.join.nursingworld.org/MainMenuCategories/ANAMarketplace/ANAPeriodicals/OJIN/TableofContents/Vol-22-2017/No1-Jan-2017/Articles-Previous-Topics/Implementing-the-New-ANA-Standard-8.html

Project Implicit. *Harvard implicit bias test.* https://implicit.harvard.edu/implicit/takeatest.html

National League for Nursing Diversity & Cultural Competence. Retrieved from www.nln.org/docs/default-source/nln-reports/summer15nlnreport.pdf?sfvrsn=2

Transcultural Nursing Society. Retrieved from www.tcns.org

Cultural Competency Models and Guidelines

Gloria Kersey-Matusiak

The only place where true change can occur and where the past can be dissolved is the Now.

—ECKHART TOLLE

LEARNING OBJECTIVES

After this chapter, the reader will be able to
1. Describe the rationale for utilizing a patient-centered cultural assessment model.
2. Describe selected cultural assessment models developed specifically for nurses.
3. Discuss the components of a selected group of cultural assessment models used for other health professionals.
4. Utilize an appropriate cultural assessment model to enhance communication when delivering care to culturally diverse patients.
5. Integrate cultural assessment fondings in care planning for culturally diverse clients.
6. Examine the models of cultural competence that may be utilized to assess organizations and institutions.

KEY TERMS

Biocultural ecology	Culture Care Diversity and Universality
Conscious competence	Cultural incapacity
Conscious incompetence	Cultural precompetence
Cultural assessment	Generic or folk systems
Cultural blindness	Intercultural competence
Cultural competence	Patient assessment
Cultural destructiveness	Self-assessment
Cultural encounter	Sunrise Model
Culturally congruent	Unconscious competence
Culture care	Unconscious incompetence

CULTURAL COMPETENCY MODELS AND GUIDELINES

Introduction

We begin this chapter highlighting the key concepts of Chapter 1 that we wish to expand on in the current chapter. First, in Chapter 1, we acknowledged the visionary leadership of Madeleine Leininger, who first established the goal for nurses to view the patients' healthcare situation through that patient's own cultural lens. Second, nurses are encouraged by the authors and by past and present nurse leaders to address the existing healthcare disparities and ensure safe, equitable, quality care for all patients. Third, and most importantly, in today's climate of civil, political, and social unrest, nurses are encouraged to be exemplary in redressing societal ills like racism, homophobia, ageism, sizeism, and the like that exist in the larger society. Why? Because these "isms" have been documented in the medical literature to negatively impact the quality of care patients receive; ultimately, they contribute to disparities in healthcare access and outcomes. Ludwig-Beymer (2022) in an editorial in the *Journal of Transcultural Nursing* described the role of the transcultural nurse in the future of nursing. Nurses are challenged by the American Association of Colleges of Nursing (AACN; 2021) and the *Future of Nursing 2020–2030* report to promote health equity and social justice by improving healthcare access and quality for all.

As racial, cultural, and ethnic diversity increase in the United States, to be effective in achieving these goals, nurses and all healthcare professionals will need to develop an arsenal of strategies to support these efforts. Such strategies assist their patients in overcoming power imbalances that impact social determinants of health; lead to healthcare disparities; and negatively affect racial minorities, immigrants, and other socially oppressed groups. To begin this process, it is critical that nurses gain cultural knowledge and understanding of the patients they serve. In Chapter 1, nurses are reminded to build on cultural knowledge about themselves as well as that of their patients and to think critically about their patients' identified needs and the potential for cultural conflicts or barriers to care. Medical and healthcare literature tell us that the best way to gain that knowledge is through our interactions with culturally diverse groups and individuals (Rukadikar et al., 2022). However, having a structured, organized plan to direct nurses in that effort is a more effective way of achieving success. In a discussion about enhancing cultural competency and humility in personality assessment, Lui (2022) stated, "personality assessment requires assessors' training and competency to engage in a systematic process of information gathering" (p. 19). The same is true for nurses hoping to gain cultural information about their patients.

A review of the literature revealed numerous cultural competency models and frameworks. Each model either attempts to describe or explain cultural competence, or determine an individual's or organization's level of achievement in this regard.

Models and Guidelines

Over the last several decades, researchers and writers have developed a variety of cultural competency models that provide guidance for nurses and other healthcare professionals. These models and frameworks may be categorized as those intended for use when conducting cultural **self-assessments** for healthcare professionals, patient assessments, and organizational assessments. One of the earliest models of this kind, developed by Cross and colleagues (1989), focused on the treatment of children. The paper explained how cultural differences can lead to inequitable care. In this paper, Cross and colleagues (1989) and a group of mental health researchers described the Cultural Competence Continuum, a framework that posits cultural competency occurs over six stages: cultural destructiveness, cultural incapacity, cultural blindness, cultural precompetence, cultural competence, and cultural proficiency. This model was the inspiration for the Staircase Self-Assessment Model developed by the author of this text in 1991, but first published in 2001 in an action plan for nurses that was introduced in this edition in Chapter 1. It is easy to see how the continuum framework could be utilized to assess the cultural competency status or level of an institution or an individual. Other researchers focused similarly on either a self-assessment of one's level of cultural competency or guidelines for determining patients' cultural characteristics. For example, Purnell (2013, 2019) developed the Purnell Theory and Model for Culturally Competent Health Care. The Purnell model has been revised and updated over the years since its inception and used globally as a way of assessing diverse cultural groups. According to Purnell, the model is based on assumptions, such as that one culture is not better than another; they are just different. Another assumption is that culture has a powerful influence on one's interpretation of and responses to healthcare; and everyone has the right to be respected for their uniqueness and cultural heritage. Purnell identified 12 domains, which are suitable in their totality for conducting a comprehensive cultural assessment of a patient. Readers are encouraged as they read the case scenarios at the end of each chapter in this text to consider using this model by including the domains that are applicable to the situation when culturally assessing their patients.

Other Assessment Models

Some models discussed in this chapter are intended to assist nurses and other health professionals in teaching students or health professionals the process of becoming culturally competent. Like the Staircase Self-Assessment Model in Chapter 1, some of these schematics, theoretical models, and conceptual frameworks are focused on describing the characteristics of the culturally competent individual or organization (Cross et al., 1989; Kersey-Matusiak, 2019). The aims of these models are to foster ongoing self-reflection, to help nurses and other health professionals determine where they are in the journey to becoming culturally competent, to minimize the potential impact of biases, and to guide them through the process.

Other models focus on **patient assessment** and nurses gaining knowledge about diverse cultural or ethnic groups and their characteristics. While some of these models originated in nursing, others are products of other disciplines, including social work, psychology, and medicine. For example, Hordijk and colleagues (2019) developed a framework consisting of 10 competencies that were viewed as essential for all medical teachers. Included among the 10 competencies were (a) the ability to critically reflect on one's own values and beliefs; (b) the ability to communicate about individuals in a nondiscriminatory, nonstereotyping way; and (c) to have knowledge of ethnic and social determinants of physical and mental health. Despite their origin, if used in an appropriate setting, each selected model can enhance nurses' and other health professionals' ability to deliver patient-centered and **culturally congruent** care. Among the models presented here are those specifically intended for nurses, which can be found in texts by their respective authors (Andrews & Boyle, 2021; Giger & Davidhizar, 2008; Leininger, 1978; Purnell, 2013, 2019; Spector, 2021). These models assist nurses in providing care that is culturally congruent with the patients' own values and beliefs.

Nonnursing assessment models, such as the BATHE (background, affect, trouble, handling, and empathy), GREET (generation, reason, extended family, ethnic behavior, and time), ETHNIC (explanation, treatment, healers, negotiation, intervention, and collaboration), and LEARN (listen, explain, acknowledge, recommend, and negotiate) models, also lend themselves to the provision of culturally sensitive care and are discussed briefly in this chapter.

Since nurses themselves represent a diverse group of health professionals who practice in a variety of care settings and encounter numerous patient contexts, it is helpful to have various models from which readers can select the most appropriate model for their use at a given time. It is also important for nurses to become familiar with an approach with which they are most comfortable and able to readily apply in their practice when needed.

Communication between the nurse and culturally diverse patients is integral to overcoming language barriers and differences in communication styles, as well as to becoming culturally competent. Therefore, models that identify strategic ways of strengthening communication between the patient and the nurse are also included in this chapter. For example, the PEARLS (partnership, empathy, acknowledgement, respect, legitimization, and support) statements and the Guidelines on Validating Patients are examples of models that, while not developed by or for nurses specifically, can facilitate nurse–patient communication; therefore, they have been added to this discussion. To help nurses understand the evolution of cultural competence in the literature, two early models that have application for use either by individuals or organizations that were developed by Howell and Fleishman (1982) and Cross (2012) and colleagues (1989) are discussed in this chapter.

Nurses can use one or more of the models presented in this chapter as tools to enhance their knowledge, attitude, and skills in their quest for cultural competence. However, no matter which model one uses or how skillful the nurse becomes at using it, caring for all patients with dignity and respect is most important. Also important is remembering that the journey is ongoing and the ultimate goal of the process of developing cultural competence skills is to build a relationship between the patient and the nurse that facilitates the attainment of the patient's healthcare goals.

EARLY MODELS OF CULTURAL COMPETENCE

The Stages of Intercultural Competence, by William Howell (1982)

Source: The Stages of Intercultural Competence. C Ward Intercultural Communication, LLC. https://cwardintercultural.com/2016/02/11/the-stages-of-intercultural-competence/

1. **Unconscious incompetence** is when people are not yet aware that they lack a particular skill. They tend to believe that their own way of doing things is the only way of doing things.
2. **Conscious incompetence** is when people know that they want to learn something, but are incompetent at doing it. They start to notice differences, but are unsure about how to cope with them.
3. **Conscious competence** is when people are able to perform tasks competently, but not without being highly conscious of their behavior; they are hyperaware and often worry about making mistakes.
4. **Unconscious competence** is when people have mastered the skill to the degree that they can perform it without thinking about it; they do it naturally.

Source: Adapted from The Cultural Competence Continuum By T. Cross et al., Georgetown University (1989)

This framework describes six levels of personal growth, from cultural destructiveness to cultural competence: These levels are applicable to individuals or organizations.

Cultural destructiveness is characterized by attitudes, policies, structures, and practices within a system or organization that are destructive to a cultural group.
Cultural incapacity is the lack of systems or organizations to respond effectively to the needs, interests, and preferences of culturally and linguistically diverse groups; and may involve bias, discrimination, and/or subtle messages that some groups are valued over others.
Cultural blindness is expressed as a philosophy of treating all groups the same without regard for cultural differences.
Cultural precompetence is having a level of awareness of strengths and areas for growth to respond effectively to culturally and linguistically diverse populations and to support

diversity; and the tendency for token representation on boards and no clear plan for achieving organizational cultural competence.

Cultural competence is to demonstrate an acceptance and respect for cultural differences. Among other behaviors, systems and organizations that exemplify cultural competence identify, use, and/or adapt evidence-based and promising practices that are culturally and linguistically competent.

In reviewing each of the two previous models, one might ask, "Where do I see myself on either or both of these continuums? How does my placement impact my ability to provide culturally competent care to the diverse patients I encounter?"

SELECTING A CULTURAL ASSESSMENT TOOL

Opportunities to conduct **cultural assessments** occur each time there is contact between the patient and the nurse or other healthcare provider. These encounters may occur face to face, but can also occur during phone conversations, teleconferences, or other means through which there is interaction between the client and the nurse. Each encounter is an opportunity for the nurse to establish or affirm a trusting, supportive relationship with the patient. It is also an opportunity for nurses to gain insights about their patients' culture, health attitudes, and beliefs, and to explore the entire situation or context in which the patient's cultural health beliefs exist. Armed with this knowledge, the nurse can partner with the patient to establish mutually agreed on and culturally congruent goals for care. It is important to note here that no one is expected to learn all there is to know about any culture during a single, brief clinical encounter. However, the nurse must place emphasis on learning about what is deemed most significant from a cultural perspective from the patient's point of view. The nurse must also recognize that there may be differences about what is culturally important between members of the same group. Using a cultural assessment model, the nurse can explore how the patient feels about a variety of factors that impact health. These include, but are not limited to, the patient's beliefs about the illness; hospitalization; Western medicine; healthcare decision-making; nutrition; medications; and values and beliefs about life, death, and spirituality. It may not be possible to have extended periods during which to gather important cultural information, so the nurse is encouraged to use each opportunity during which there is interaction with the patient to seek this information.

Besides Purnell's model, discussed at the beginning of this chapter, there are many cultural assessment models found in the nursing literature; for example, Madeleine Leininger's Sunrise Model, which was developed in 1960. Leininger was the first to develop a theory in the field of transcultural nursing, entitled Culture Care Diversity and Universality. The model explores diverse cultures and examines multiple factors impacting health. Giger and Davidhizar's Transcultural Assessment Model developed in 1988 to provide an assessment tool for student nurses to assess patients' cultural values and their impact on health. The model uses six cultural phenomenon to conduct a cultural assessment: communication, space, time, social organization, environmental control, and biological variations. This assessment model developed to assess cultural values and their impact on health and disease behavior. The Andrews and Boyle Transcultural Interprofessional Practice (TIP) Model offers a five-step, systematic, scientific problem-solving process-assessment. In Spector's (2021) Cultural Diversity in Health and Illness, the author includes cultural care, cultural heritage, and ethnocultural community assessment guidelines.

In addition, Jeffreys (2006, 2021) offers a model to guide cultural competence education. Each model offers its own constructs and/or parameters to use as a basis for either determining one's own level of cultural competency or performing a cultural assessment. The author of this text encourages nurses to use a model that is most suitable for their communication style, care setting, and patient situation. By learning about many of the models and frameworks currently available, the nurse builds an arsenal of strategies to use at the appropriate time to meet the situation at hand. The purpose of this text is to assist nurses in practicing cultural competency skills routinely, when giving nursing care. A description of various cultural assessment models is presented here that may be applied to actual clinical practice. Case scenarios are presented at the end of the chapters to provide the reader with practice opportunities using the models. A specific assessment model is suggested for the application to each of the cases throughout the text.

Many of the models found in the literature are specifically intended to assist nurses in integrating cultural information into their clinical nursing assessments and care planning. Stein (2010) also identified assessment models such as ETHNIC, LEARN, BATHE, and GREET that, although not initially developed for nurses, are applicable in patient-care situations and therefore may be useful to nurses.

Before beginning any cultural assessment, the nurse must first be motivated to engage in the assessment process. Nurses at Step 1 of the Staircase Self-Assessment Model (discussed in Chapter 1) may believe that having knowledge of the patient's physiologic needs, which the nurse discovers during a health and/or physical assessment, is all that is needed. However, obtaining a cultural assessment is an essential cultural competency skill that nurses must practice to gain cultural information and to become proficient at doing so.

Fortunately, the more nurses interact with patients from culturally diverse groups, the more likely they are to gain an understanding of differences and similarities that exist between themselves and their patients. Nurses who are able to overcome cultural differences can provide care that is holistic and patient centered.

Some institutions incorporate cultural assessment questions within the nursing history questionnaires used during patient admission surveys. When assessing the patient's cultural values, attitudes, and beliefs, the nurse considers the patient's worldview or how that individual views the world. One's thoughts on morality, esthetics, and social behavior would reflect one's worldview. Worldview is influenced by regional and national values, which is why it is important for the nurse to consider the patient's geographical region of origin. One's gender, familial values, and degree of religiosity or spirituality also influence a person's worldview.

Although many persons from the same cultural or ethnic group generally share a worldview, there are differences within the same ethnic group based on life experiences. Each person is unique, so when conducting a cultural assessment and planning care, nurses must identify the specific beliefs, attitudes, and needs of that individual. As observed previously, all patients present with visible and invisible aspects of culture. Much like an iceberg, at the visible tip one can observe some characteristics easily. Skin color, dress, language usage, gender, age, communication style, and body size may be apparent, while other traits, such as values, political views, spiritual needs, health beliefs, and sexual orientation, are often hidden below the surface. For this reason, nurses act as detectives uncovering that which is unknown to ensure that healthcare decision-making is congruent with the patient's values, health beliefs, and wishes. Cultural assessment models assist the nurse in accomplishing this task. An overview of selected cultural assessment models follows.

NONNURSING MODELS

In the cultural competency learning module, Think Cultural Health, the author explains Kleinman's (1992) model. One of the earliest frameworks for a cultural assessment was developed by Kleinman (1992), who posed eight questions for physicians to guide the process of appraisal in counseling; it was one of the first models to include the client in the problem-solving approach (U.S. Department of Health and Human Services [US DHHS], Think Cultural Health, n.d.). Using this explanatory model, the nurse or other healthcare provider explores the personal and social meaning the illness has for the patient, as well as the expectations about the appropriate treatment, goals for care, and the expected outcomes. The model also enables the clinician to determine if there are areas of conflict to be addressed through collaboration and negotiation with the patient. The model is useful in a variety of healthcare situations. Kleinman's explanatory model includes several open-ended questions and is useful in various situations:

1. What do you call your problem?
2. What do you think has caused your problem?
3. Why do you think it started when it did?
4. What do you think your sickness does to you? How does it work?
5. How severe is it? Will it have a short or long course?
6. What do you fear the most about your sickness?
7. What are the chief problems your sickness has caused for you?
8. What kind of treatment do you think you should receive? What are the most important results you hope to receive from this treatment?

Taking this approach affords the nurse or other health provider a baseline from which to begin a collaboration with the patient. The nurse is able to share health information based on the patient's understanding and healthcare beliefs.

The ETHNIC Model

The ETHNIC Model of culturally competent care was developed in 1997 by Steven J. Levin, Robert C. Like, and Jan E. Gottleib. ETHNIC stands for *explanation, treatment, healers, nego-tiation, intervention,* and *collaboration*. This model allows the nurse to determine what the client expects to happen during the illness, based on that person's cultural beliefs. The model also affords a collaboration between the nurse and the client in planning culturally appropriate care. An example of a question the nurse might ask when using this approach is: "Do you receive advice about your care from persons outside of the medical profession, such as traditional healers?"

The LEARN Model

The LEARN Model enables the nurse to overcome the barriers in communication between the patient and the nurse. This model was developed in 1983 by Elois Ann Berlin and William C. Fowlkes Jr. The acronym LEARN represents *listen, explain, acknowledge, recom-mend,* and *negotiate*. Nurses using this model will acknowledge and discuss the similarities and differences between the patient's explanation and the clinical or medical explanation of that patient's illness. The authors of this model suggest that the provider *listen* with a sympathetic ear and then *explain* their perceptions of what the patient is saying. This process is also referred to as *reflective* or *active listening*, which originated in the field of counseling psychology. Reflective listening is associated with Carl Rogers's "client-cen-tered" approach to therapy, which involves restating or clarifying, and responding with acceptance and empathy to what the speaker is saying (People Communicating, 2014). (For more information about active listening, see www.analytictech.com/mb119/reflecti.htm.) At that point, the provider attempts to identify the differences and similarities in percep-tions between the patient and provider, and *recommends* treatment. The idea of recom-mending treatment suggests that the nurse or other healthcare provider finally *negotiates* the treatment plan with the patient and offers clinical options based on the patient's values and goals for care, rather than have them imposed by the provider.

The BATHE Model

The BATHE Model was developed by Marian Stuart and Joseph Lieberman in 2002 for use by psychotherapists. The acronym refers to *background, affect, trouble, handling,* and *empathy*. This model seeks to enhance communication between the client and care provider by focusing on the psychosocial context of the client. When exploring the *background*, the nurse attempts to gain knowledge of the circumstances surrounding the patient and influence the patient's perceptions of the illness. *Affect* refers to the feelings the patient has related to the illness or condition. Asking the patient what is *troubling* about the illness is an attempt to explore how the illness is impacting the patient's life. It also helps the provider determine an area to focus attention in planning care. The patient is then asked about how they are *handling* the illness. *Empathy* refers to the statements that the provider uses to affirm or legitimize what the patient has said in an effort to provide psychologic support (Lieberman & Stuart, 1999). Although the model was intended originally for mental health physicians, one can see the potential benefits for using the models in nursing.

The GREET Model

The GREET Model is specifically intended for nonnative patients (Stein, 2010). GREET signifies *generation, reason, extended family, ethnic behavior,* and *time* living in the United States. Learning when and why the patient has come to the United States and what supports the individual has available are all important pieces of information to ensure effective cross-cultural information.

Each of these models illustrates strategies for ensuring enhanced cross-cultural communication. The provider must first understand patients' situations or circumstances, perceptions of their illness, and be willing to collaborate and negotiate with them to determine the goals and interventions that are culturally congruent.

NURSING MODELS

Any discussion of nursing models begins with Madeleine Leininger's **Sunrise Model** and Theory of **Culture Care Diversity and Universality**. A cultural anthropologist and nurse, Leininger, founder of transcultural nursing, conceptualized **culture care** as early as the 1950s. These concepts mean providing care that is congruent with the cultural values of the patient. Leininger described several dimensions of culture and social structure that influence caring practices, well-being, and the experiences of health and illness among individuals, families, and groups. These dimensions or factors include cultural values and life ways, political factors, economic factors, educational factors, technological factors, religious and philosophical factors, kinship, and social factors. Patients engage in diverse health systems, including **generic or folk systems** and professional systems. The Sunrise Model illustrates three ways in which nursing may provide culturally competent care through culture care preservation and/or maintenance, culture care accommodation and/or negotiation, and/or culture care repatterning and/or restructuring.

Among those who have been recognized with Leininger as leaders in the field of transcultural nursing are Spector (2021), Giger and Davidhizar (2008), Andrews and Boyle (2021), and Purnell (2013). Each has made a distinct contribution to the transcultural nursing body of knowledge, and references to their work will be made throughout the text where appropriate. When conducting physical assessments, nurses must also apply their cultural knowledge about physical, physiological, and biological variations that may influence the interpretation of results.

One model that is particularly useful to include in the physical assessment of clients is Giger and Davidhizar's Transcultural Assessment Model. In this model, there are six essential cultural phenomena that address *communication, space, social orientation, time, environmental control,* and *biological variations*. The phenomenon of biological variations is used by the nurse when conducting a full physical assessment (Giger & Davidhizar, 2008). The authors have identified several questions to determine culture-specific biologic information. For example, when examining lab work and reviewing the hemoglobin results, the nurse considers the possibility of sickle cell phenomenon in the Black or Mediterranean client (Dayer-Berenson, 2014).

Rachel Spector (2021) focuses on the relationship between one's *cultural heritage* and healthcare choices. She describes the traditional health beliefs and practices of selected North American groups and emphasizes the influence of sociopolitical changes and demographics on current perceptions of health and illness. Spector emphasizes the interconnectedness of heritage, culture, ethnicity, religion, socialization, identity, diversity, demographic change, population, immigration, and poverty. The author relates these to the concepts of health, illness, and healing. In Spector's latest text, the author suggests five steps to climb toward cultural competency. A tool for conducting a heritage assessment is also provided.

In another model, Andrews and Boyle (2019) apply principles of transcultural nursing across the life span and in various healthcare settings. These authors focus on seven components to include in a cultural assessment: *family and kinship systems, social life, political systems, language and traditions, worldview, value orientations,* and *cultural norms, religion, health beliefs, and practices*. They also discuss the transcultural aspects of pain among other nursing considerations, and offer culturally appropriate interventions.

Purnell (2019) offers a cultural competency assessment model utilizing 12 domains that are applicable to all cultures when performing a cultural assessment. The Purnell Model for Cultural Competence and its organizing framework is applicable to all healthcare providers and disciplines. Purnell's domains include *localities and topography, communication, family roles and organization, workforce issues,* **biocultural ecology,** *high-risk health behaviors, nutrition, pregnancy and child-bearing practices,* and *death rituals*. These constructs may be used to assess both the healthcare client and the provider.

A text by Marianne Jeffreys (2021) provides a resource for faculty and graduate nurse educators in teaching cultural competency skills in schools of nursing. A model of learning outcome assessment is also provided in her text and may be used with the author's permission.

MODELS FOR ENHANCING COMMUNICATION IN BUILDING CULTURAL COMPETENCE

Source: Hewson (2005).

PEARLS Statements

One model found in the literature focuses on building relationships and communicating positive regard for the person with whom you are communicating. This approach demonstrates a desire to establish and maintain a mutually respectful relationship. This model uses the mnemonic PEARLS for *partnership, empathy, acknowledgement, respect, legitimization,* and *support* (Suchman & Williamson, 2011). It is easy to see how nurses might apply this approach to their communication with patients. This model is especially useful when the nurse feels challenged or anxious about a particular nurse–patient interaction.

Use of Validation

In an effort to provide "family-centered care" when the nurse encounters "family member behavior, choices, attitudes, or emotions as difficult, or challenging to deal with," Harvey and Ahmann (2016), in a discussion about pediatric nurses interacting with family members, described the skill of "validation" (p. 61). Nurses can use this therapeutic technique to empower themselves and the patient when these situations arise. Use of the model enables the nurse to focus on behaviors rather than personality traits, and to develop new skills that enhance interaction with patients and their family members. The authors describe validation as a way for the nurse to express an understanding of how the patient feels without necessarily agreeing with the patient. The nurse accepts the patient/family members' thoughts and feelings as being understandable for them at that time (p. 61). This approach reassures the patient that the nurse is listening and that the relationship matters. By using this approach, patients or family members are more likely to be open to listening to what the nurse has to say. Therefore, validation offers an opportunity for a reciprocal exchange of information and facilitates optimum care delivery.

Harvey and Ahmann (2016) identified several ways that nurses can demonstrate validation: being present, reflecting or paraphrasing what the patient has said, articulating nonverbalized emotions, and restating information about the patient's past history. These authors also warned nurses against making statements that are dismissive of patients' feelings or emotions or that trivialize the patient's point of view, such as, "calm down or do not worry, saying that you understand, or expressing judgments that include words such as should, must, or inappropriate" (p. 64). Among the tips offered by the author for making validation easier are "calming yourself, realizing that someone else's feelings are really about themselves, asking questions, listening for answers without judging, and being mindful of nonverbal signals" (p. 64).

In light of the nation's increasing cultural diversity and the persistence of healthcare disparities, healthcare providers need to be able to deliver care using an efficient and effective approach to communicating with all patients. The literature offers many models and conceptual frameworks from which nurses might choose one best suited for their clinical situation. Some of those models have been presented here for application in practice or real-life situations.

The author hopes to encourage nurses to approach **cultural encounters** in a new and creative way with the help of a guiding framework to facilitate communication between the nurses and their clients. As nurses develop a greater understanding of what it means to become culturally competent and refine their skills in self- and patient-focused cultural assessment, they become better able to provide culturally sensitive care. As nurses' confidence in their ability to deliver culturally competent care increases, so, too, does their desire to experience newer and more challenging multicultural patient-care encounters. Those who reach this level of confidence as culturally competent nurses will help reduce the disparities that exist between groups and serve as role models and mentors for other nurses.

IMPORTANT POINTS

- In addition to a self-assessment, culturally competent nurses must assess their patients/clients based on cultural criteria and the situation or context in which the nurse finds the patient.
- The nursing literature provides a variety of nursing and nonnursing cultural assessment models.
- The nurse should select a model that is appropriate for the nurse's communication style, the patient's situation, and the clinical setting.
- Data gathered through the cultural assessment is used to inform patient care planning.

A male nurse admits a 40-year-old woman, Mrs. V, of Asian Indian descent, to the medical–surgical unit. The patient had sustained a head injury and was confused and somewhat disoriented. Her husband, who spoke some English but had a heavy Indian accent, accompanied her. While the patient was very quiet, the husband, who answered all questions addressed to his wife, seemed very anxious and annoyed. The nurse attempted to reassure Mr. V that everything was going to be okay. Nevertheless, he insisted on seeing a doctor right away and stated, "I don't want to keep speaking to a nurse, I need to speak with the doctor." The admitting nurse explained to the patient that the doctor would be in as soon as possible, but in the meantime decided to conduct a cultural assessment. During the assessment, the nurse learned that the husband was a recent immigrant to the United States from India and was not used to, and therefore uncomfortable with, the idea of his wife having a male nurse. The nurse later explained to the patient and her husband that he would remain the nurse primarily in charge of the patient's care, but that he would have a female assistant nurse provide her personal care. Mr. V was satisfied with this arrangement, but, with the staff's permission, remained at the bedside throughout her hospitalization.

SELECTED CULTURAL CONSIDERATIONS USING THE GIGER AND DAVIDHIZAR TRANSCULTURAL ASSESSMENT MODEL

Relevant aspects of this model are selected for this case. The nurse selects this cultural assessment model by Giger and Davidhizar and focuses on the following seven parameters when interviewing the patient and her spouse:

Communication: The patient is unable or unwilling to communicate verbally; husband answers for patient, has good English command, but heavy accent. Both husband and wife speak Indian dialect in the home. Patient tends to defer to husband when questioned. Nurse may need to investigate need for a medical interpreter.

Space: Both the patient and the nurse seem comfortable with close personal space, but do not like touching or close contact unless necessary for clinical procedures. Cross-gender touching is culturally unacceptable to the patient and her spouse.

Social orientation: There is an obvious gender role difference in expectations between what the nurse expects and what the patient's spouse expects in terms of spousal roles. This husband is very attentive and protective of Mrs. V and chooses to always stay with his wife. The nurses will need to be creative in planning to incorporate Mr. V in the care of this patient.

Time: Since Asian Indians are believed to be present, past, and future oriented, the nurse will need to assess the specific orientation of the patient and family during the patient–nurse encounter.

Environmental control: During the cultural assessment, when asked what Mr. V believes is a cause of this illness, he responds, "This is what God wants and we must always obey His will."

Biological variations: Because Mrs. V has sustained a head injury, the nurse will need to include various components of a neurologic assessment, monitoring Mrs. V for skin color changes, indications of inadequate breathing patterns, ineffective airway clearance, and impaired gas exchange. Mrs. V is Indian and is dark skinned. The nurse will need to observe the patient's normal skin tone to establish a baseline and compare later skin assessments to her own norm.

Plan: Using this model, the nurse will establish the following culturally competent goals for the patient. This is not an exhaustive list.

Goal 1: The patient will be able to communicate clearly with staff and staff will provide needed materials in a language the patient clearly understands. A medical interpreter can help with clarifying information that the patient or family attempts to convey. The interpreter can also make sure that the patient and her spouse understand the staff.

Goal 2: The patient's spouse will be included in patient's care and be encouraged to stay with her as much as is possible.

Goal 3: The patient will be treated with respect regarding cultural preferences regarding issues of personal privacy, touching, and so on. A female nurse will administer personal care.

Goal 4: The patient will have spiritual care based on her expressed wishes.

Goal 5: The patient will have adequate gas exchange. Among the assessment parameters monitored, the nurses will provide appropriate skin assessments based on the patient's norm.

NCLEX®-TYPE QUESTIONS

1. A nurse selects a cultural assessment model when performing a nursing history of a newly admitted recent immigrant from Cambodia. The primary reason for selecting the model is to
   A. Determine the nurse's ability to provide culturally competent care
   B. Assess the patient's ability to communicate in English
   C. Gain cultural knowledge about factors that may influence the patient's healthcare decision-making
   D. Determine the patient's readiness to utilize Western medicine

2. When using Purnell's 12 domains to perform a cultural assessment, the culturally competent nurse understands that the term *biocultural ecology* refers to
   A. Physical, biological, and physiological variations, such as skin color
   B. Differences in geographic location
   C. Attitudes toward preserving the environment
   D. One's country of origin

3. When performing a cultural assessment, the nurse utilizes Giger and Davidhizar's Transcultural Assessment Model. When assessing the construct of space, the nurse considers the patient's
   A. Visual depth perception
   B. Comfort level regarding social distance
   C. Adequacy of the patient's prior reception
   D. Sense of physiologic balance

4. In Leininger's Sunrise Model, "generic or folk systems" refers to
   A. Western medicine
   B. Systems of medicine that are antiquated and no longer useful
   C. Health practices of older adults
   D. Traditional healthcare practices and belief systems used as alternatives to Western medicine

5. The culturally competent nurse recognizes that the most appropriate time for performing a cultural assessment is
   A. When obtaining a health history
   B. After the nurse has met with the patient and the family
   C. During each patient–nurse encounter
   D. During the physical examination

6. The model that allows the nurse to express an understanding of how the patient feels without necessarily conveying agreement is called
   A. The Sunrise Model
   B. PEARLS
   C. Validation
   D. Kleinman's Explanatory Model

7. The nurse discovers that a newly admitted patient is unable to speak or understand English. In taking a patient-centered approach to care, what is an appropriate goal of care? *Select all that apply.*
   A. The patient will understand the diagnosis and treatment plan in their own language.
   B. The patient will learn some English to communicate with the staff.
   C. The patient's family will be included in the care planning as the patient desires.
   D. The patient's children will be utilized to translate to minimize the need for a medical translator.

8. The culturally competent nurse uses Kleinman's Explanatory Model during a cultural assessment. This model was selected because the nurse wants the patient to focus on
   A. The patient's perceptions about their illness
   B. The patient's allegiance to their family
   C. The patient's concerns about their spiritual beliefs
   D. The patient's concerns about the hospital staff

9. When using any of the cultural assessment tools, the culturally competent nurse employs a particular type of listening technique that requires the nurse to
   A. Question the patient's comments
   B. Restate and clarify
   C. Discuss the situation from the nurse's point of view
   D. Offer advice based on the nurse's medical knowledge

10. The ETHNIC Model affords the nurse an opportunity to learn about the patient's
    A. Genetic predispositions to diseases
    B. Socioeconomic problems
    C. Health beliefs, practices, preferences, and expectations
    D. Racial background

11. According to the stages of intercultural competence, a person who believes that their way of doing something is the only way may be viewed as being at what stage of competence?
    A. Unconscious incompetence
    B. Conscious incompetence
    C. Conscious competence
    D. Unconscious competence

12. Which statement best describes Cross's concept of cultural blindness?
    A. Attitudes that are destructive of cultures
    B. Attitudes that involve bias and discrimination
    C. Levels of awareness and an effective response to diverse populations
    D. A belief in treating all groups the same without regard for differences

ANSWERS TO NCLEX-TYPE QUESTIONS

1. C	5. C	9. B
2. A	6. C	10. C
3. B	7. A and C	11. A
4. D	8. A	12. D

AMERICAN ASSOCIATION OF COLLEGES OF NURSING COMPETENCIES ADDRESSED IN THIS CHAPTER

1. Apply knowledge of social and cultural factors that affect nursing and healthcare across multiple contexts.
2. Use relevant data sources and best evidence in providing culturally competent care.
3. Participate in continuous cultural competence development.

 A robust set of instructor resources designed to supplement this text is located at http://connect.springerpub.com/content/book/978-0-8261-8302-6. Qualifying instructors may request access by emailing textbook@springerpub.com.

REFERENCES

American Association of Colleges of Nurses. (2021). *The essentials: Core competencies for professional nursing education.* https://www.aacnnursing.org/Portals/0/PDFs/Publications/Essentials-2021.pdf

Andrews, M. M., & Boyle, J. S. (2019). The Andrews/Boyle Transcultural Interprofessional Practice (TIP) model. *Journal of Transcultural Nursing, 30*(4), 323–330. https://doi.org/10.1177/1043659619849475

Andrews, M. M., & Boyle, J. S. (2021). *Transcultural concepts in nursing care* (8th ed.). Wolters Kluwer.

Cross, T. (2012). Cultural Competence Continuum. *Journal of Child and Youth Care Work, 24*, 83–85. https://doi.org/10.5195/jcycw.2012.48

Cross, T. L., Bazron, B. J., Dennis, K. W., & Issacs, M. R. (1989). *Towards a culturally competent system of care: A monograph of effective services for minority children who are severely emotionally disturbed.* Georgetown University, Child Development Center. https://spu.edu/~/media/academics/school-of-education/Cultural%20Diversity/Towards%20a%20Culturally%20Competent%20System%20of%20Care%20Abridged.ashx

Dayer-Berenson, L. (2014). *Cultural competencies for nurses* (2nd ed.). Jones & Bartlett Learning.

Giger, J., & Davidhizar, R. E. (2008). *Transcultural nursing: Assessment and intervention* (5th ed.). Mosby/Elsevier.

Harvey, P., & Ahmann, E. (2016). Validation: A family-centered communication skill. *Nephrology Nursing Journal, 43*(1), 61–65. https://www.ncbi.nlm.nih.gov/pubmed/27025151

Hewson, M. G. (2005). It takes two to communicate: A review of the PAIR model and PEARLS statements. *Ophthalmology Management.* https://www.ophthalmologymanagement.com/issues/2005/october-2005/it-takes-two-to-communicate

Hordijk, R., Hendrick, K., Lanting, K., Macfarlane, A., Muntinga, M., & Suurmond, J. (2019). Defining a framework for medical teachers' competencies to teach ethnic and cultural diversity: Results of a European Delphi study. *Medical Teacher, 41*(1), 68–74. https://doi.org/10.1080/0142159x.2018.1439160

Howell, W. C. & Fleishman, E. A. (1982). *Human Performance and Productivity.* Vol. 2: Information Processing and Decision-making. Accessed at https://www.surgeons.org/-/media/Project/RACS/surgeons-org/files/professional-development/pap2010-09-23_stages_of_learning.pdf?rev=f4fb6b393fa44767b590bb3a40b8d2a9&hash=993E4B7134C1934699E984902CE64D4

Jeffreys M. R. (2006). *Teaching Cultural Competence in Nursing and Health Care.* Springer Publishing Company.

Jeffreys, M. R. (2021). *Teaching cultural competence in nursing and health care* (3rd ed.). Springer Publishing.

Kersey-Matusiak, G. (2019). *Delivering culturally competent nursing care: Working with diverse and vulnerable populations* (2nd ed.). Springer Publishing Company.

Kleinman, A., Eisenberg, L., & Good, B. (1978). Culture, illness, and care: clinical lessons from anthropologic and cross-cultural research. Annals of internal medicine, 88(2), 251-258.

Leininger, M. (1978). *Transcultural nursing: Theories, concepts and practices.* John Wiley & Sons.

Lieberman, J. A., & Stuart, M. R. (1999). The BATHE Model. *The Primary Care Companion to the Journal of Clinical Psychiatry, 1*(2), 35–38. https://www.ncbi.nlm.nih.gov/pmc/articles/PMC181054

Ludwig-Beymer, P. (2022). The role of transcultural nurses in the future of nursing. *Journal of Transcultural Nursing, 33*(3), 257–258. https://doi.org/10.1177/10436596221095065

Lui, P. P. (2022). Whose evidence? Enhancing cultural competency and humility in personality assessment: Commentary on Krishnamurthy et al. (2022). *Journal of Personality Assessment, 104*(1), 19–22. https://doi.org/10.1080/00223891.2021.2006674

People Communicating. (2014). *Reflective listening to improve communication skills.* http://www.people-communicating.com/reflective-listening.html

Purnell, L. D. (2013). *Transcultural health care: A culturally competent approach* (4th ed.). F. A. Davis.

Purnell, L. (2019). Update the Purnell theory and model for culturally competent health care. *Journal of Transcultural Nursing, 30*(2), 98–105. https://doi.org/10.1177/1043659618817587

Rukadikar, C., Mali, S., Bajpai, R., Rukadikar, A., & Singh, A. K. (2022). A review on cultural competency in medical education. *Journal of Family Medicine and Primary Care, 11*(8), 4319–4329. https://doi.org/10.4103/jfmpc.jfmpc_2503_21

Spector, R. (2021). *Cultural diversity in health and illness* (9th ed.). Pearson, Prentice Hall.

Stein, K. (2010). Moving cultural competency from abstract to act. *Journal of the American Dietetic Association, 110*(2), 186–187. https://doi.org/10.1016/j.jada.2009.12.007

Suchman, A., & Williamson, P. (2011). Principles and practices of relationship-centered meetings. In A. Suchman, D. Sluyter, & P. Williamson (Eds.), *Leading change in healthcare: Transforming organizations with complexity, positive psychology and relationship-centered care.* Radcliffe Publishing. https://www.acgme.org/globalassets/PDFs/Symposium/Suchman_Appendix-2---Principles-and-Practices-of-Relationship-Centered-Meetings.pdf

U.S. Department of Health & Human Services. Think Cultural Health. (n.d.). *Culturally competent nursing care: A cornerstone of nursing.* https://ccnm.thinkculturalhealth.hhs.gov

IMPORTANT WEBSITES

For information about diseases, conditions, health risks, fact sheets, and what to do.

Agency for Healthcare Quality and Research. Retrieved from innovations.ahrq.gov/ qualitytools/providers-guide-quality-culture
Centers for Disease Control. Retrieved from www.cdc.gov
National Institute of Health. Retrieved from www.nih.gov
Office of Minority Health. Retrieved from www.minorityhealth.hhs.gov
Think Culture Health DHHS. Nurses - Think Cultural Health. Retrieved from https:// thinkculturalhealth.hhs.gov/education/nurses

3

Embracing the Diversity
Among Our Ranks

Gloria Kersey-Matusiak

Everything that irritates us about others can lead us to an understanding of ourselves.

—CARL JUNG

LEARNING OBJECTIVES

After this chapter, the reader will be able to
1. Identify personal barriers to effective communication between culturally diverse coworkers.
2. Describe linguistic barriers that interfere with effective communication between domestic nurses and nurses educated outside of the United States.
3. Develop strategies for enhancing positive interactions between culturally diverse coworkers.
4. Recognize institutional barriers to positive interactions between culturally diverse colleagues.
5. Develop strategies for addressing institutional barriers to enhance interaction between culturally diverse coworkers.
6. Determine methods of eliminating discrimination, racism, and horizontal and lateral violence in the workplace.

KEY TERMS

Acculturated	Racism
Discrimination	Workplace bullying
Horizontal or lateral violence	

OVERVIEW

Issues of diversity in healthcare go beyond relationships between the patient and the nurse. They include nurse-to-nurse as well as nurse-to-other members of the health team. Today, as the diversity of the nation's population increases, many are touting the benefits of a multicultural and diverse workforce (Barr & Dowding, 2022; Brown, 2021; Eze, 2020; Hendricks & Cope, 2013). In Chapter 1, and throughout this text, diversity is defined broadly and refers to attributes that include such characteristics as age, ability, culture and ethnicity, gender, race, religion, and sexual orientation, among others. For the benefit of the institution, organizational leaders are encouraged to maximize the advantages of the unique talents and varied experiences that a diverse workforce has to offer. In addition, the literature also stresses the importance of collegial solidarity in the healthcare environment as a means of ensuring patient safety and optimum health outcomes (Kiliç & Altuntaş, 2019).

As members of the largest group of caring health professionals, most nurses pride themselves on caring for others. Additionally, in Gallups' most recent rankings of the most revered professions, nurses ranked highest for being the most honest and ethical for the 20th straight year (Saad, 2022). As one writer observed, "nurses have more than earned that position during the COVID-19 pandemic, risking their lives, working longer shifts to meet patient demands" (Carson-Neumann University, 2022). These findings are significant because having patients' trust and confidence in nurses is critical to establishing and maintaining caring relationships in which quality care and patient outcomes are optimized. Trust is also viewed as an ethical norm within nursing practice (Dinc & Gastmans, 2013). Yet, too often nurses encounter challenges to maintaining trust among one another due to a variety of factors that influence their ability to effectively interact and collaborate with one another on patients' behalf. In 21st century nursing, these factors include the increasing diversity among patients and nursing staff, potential language barriers, increasing technological demands, workplace incivility, variations in nurses' leadership, and hospital and unit policies to address issues that threaten the maintenance of a culture of collegiality and unity in clinical settings. In recent years, the COVID-19 pandemic also played a role in challenging nurses' ability to present a cohesive and united front.

Increasing Emergence of International Nurses

To respond to the increased need for nurses due to the nurse shortage during the COVID-19 pandemic, international nurses began filling frontline roles in critical care areas at a greater rate than U.S. nurses (Nurse Journal, 2023). According to a survey conducted by O'Grady Peyton (2021, p. 3), a division of AMN Healthcare, about 8% of all nurses providing care in the United States are internationally trained; of these nurses, 19% surveyed work in ICUs, 8% in EDs, and 11% in psychiatric care settings. "Most (77%) of the nurses are from one of three countries: the Philippines, Jamaica, and India, with 10% from Africa." This survey indicates that the levels of preparation and training of these nurses is greater, with 90% of international nurses holding a BSN or higher degree, whereas 56% of U.S. nurses hold a BSN or higher degree. Many of these nurses also have multiple years of work experience before coming to the United States as well. Although most international nurses in the study reported feeling accepted by patients, other nurses, and physicians, 36% said they have often or many times experienced **discrimination** based on their country of origin or ethnicity. While many international nurses speak English fluently, others struggle with a language barrier or are perceived as not speaking or understanding English well because of having an accent. Like all nurses, international nurses are subject to high levels of burnout.

Besides the professional contributions that help to offset the shortage in nursing, these nurses also enrich the cultural diversity of the nursing workforce. During the most significant nursing shortages in the past, nurses from the Philippines readily sought to address that gap as there was an abundance of nurses in that country, but fewer jobs available. Immigration of these nurses to the United States met the needs of both countries. Unfortunately, the literature reveals that nurses recruited from foreign countries often experience more challenges to their employment survival than are even usually discussed (Ali & Johnson, 2017; Baptiste, 2015; Okougha & Tilki, 2010; Seo & Kim, 2016; Wagner et al., 2015). Stories of these nurses' experiences highlight problems that range from foreign-born nurses feeling misunderstood to feelings of discrimination, mistreatment, and oppression on the part of domestic nurses. These perceptions are supported by reports of complaints from physicians, nurses, and patients to administration about problems they have with foreign-born nurses. Patients often complain about being assigned a foreign-born nurse to care for them, reporting that they have difficulty communicating with the nurse. Consequently, as Baptiste (2015) discussed, a negative relationship exists between nurses' job satisfaction, patient satisfaction, and perceptions of the quality of care patients receive.

Baptiste (2015) and a study by NYU Rory Meyers College of Nursing (2020) stated that internationally educated nurses (IENs) are essential to the U.S. healthcare system. According to the Health Resources and Services Administration (HRSA), 68% of IENs hold a BSN, compared to 49.2% of U.S.-educated nurses. Yet, discrimination in the work environment remains an issue of concern. Baptiste (2015) described discriminatory behavior in the workplace as being overt or subtle, conscious or unconscious, but born of "irrational, stereotypical beliefs related to different ethnic, cultural, or religious groups." These behaviors impact a target's "well-being, job turnover, or desire to leave an employment situation" (p. 8). Moreover, while not often discussed, workplace discrimination against IENs can be found in the literature as an additional source of psychologic stress for these nurses, adding to the stressors of acculturating to an entirely new environment and adapting to the nuances of a new societal and workplace culture. According to Baptiste, nurses leaving their homelands to work abroad are motivated by economic, social, professional, personal, and political factors. The process for gaining entry to the United States is both lengthy and challenging. In this study, Baptiste identified the countries, continents, and regions from which nurses come to the United States: the Philippines (50.1%), Canada (11.9%), India (9.6%), the United Kingdom (UK) (6%), South Korea (2.6%), Nigeria (2.1%), other Asia/Australia (6.7%), other North/South America/Caribbean (5.6%), other Europe (3.3%), and other Africa (2%).

According to this research, employees who are targets of discriminatory behavior disengage and experience burnout prior to physical withdrawal. Ma et al. (2020) suggest IENs may be helped to integrate into the U.S. workforce through training; workshops on culture, communication, and teamwork; and by recognizing these nurses' contributions to care provision. Although many IENs are English-speaking, those nurses who encounter a language barrier should be assisted with English as a second language (ESL) training when needed.

Diversity in Nursing

A 2020 survey of the nursing workforce conducted by the National Council of State Boards of Nursing (NCSBN) reported that the RN population is comprised of the following ethnic groups: 80.6% White/Caucasian, 6.7% Black/African American, 7.2% Asian, 0.5% American Indian/Alaskan Native, 0.4% Native Hawaiian/Pacific Islander, 2.1% two or more races, and 2.5% other nurses. In this same survey, 5% of RNs reported their ethnic identity as Hispanic. While the gradually increasing racial and ethnic diversity within nursing's workforce is viewed as a strength that enhances the potential to deliver more culturally sensitive care, it also poses the challenge of sometimes presenting obstacles to nurse-to-nurse interaction. For example, differences in patterns and styles of communication can sometimes lead to miscommunication or delayed communication between nurses and other healthcare workers. According to this survey, the number of men in nursing has been slowly increasing; however, women continue to dominate the profession, with men accounting for only 9.4% of RNs.

Besides the disparities that exist between the percent of minority members in society (40%) and those who are represented in the nursing workforce (19.4%; Eze, 2020), the lack of diversity leadership in healthcare in general, as well as in the nursing workforce, is reflected by data revealed in a study by the Institute for Diversity and Health Equity that reported minorities comprise only 14% of hospital board members, 11% of executive leadership positions, and 19% of first and mid-level managers. That same study reported that minorities made up 32% of patients in the responding hospitals. According to Korn Ferry

(2019), women hold 80% of healthcare jobs, but only 4% of healthcare organizations are run by women.

More senior-level positions are held by White women than minority women, and the gap between the two continues to increase; minorities hold only 9% CEO positions in hospitals and health systems in the United States. Financial need was cited as the reason why 29% of minorities compared to 15% of Whites took a less desirable position, and 38% of Blacks compared to 24% of Whites cited lack of opportunity as the reason they took less desirable positions (Eze, 2020).

In a policy statement titled "Increasing and Sustaining Racial/Ethnic Diversity in Healthcare Leadership," the American College of Healthcare Executives (ACHE) encourages organizations and executives to address areas of recruitment, promotion, and advocacy to improve the representation and equitable treatment of those in healthcare leadership (Health Stream Resources, 2021). Researchers agree that having a culturally diverse mix of healthcare team workers matters in providing culturally competent care (Barr & Dowding, 2022; Brown, 2021; Kennedy et al., 2022). In addition, many indicate that the need for culturally diverse leaders in healthcare is equally important. As one writer observed, "to provide truly compassionate person,-centered care, it is important to be aware of patients' cultural, religious beliefs and traditional customs, and more importantly their feelings when they are decision making regarding care and treatment" (Barr & Dowding, 2022, p.45). Therefore, having a culturally diverse mix of health team workers and team leaders at every level of management provides the human resources to achieve that goal.

Barriers to Cross-Cultural Interaction

Since 1986, the American Nurses Association (ANA) has made a commitment through its mission, position statements, and strategic planning to enhance diversity in nursing, yet progress remains slow. This lack of progress is due to a number of obstacles or institutional barriers to positive group interaction, including a limited number of culturally diverse nurses, a lack of gender diversity, cultural differences, racial discrimination, differences in interaction styles, and a lack of cultural self-awareness and sensitivity by many nurses from all cultural groups. Nevertheless, nursing departments are increasingly made up of individuals with diverse racial, ethnic, and gender backgrounds. These individuals have been born and educated both within and outside of the United States. Therefore, despite nurses' shared membership in the nursing profession, all nurses bring with them their own unique set of values and behaviors that are products of their racial, cultural, ethnic, and gender identities.

Strategies for Promoting Positive Cross-Cultural Interactions

The commitment to promoting an inclusive environment must begin at the top with a well-communicated statement of the institution's vision and mission that is shared with management and staff. Administrators and line managers provide resources to support the staff in meeting the institution's diversity goals. Examples of activities to strengthen diversity include mentoring of culturally diverse staff as well as diversity staff development for all nurses. These activities are aimed at enhancing cross-cultural understanding between groups. Evaluation and promotion prerequisites should include documentation of demonstrated achievement of the institution's or unit's diversity goals.

When working with culturally diverse colleagues, nurses should begin by becoming aware of their own attitudes, beliefs, and behaviors and being careful not to take an ethnocentric perspective (i.e., believing one's own values and beliefs are superior). Both majority and minority nurses must be careful in avoiding this viewpoint and aim toward bridging any cultural gaps. One strategy to help minority group members establish better working relationships with members of the dominant group is by building trust through open and honest dialogue, respecting areas considered private, being willing to give others the benefit of the doubt, commanding equitable treatment for yourself and others, and by attempting to understand how your behaviors are perceived. Unit leaders can provide opportunities for nurses to share formally and informally about themselves to foster appreciation and respect for diversity. New members of the team can be familiarized with the unit's culture, norms, and work team expectations in a nonthreatening way. When communicating with one another, nurse colleagues need to seek clarification when uncertain about one another's intended message. This process is accomplished by restating the message to the speaker using "I" statements: "I believe you are saying this." It is also helpful to find a trusted colleague among the team to assist in analyzing a new nurse's personal attitudes and behaviors. An atmosphere in which there is open dialogue about one's values and beliefs also provides opportunities for nurses to validate and support one another. Staff development activities aim to reduce uncertainty about what to say or do in initial interracial encounters.

The authors of the website Master Class (2023) also note strategies for strengthening cross-cultural interaction. The five strategies they offer to hone cross-cultural skills are (a) be friendly, (b) educate yourself, (c) embrace humility, (d) keep an eye out for unconscious biases, and (e) remain adaptable.

Garcia (2020) discussed the use of the term BIPOC in describing indigenous and people of color in the literature. The literature suggests that BIPOC and White nurses can benefit by enhanced cross-cultural interaction. Diversity training can provide opportunities for nurses to practice cross-cultural interaction skills, overcome challenges, and enhance their effectiveness as members of a multicultural healthcare team.

Ageism in Nursing

Nurses also differ by age group; the four generations currently in the nursing workforce are Traditionalist/Veterans/Silent Generation (1922–1945), Boomers (1946–1964), Generation X (1963–1980), and Millenials/Gen Y (1980–2000). These differences "can prevent some team members from connecting" (Bethea, n.d., para. 1). Bethea identified several barriers to connection including communication, technology, and management style issues. As in other professions and industries, ageism can impact both new graduates and veteran nurses in the form of age discrimination. Ageism is defined by the U.S. Equal Employment Opportunity Commission (EEOC) as treating a job applicant or employee less favorably because of age. This behavior can impact recruitment, pay, job assignments, training, benefits, and promotions. In a poll of healthcare professionals, 59% said they have been passed over for an employment opportunity due to age; 42% of nurses said they have been more stereotyped by age than physicians, pharmacists, and other clinicians (Duquesne University, School of Nursing, 2020).

To offset this phenomenon, an effective leader will need to identify ways to keep experienced nurses on the floor as they hire new, less experienced nurses and manage the unique set of traits and attributes of each generational group, while promoting engagement between them (Bethea, n.d.). This author recommended "BRIDGE," a corporate training strategy, as one way to facilitate work between people of multiple generations. This strategy includes forgetting preconceived notions about others, using one's experience to empower others, keeping the goal of caring for patients in mind, and creating a sense of collaboration and unity.

Incivility, Horizontal Violence, and Racism in Nursing

Incivility in nursing can be expressed in various forms through nurse-to-nurse, patient-to-nurse, and healthcare professional-to-nurse interactions (Robbins, 2021; Thomas, 2022).

Over the last several years, many writers have discussed the incivility that exists between nurses; this incivility can lead to low intensity behaviors with unclear intention that harm and disrupt the climate of mutual respect in the workplace (Alquwez, 2023; Kile et al., 2018; Layne et al., 2019; McPherson & Buxton, 2019; Sherman & Cohn, 2023). Contrasted with incivility, bullying is defined as a more targeted set of behaviors aimed at directly impacting an identified individual or group. According to Green (2020), bullying can be associated with race, culture, sex, gender, ageism, religion, or socioeconomics, and may occur because of discrimination or professional jealousy, among other situations. "Uncivil conduct can include superficial listening, rudeness, intentional withholding of information, blaming others, verbal attacks, lack of collaboration, and condescending language; setting up the victim, shaming, lying, distorting, devaluing, betraying, and excluding" (Green, 2020, p. 434). Incivility in nursing can also occur when a patient refuses care on the basis of the race or ethnicity of the nurse assigned to care for them (Robbins, 2021), or based on gender or age as previously described.

Incivility and bullying place the affected nurses, as well as the patients being cared for by them, at risk. Nurses who are exposed to incivility or bullying feel unsafe and insecure, begin to doubt their own competence, and are more likely to make clinical errors that impact patient safety. These nurses are also more likely to experience frequent absenteeism, burnout, and may ultimately leave their positions. Strategies for combatting incivility and bullying in nursing include prevention strategies, education, leadership, and systems thinking (Layne et al., 2019). Nurses experiencing incivility should consider seeking help from their employer including nurse managers and the Human Resource Department representatives to resolve the incivility (Green, 2020). These authors suggest that nurse educators also have a role to play in educating student nurses about the consequences of incivility and bullying on an individual's psychologic well-being, as well as the ultimate impact it has on patient care.

Racism

The 2020 murders of Breonna Taylor in March and George Floyd in May sparked protests across the nation and the world, fuelled by a new perspective of racism in the United States. For many, these events provided a fresh realization that blatant discrimination and racism existed and could often result in loss of life, especially for persons of color. Attempts to confront racism in healthcare were made by various organizations following these events. For example, The Joint Commission (TJC, formerly known as the Joint Commission on Accreditation of Healthcare Organizations [JCAHO]) has stated that it has "no tolerance for bias or discrimination in its organizations" (The Joint Commission, 2021). The board of the Massachusetts Nurses Association (MNA) approved an anti-racism position statement that acknowledges the impact of racism on patients and communities (Massachusetts Nurses Association, 2021). Other national efforts included the report of the National Commission to Address Racism in Nursing (ANA, 2022a) that documented the history of racism and its harmful consequences for all nurses of color. As Thomas (2022) observed, "… substantial racism in the work environment continues to affect their well-being today" (p. 705). In July 2022, the voting members of the ANA unanimously adopted a Racial Reckoning Statement, an acknowledgement of the organization's "past actions that have negatively impacted nurses of color and perpetuated systemic racism" (ANA, 2022b). These actions by the ANA and those of the ACHE that encouraged healthcare organizations and executives to address the equitable treatment of those with diverse racial and ethnic backgrounds in healthcare leadership are welcomed first steps in reconciliation between White nurses and nurses of color. However, issues of systemic racism and discrimination are not unique to the United States. Cooper Brathwaite and colleagues (2022) discussed racism in Canadian academic and healthcare settings that was directed toward Black nurses and students in Ontario. The researchers in this study defined racism "as a system of structuring opportunities and assigning value based on phenotype (race) that unfairly disadvantages some individuals and communities while unfairly advantaging other individuals and communities" (p. 21). In this study, the authors suggested the implementation of multilevel, multipronged interventions in workplaces to create a healthy work environment for all members of society. They also explained that "people who experience racism need healing, support, protection, including trauma-related services." In 2020, the Registered Nurses' Association of Ontario (RNAO) led a broad initiative to address anti-Black racism in nursing. In their review of the literature, these researchers found "that African American nurses' accents and race were factors prohibiting them from being hired into management and faculty positions in the United States, as well as creating high turnover rates of ethnic minorities in nursing leaders, educators, and staff."

In the United States, nursing is a microcosm of American society, so it should not be surprising that one of America's societal ills, racism, a by-product of slavery, has existed for a long time within the profession of nursing as it does in other professions and institutions in the nation. Many have described various events that substantiate that claim. For example, a case exemplar offered by Robbins (2021) provides an example of discrimination of a nurse by a patient who refused care by a particular nurse based on race. Camelo and Lim (2021) suggest that when a patient refuses a nurse assignment, nurse leaders should develop a plan that addresses the refusal and supports the staff. While this problem, and discrimination in general toward nurses of color, has long existed in nursing, Robbins observed that the COVID-19 pandemic exacerbated that situation and heightened society's awareness of health inequities (Robbins, 2021). While all nurses and other frontline workers were finally recognized for the critical roles they play in addressing health crises like the pandemic, BIPOC nurses and other health workers faced the added burden of being more likely to become seriously ill and die from COVID-19, to be more likely to be on the frontlines of care, and to be more economically dependent on their positions to support their families (Lopez & Wu, 2022).

The authors of this text are choosing to use the term BIPOC in this context to be inclusive of the indigenous people of North America, including Indian Nations (many of whom have borne the greatest burden of the COVID pandemic), Native Alaskans, and Hawaiian and Pacific Islanders (Garcia, 2020). Racism is but one of several -isms discussed in this text that threatens collegiality and unity between members of the nursing profession, although, other -isms may impact nurse solidarity to a lesser degree. Nevertheless, all of the -isms represent societal problems that can lead to a toxic work environment for nurses and other healthcare professionals, making it difficult for the targeted individuals to focus on the care they must provide to their patients.

Therefore, incivility of any kind, especially racism in the healthcare workplace, prohibits nurse-to-nurse collaboration, threatens collegiality and nurses' psychologic well-being, and jeopardizes patient safety. By so doing, racism minimizes the capacity of nursing to be a helping profession. Conversely, in a study that examined the impact of nurse solidarity, researchers found that "the situation in which the nurses help each other and are supported by the managers provided a better working environment, increases the confidence of the nurses, and increases the common power for the profession" (Kiliç & Altuntaş, 2019, p. 357).

To mitigate the long-standing effects of systemic racism in the healthcare workplace and promote a climate of unity between White nurses and all BIPOC nurses, there needs to be a transformation of the healthcare environment. Because there is no monolithic group of White nurses or nurses of color, members of both groups will need to determine the ways they can contribute to this transformation at the individual, interpersonal, or institutional level. That transformation will depend upon specific actions by nurse leaders, administrators, and staff; most importantly, however, all nurses regardless of their role will need to take responsibility for their own actions, attitudes, and beliefs.

For example, BIPOC nurses who have lost faith in the nursing profession's readiness to treat them equitably or without discrimination can choose to raise their expectations and adopt a can-do attitude and belief in their own capacity to excel in whatever roles they choose to seek for themselves. Despite any barriers these nurses may encounter, they can consistently strive toward being the best that they can be throughout their careers and command the positions and leadership roles they desire. BIPOC nurses who are already practicing with a full recognition of their talents and potential can serve as role models and mentors for others.

White nurses who already understand and appreciate the benefits of having a racially and ethnically diverse workforce can continue to promote the ideals expressed in ANA's Racial Reckoning Statement and maintain collaborative, collegial partnerships with nurses of color to ensure patient safety and positive patient outcomes. Others who have been influenced, misguided, or conditioned by historically racist views can begin to consider that the opportunity to serve optimally as a nurse or nurse leader at various levels in nursing is a privilege earned through one's hard work, interpersonal skills, education, and self-development, irrespective of one's skin color or ethnic background. Having an attitude of acceptance and a desire to build intercultural relationships promotes collegiality, facilitates collaboration, and contributes to the quality of patient care.

The increasing cultural, generational, racial, and ethnic diversity of the nursing workforce affords nurses many opportunities to provide culturally sensitive and appropriate care to a diverse population of patients. However, the benefits of diversity also create a need for nurses to identify effective ways of building positive working relationships with one another. This is especially critical during times when nurses and other health team members are already challenged by the consequences of COVID-19 and have to contend with lateral/horizontal violence, staffing problems, burnout, and job dissatisfaction to the extent that many are "not staying long at the bedside in the hospital setting. . . . [N]ew graduate nurses are seeking to further their educate themselves and leave bedside patient care early" (p. 435). Based on trends in RN supply and demand in the United States, the U.S. Department of Health and Human Services (DHHS), Health Resources and Services Administration (HRSA), National Center for Health Workforce Analysis (NCHWA, 2017) reported that despite increasing numbers of graduates from schools of nursing entering the workforce, there will be a decline in RN full-time employees, as the workforce continues to age and nurses retire. As a result, there is a projected demand for RNs in many states that will exceed the supply. The DHHS predicts an increased demand of 776,400 RNs by 2030 (DHHS, HRSA, NCHWA, 2017). While the American Association of Colleges of Nursing (AACN) reported schools of nursing had a 3.6% enrollment increase in entry-level BSN programs in 2016, it has not been sufficient to meet the growing demand for nursing services (AACN, 2022). For all of these reasons, hospitals and other care facilities have sought the expertise of nurses from outside the United States to aid in addressing this shortage.

Strategies for Promoting a Healthy Work Environment

So, what can nurses do to create a more supportive work environment where all nurses thrive and are able to do their best work for the sake of ensuring quality care for all patients? Several strategies are discussed in the literature and suggest a need for a concerted effort on the part of all nurses including students, faculty, practicing nurses, nurse managers, university and hospital administrators, and nurse leaders. As previously stated, the ANA has taken a stand to redress past acts of discrimination and racism toward nurses of color in its publication of the Racial Reckoning Statement, which encourages collaboration and collegiality between nurses. A study that examined the presence and source of incivility (Layne et al., 2019) concluded that nurses working in high-risk clinical settings may benefit from "targeted training in communication skills and conflict resolution to minimize experiences of incivility" (p. 1511). Universities, while continuing to recruit students of color to their nursing programs, should also offer content on the benefits of diversity, equity, and inclusion within their curricula. Students can also benefit by having opportunities to assess their biases even before entering clinical situations. Such self-learning activities can be obtained through the Implicit Association Test (IAT), available through Harvard's Take a Test website (https://implicit.harvard.edu/implicit/takeatest.html). Nursing curricula can also provide opportunities for diverse groups of students to share meaningful learning activities and promote contact between them. According to Tropp and Barlow (2018), contact "encourages members of advantaged racial groups to become psychologically invested in the perspectives, experiences, and welfare of members of disadvantaged groups" (p. 194).

When there are issues between patients and staff nurses, such as when patients refuse care by a nurse based on race or ethnicity, colleagues and nursing management can first assess the patient's rationale for the refusal, and then support the staff by reassuring the patient of the nurse's qualifications. The last resort should be reassigning the nurse, and this should only occur when resources are available. However, if the request by the patient is due to cultural or religious norms (e.g., a request due to prohibitions related to gender norms), these norms should be accommodated (Robbins, 2021). The authors provide an algorithm for patient refusals to assess patients' medical stability in these situations (Table 3.1). Finally, workplace bullying and other forms of horizontal violence can be addressed by clinical nurse leaders who (Green, 2020, p. 433) "educate and empower nurses to have an expectation of a healthy work environment for all nurses." All nurses should have a zero tolerance for incivility of any kind as it jeopardizes collegiality, threatens our status as professionals, and ultimately impacts patient safety. No one should stand by when acts of incivility occur in the workplace. Every nurse should be willing to speak up against all behavior that threatens a healthy work environment for the sake of our profession and our patients.

TABLE 3.1 ▪ STRATEGIES FOR PROMOTING A HEALTHY WORK ENVIRONMENT

1. Follow the ANAs Racial Reckoning Statement.
2. Provide targeted training for all nurses in communication skills and conflict resolution.
3. As universities recruit diverse students and maintain student diversity, they should also provide programs that promote diversity, equity, and inclusion within their curricula.
4. Have nursing faculty facilitate contact between students of different socioeconomic levels by providing learning opportunities for diverse students to interact with one another.
5. Address a patient's refusal of a nurse's care based on race or ethnicity in a way that is supportive of staff; the facility should assess the patient's rationale for the request, and reassure the patient of the nurse's qualifications; other staff members should also be supportive of their coworkers.
6. Have clinical nurse managers and other clinical leaders educate and empower nurses to have an expectation of a healthy work environment for all.
7. Support IENs through workshops on culture, communication, and teamwork, and provide ESL classes when needed.
8. Encourage all nurses to have zero tolerance for horizontal violence of any kind in the workplace and be willing to speak up against it in support of promoting quality care to patients.

IMPORTANT POINTS

- Since 1986, the nursing profession, through the ANA, has made a commitment to diversity, yet progress has been slow. In the workforce, 19.4% of nurses have minority backgrounds, and males represented only 9.4% of the nursing workforce in 2020.
- Increasing numbers of IEN nurses are helping to alleviate the nursing shortage.
- 77% of IEN nurses come from the Philippines, Jamaica, and India, with 19% coming from Africa.
- Researchers agree that having a cultural mix of healthcare team members and healthcare leaders is equally important.

(continued)

- Gender differences can prevent some team members from connecting.
- Every member of the work team, as well as institutional administrators, are responsible for maintaining a welcoming and supportive institutional culture and work environment.
- Variations in worldviews, values and beliefs, and patterns and styles of communication exist between workgroup members from culturally diverse groups.
- New members of the workforce must strive to acclimate to the new cultural environment through open and honest dialogue.
- Differences in values, attitudes, and beliefs between the dominant and minority group members should be addressed through planned opportunities for making contact with one another and cultural sharing.
- Nurse managers must find strategies to facilitate work between generationally diverse team members.
- Barriers to cross-cultural interaction include low numbers of culturally diverse health team members, low gender diversity, differences in interaction styles, and lack of cultural sensitivity and awareness by many nurses in all groups.
- When working with culturally diverse coworkers, active listening and seeking clarification through "I" statements are important strategies for effective communication.
- Considering the nurse shortage and the need for a multicultural workforce, all nurses should strive to support IENs to enhance patient safety and culturally competent care delivery.
- Nurses and nurse leaders should ensure a no-tolerance policy regarding lateral/horizontal violence discrimination and racism in the workplace.
- Only 4% of healthcare organizations are run by women; senior level positions are largely held by White women.
- Minorities hold only 9% of CEO positions in hospitals and healthcare systems.
- The ACHE encourages organizations to improve representation and equitable treatment of racial, ethnic diversity in their leadership.
- Incivility and bullying harms and disrupts the climate of mutual respect in the workplace.
- Strategies to promote positive cross-cultural interaction include forgetting preconceived notions about one another, using one's experience to empower others, keeping the goal of patient care in mind, and creating unity and collaboration.

CASE SCENARIO

Kim is a shy, 23-year-old RN who was born in Vietnam. At age 12, she immigrated with her parents as a refugee to the United States from Cambodia. While in Cambodia, Kim learned to speak English moderately well, but she still has a strong accent and sometimes, when anxious, forgets the appropriate word to use. After coming to the United States, Kim attended high school with a small group of other Cambodian refugee students whose families had also recently come to America. This small group became Kim's social network while in high school. Kim continued to strengthen her language skills through an ESL program. After graduating from high school, Kim attended a BSN program, from which she recently graduated.

Throughout her education, Kim, although very bright, has been uncomfortable with her English when she is around a group of native English speakers, and finds it difficult to contribute to group discussions.

The nurses on a busy surgical unit have been complaining for some time about the staffing shortage, high patient acuity, and the rapid patient turnover rates. They are concerned that the quality of care is being compromised. In response, the administration has recently added an additional full-time position to the unit's budget. Kim, the Vietnamese nurse, was hired to fill the position. Since Kim's arrival, members of the staff have complained among themselves about her inability to "fit in" as a member of the group. The major problem, as they see it, is Kim's poor language skills. Kim says little in communicating with other staff members. One of Kim's patients has even requested to have "another nurse, someone who speaks better English." On the other hand, many of Kim's other patients say that she is a caring and conscientious nurse. Some staff members complain, "Why can't these people learn the language if they want to work here?" One colleague laments: "I don't think she knows what she's doing" and "having Kim is like having no help at all." The staff decides to discuss the matter with the head nurse.

Kim is unaware of the staff's attitudes toward her, but senses that she has not yet been fully accepted as a member of the group and does not believe her input about patient care is valued. Still, Kim tries hard to befriend members of the staff through one-on-one interactions with them. She loves her job as a staff nurse, enjoys caring for patients, and is eager to learn as much as she can about her new role. She frequently offers to work overtime and to assist others as needed during her scheduled shifts. Kim wants so much to be accepted by the group and to make her mother and father proud of her success as a member of this nursing staff.

WHAT NURSES NEED TO KNOW ABOUT THEMSELVES

Application of the Staircase Self-Assessment Model: Self-Reflection Questions

1. Where am I on the Cultural Competency Staircase? How can I progress to the next level? (See Chapter 1 progression.)
2. How many encounters with people from Kim's background have I had to prepare me for interactions with Kim?
3. What do I know about members of this specific Asian group, Vietnamese or Cambodian?
4. What assumptions, stereotypes, or generalizations underlie my beliefs about Kim or about other members of Kim's cultural group? Am I prejudiced toward her?
5. What do I really know about Kim's attitudes, values, health beliefs, and work ethic, and how do these differ from my own?
6. How much have I tried to communicate with Kim personally?
7. How willing am I to extend myself to establish a positive and collegial rapport with this new member of the nursing staff?
8. What are some potential interpersonal problems or potential cultural conflicts based on this case scenario?
9. How can I overcome them?
10. Are there any legitimate patient-care issues that may be addressed through staff development, such as mentoring?

Please note: The selection of a nurse of Vietnamese heritage is a prototype; these questions may also be applied to encounters with other cultural groups.

Responses to Self-Reflection Questions 3, 4, 5, 6, 7, and 10

Response: What do I know about members of this specific Asian group, Vietnamese or Cambodian?

Many of the sources discussed in Chapter 1 offer culture-specific information about various cultural groups. A brief overview, such as the one that follows regarding Vietnamese culture, might assist nurses in having a better understanding of Kim and other nurses who are immigrants to the United States.

Vietnamese Culture

As of 2019, 1.4 million Vietnamese have emigrated to the United States since 1975 (Harjonto & Batalova, 2021), with many seeking asylum from war, persecution, or fear of death. The number of refugees that fled to the United States in 1975 (125,000) has since doubled every decade between 1980 and 2000. The 1.4 million Vietnamese refugees represent the fourth largest Asian group living in America (Harjonto & Batalova, 2021).

Like other immigrants, the Vietnamese are not a monolithic group. The earliest South Vietnamese immigrants who came to America between 1975 and 1977 were business people, military officers, and professionals from urban areas who had knowledge of American culture and the ability to speak English. Later immigrants (1980–1986) came from less fortunate circumstances, were unable to speak English, and had little understanding of Western culture. These "boat people," as they were often called, came to escape communism (Nowak, 2003). However, of those who survived the refugee camps or the perilous trip to America, many remained unemployed or in menial jobs. These groups had much more difficulty acculturating to the United States. Although some of the Vietnamese practice Christianity, the majority practice Buddhism, Confucianism, or Taoism. Vietnamese religious practices and traditions are based on these ancient philosophies.

A dominant force for most Vietnamese is that they wish to bring honor and prosperity to the family, which is the central reference point for the individual throughout their life (Giger & Davidhizar, 2004; Nowak, 2003; Purnell & Paulanka, 2005). The family may be nuclear or extended, with many generations living together. Among Vietnamese, an individual's responsibility to family transcends all others. Traditionally, men serve as the decision-maker, while women care for the children and the household. Children are expected to honor and obey their parents and respect the older adults.

Although emphasis is placed on the family and its needs, most Vietnamese values enable them to be successful in the workplace. They have a high regard for authority and are willing to work hard and to sacrifice comforts to maintain a steady income. They also value a harmonious work environment in which they readily adapt to work cooperatively with their peers. Purnell and Paulanka (2003) noted that "They may be less concerned about such factors as punctuality, adherence to deadlines, and competition" (p. 332). It is important to keep in mind that this statement may be true for some Vietnamese, but not necessarily all of them.

Communication

Vietnamese Americans usually speak one or more of four languages. The first, Vietnamese, is similar to Chinese, and has many dialects reflecting the geographical origin of the speaker. Vietnamese immigrants may also speak Chinese, French, or English. However, despite having knowledge of the English language, most Vietnamese do not feel competent when speaking English. Language variations may make it difficult for individuals from one part of Southeast Asia (e.g., Vietnam) to understand the language of people who come from another (e.g., Cambodia; Nowak, 2003; Yoder Stouffer, 2004).

Vietnamese Americans differ from mainstream Americans in their style and patterns of verbal and nonverbal communication. As compared to the dominant group, Vietnamese people are often considered passive. Generally speaking, they are nonconfrontational and they communicate in a soft-spoken tone of voice. Overt expressions of emotions, such as raising one's voice or verbally expressing disagreement, are typically avoided. The Vietnamese consider these behaviors to be disrespectful and inappropriate. Vietnamese do not usually discuss their personal feelings, but are more likely to open up in a one-on-one basis. Women typically avoid discussions about sexuality, childbirth, and sensitive topics of this nature in the presence of males (Purnell & Paulanka, 2005; Yoder Stouffer, 2004).

In observing nonverbal communication with Vietnamese American colleagues, it is important to recognize that avoiding eye contact while interacting with others is a demonstration of respect for those of "higher status." Vietnamese consider age, education, and gender, as well as nurses, doctors, and other professionals, with high regard. A quiet smile may reflect a variety of emotions, including joy, acknowledgment, or an absence of feelings entirely. Nodding one's head may not necessarily indicate an affirmation; rather, it may represent an acknowledgment of what has been heard (Yoder Stouffer, 2004).

Vietnamese Americans prefer a more extended social distance or space when communicating than do Euro-Americans (Nowak, 2003). Demonstrations of affection are limited to inside the home, and it is considered an insult for a man to touch a woman in the presence of others. However, holding hands with members of the same gender is considered appropriate among Vietnamese. For Vietnamese, the head of the body is considered sacred and should not be touched. The feet, as the lowest part of the body, should not be placed on a desk or table, as this would be considered a sign of rudeness and disrespect. Pointing one's fingers at someone or motioning with the finger to summon an individual are also considered signs of disrespect (Nowak, 2003).

Using this general overview of Vietnamese culture, nurses can begin to build cultural knowledge and gain some insight into Kim's dilemma in attempting to acculturate to this nursing unit. This knowledge is useful to those seeking to identify appropriate ways of assisting her in orienting to the unit and in assuming her new role as a staff nurse.

Response: What assumptions, stereotypes, or generalizations underlie my beliefs about Kim or about other members of Kim's cultural group? Am I prejudiced toward her?

The nurses have communicated to one another their frustration regarding Kim's inability to communicate effectively with them in the statement, "Why can't these people learn the language if they want to work here?" They have also indicated a general mistrust in Kim's ability to function as a staff nurse. This is evident in their statements, "I don't think she knows what she's doing" and "Having Kim is like having no help at all." These feelings expressed by the nurses may be based on the legitimate observations of Kim's performance in clinical situations.

However, it is possible that these feelings are based on the staff's inability to get to know Kim and to gain a sense of trust and confidence in her. Anxiety about Kim may also come from the fear of what is unknown about Kim as an individual who comes from a foreign background. Some nurses may have an unconscious bias toward Asian nurses, or may view nurses from foreign countries or non-Caucasian backgrounds as being inferior to nurses from the dominant group. This is an opportunity for nurses facing this situation or a similar one to take the IAT on Harvard's Take a Test website (harvard.edu).

Kim and her colleagues must be willing to acknowledge the cultural differences that exist between them, as well as those between Kim and some of her patients. As members of the healthcare team, nurses are encouraged to respect all people. This requires that they develop an open mind, seek cross-cultural relationships, recognize the stereotypes that they may have accepted as true or partially true about certain groups, and make an effort to free themselves of these influences.

Although the nurses can do little to change the attitudes of their patients toward Kim, they can demonstrate their acceptance and collegial respect for Kim as a professional nurse and, by setting an example of acceptance, foster in patients a greater degree of confidence in Kim's ability to care for them.

Response: What do I really know about Kim's attitudes, values, health beliefs, and work ethic, and how do these differ from my own?

It is important for nurses to realize that the answer to this question can only be found through frequent encounters with Kim. Despite having a general knowledge about Asian or Vietnamese culture, one cannot assume that Kim adopts all of these cultural values and beliefs. There is much intracultural diversity between members of the same group. Much will partly depend on when Kim actually immigrated to America and whether she has acculturated to American norms. Perhaps during lunch, the nurses might encourage Kim to talk about her background, her nursing preparation, and her general experiences as an immigrant to the United States. Members of the larger group might also share their own backgrounds and experiences in diversity with her. Later, as Kim becomes more comfortable with the staff, she might be asked to share her learning experiences in an open forum with other nurses throughout the hospital. By sharing cultural knowledge, both she and the staff can begin to identify cultural conflicts or patient-centered problem areas and strategies for addressing them.

Response: How much have I tried to communicate with Kim personally?

Kim, the nurse manager, and the nursing staff, as well as the staff development department, share the responsibility for facilitating Kim's transition to her new role as staff member. As the newest member of the nursing team, Kim also has a responsibility to develop strategies for assessing the new culture (the nursing unit) she has entered. In cooperation with her nurse manager, she will need to determine effective ways of acculturating to it.

Response: How willing am I to extend myself to establish a positive and collegial rapport with this new member of the nursing staff?

Without the sincere motivation to work cooperatively with members of culturally diverse groups, it is impossible to overcome the many barriers to cross-cultural communication that cultural differences in values, beliefs, attitudes, and behaviors can create. Accomplishing this goal requires a joint effort by Kim and the staff. Bridging the cultural gap serves the best interest of both the individual who is attempting to assimilate as a new member of the group and the nursing team that benefits from the addition of a more culturally competent and better-prepared team member. Most importantly, through the achievement of these goals, patient care is ultimately enhanced.

Response: Are there any legitimate patient-care issues that may be addressed through staff development, such as mentoring?

In this case, a culturally competent nurse manager might assign a nurse mentor to determine effective methods of bridging the existing cultural gaps between Kim and the staff. The individual assigned to act as a mentor for Kim would be able to give her honest feedback about her ability to communicate with patients and to address their patient-care needs.

This approach would assist in promoting Kim's growth and productivity as a professional nurse. The resultant close, one-on-one relationship with a mentor who is also a native speaker of English would assist Kim in strengthening her language skills as well. Kim might also benefit from an ESL program to enhance her English language skills.

WHAT NURSES NEED TO KNOW WHEN WORKING WITH CULTURALLY DIVERSE COLLEAGUES

Selecting a Cultural Assessment Model

Apply a cultural assessment model to help identify cultural information about Kim that could be used to establish more effective communication with her. One cultural assessment model that might be appropriate in this situation is Andrews and Boyle's Assessment Guide for Individuals and Families. This model includes multiple components that are to be evaluated within "context": docplayer.net/33034972-Andrews-boyle-transcultural-nursing-assessment-guide.html (see Chapter 4). In Kim's case, the context to be taken into consideration is the professional work environment.

ASSESSMENT QUESTIONS FOR GAINING RELEVANT CULTURAL INFORMATION

1. What is Kim's country of origin?
2. What is her immigration status? Is she a new or longer-established immigrant?
3. What are her family network and other social supports in the United States? Who does Kim live with? What is her marital status?
4. What language does Kim speak in the home? What English language problems does Kim have? Are the staff members able to communicate with her effectively? If not, what resources are available to assist Kim in overcoming the language barrier? What strategies can I use to enhance my communication with Kim?
5. Does Kim have a collectivist or individualistic perspective? How does Kim view her role as a member of this healthcare team?
6. Does Kim hold values and beliefs or healthcare practices that differ from my own?
7. What cultural information can I learn from Kim to utilize in future cross-cultural interactions?
8. How can I assist Kim in acclimating to this unit, this hospital, and this community?

Use the information gained about Kim from these assessment questions to complete the following case exercise. Discuss your responses with a friend, a classmate, or a colleague.

CASE EXERCISE ON WORKING WITH CULTURALLY DIVERSE COLLEAGUES

A. Pretend that you are one of the nurses working with Kim. Identify three ways that you can assist Kim in acclimating to the unit.
   1.
   2.
   3.
B. Identify three ways that you can assist the patients in becoming more accepting of Kim.
   1.
   2.
   3.
C. Imagine yourself as a new member of a staff. You are the only representative member of your racial/ethnic, gender, or cultural group on the staff. What can you do to be a more effective team member?

SUMMARY

Acknowledging biases that may be based on ignorance or assumptions about persons of Asian or Vietnamese heritage, or any other ethnic group, is a first step in curtailing their influence on cross-cultural interactions. Utilizing multiple formal and informal opportunities to share cultural knowledge will strengthen the relationship between Kim and the staff. In the mutual sharing of cultural information, Kim will also be able to grow in her understanding of U.S. culture and its implications in the workplace. Staff members will gain knowledge that will assist them in caring for Vietnamese patients.

Besides knowledge and understanding, skills in communication that promote active listening and open and honest dialogue between culturally diverse groups are needed to avoid major cultural conflicts that threaten positive cross-cultural communication. Having a clear understanding of Kim's values, attitudes, health beliefs, work ethic, and interacting style will enable the nurses on the unit to identify commonalities as well as differences between them.

Establishing a trusting relationship with at least one member of the team who can serve as a provider of feedback as well as a sounding board for Kim's frustrations would be equally useful in facilitating Kim's psychologic transition and professional development in her nursing role. When Kim and the nursing staff can bridge the cultural gap that exists between them, everyone wins.

NCLEX®-TYPE QUESTIONS

1. In a culturally competent work setting, the responsibility for Kim's success as a new nurse on the unit lies with:
   A. Human resources
   B. Kim
   C. The staff
   D. Kim, human resources, and the nursing staff

2. The primary cross-cultural barrier in this case scenario is a problem due to:
   A. Kim's lack of experience in the United States
   B. Kim's educational preparation in nursing
   C. Challenges in communication
   D. Differences in worldview

3. Why is having knowledge about Kim's cultural background useful? Select all that apply.
   A. It enables the nurses to get to know Kim's cultural values and beliefs.
   B. It provides cultural information as a resource for the nurses' future encounters with patients who share Kim's ethnicity.
   C. It assists in overcoming the language barrier.
   D. It helps prevent problems in miscommunication.

4. A culturally competent nurse recognizes that cultural group members who have a collectivist perspective value:
   A. The needs of the group or team over those of the individual
   B. The needs of the individual
   C. Needs based on the circumstances
   D. The demands of the team leader

5. According to some researchers, what methods can minority group members use to establish better relationships with members of the dominant group? Select all that apply.
   A. Building trust through honest dialogue
   B. Being vigilant in watching for any signs of prejudice or bias toward them
   C. Being willing to give others the benefit of the doubt
   D. Demanding equitable treatment for themselves and others
   E. Striving to understand how their behaviors are perceived

6. When culturally competent nurses are working with diverse colleagues, the first step in the process is to:
   A. Determine the new colleague's level of communication
   B. Explore their own attitudes, beliefs, and behavior
   C. Share cultural knowledge about their own cultural background
   D. Explore cultural differences that exist between themselves and the new staff member

7. How can nurse administrators and human resources personnel help ensure the cultural acclimation of newly hired nurses from culturally diverse backgrounds? Select all that apply.
   A. Providing staff development opportunities that promote cultural sharing
   B. Orienting culturally diverse nurses to the culture of the unit and the institution
   C. Setting a deadline by which new staff must complete their orientation
   D. Assigning a mentor to work specifically with a new nurse

8. The culturally competent nurse is working with a colleague who adopts a traditional interpersonal style. The nurse recognizes that persons practicing this style are more likely to:
   A. Be willing to abandon their cultural values
   B. Find it difficult to relinquish their beliefs and attitudes
   C. Fail to recognize or acknowledge their cultural identity
   D. Take pride in their own culture while being comfortable interacting with members of another

9. Active listening is a strategy used by culturally competent nurses. This means that during communication, the culturally competent nurse:
   A. Allows the speaker to speak without ever interrupting
   B. Seeks clarification to ensure accuracy
   C. Uses nonverbal communication for emphasis
   D. Actively engages the speaker by sharing stories

10. When a patient asks to have someone other than a culturally diverse coworker care for them, culturally competent nurses can respond by:
    A. Speaking supportively about the professional competence of the nurse
    B. Agreeing to take the assignment on behalf of the nurse
    C. Insisting that the patient will have to accept the hospital's policy on nondiscrimination
    D. Refusing to care for the patient

ANSWERS TO NCLEX-TYPE QUESTIONS

1. D
2. C
3. A, B, and D
4. A

5. A, C, and E
6. B
7. A, B, and D
8. C

9. B
10. A

AMERICAN ASSOCIATION OF COLLEGES OF NURSING COMPETENCIES ADDRESSED IN THIS CHAPTER

1. Apply knowledge of social and cultural factors that affect nursing and healthcare across multiple contexts.
2. Advocate for social justice, including commitment to the health of vulnerable populations and elimination of healthcare disparities.
3. Participate in continuous cultural competency development.

 SPRINGER PUBLISHING CONNECT™ | A robust set of instructor resources designed to supplement this text is located at http://connect.springerpub.com/content/book/978-0-8261-8302-6. Qualifying instructors may request access by emailing textbook@springerpub.com.

REFERENCES

Ali, P. A., & Johnson, S. (2017). Speaking my patient's language: bilingual nurses' perspective about provision of language concordant care to patients with limited English proficiency. *Journal of Advanced Nursing, 73*(2), 421–432. https://doi.org/10.1111/jan.13143

Alquwez, N. (2023). Association between nurses' experiences of workplace incivility and the culture of workplace incivility and the culture of safety of hospitals: A cross-sectional study. *Journal of Clinical Nursing, 32*(1–2), 320–331. https://doi.org/10.1111/jocn.16230

American Association of Colleges of Nursing. (2022). *Fact sheet: Nursing shortage.* https://www.aacnnursing.org/Portals/0/PDFs/Fact-Sheets/Nursing-Shortage-Factsheet.pdf

American Association of Critical Care Nurses. (2022). *Fact sheet: Nursing shortage.* https://www.aacnnursing.org/news-data/fact-sheets/nursing-shortage

American Nurses Association. (2022a). *The National Commission to address racism in nursing reflects on nurses' vast contributions during nurses month.* https://www.nursingworld.org/news/news-releases/2021/the-national-commission-to-address-racism-in-nursing-reflects-on--nurses-vast-contributions-during-nurses-month/

American Nurses Association. (2022b). *Our racial reckoning statement.* https://www.nursingworld.org/practice-policy/workforce/racism-in-nursing/RacialReckoningStatement/

Baptiste, M. M. (2015). Workplace discrimination: An additional stressor for internationally educated nurses. *Online Journal of Issues in Nursing, 20*(3), 8. https://doi.org/10.3912/OJIN.Vol20No03PPT01

Barr, J., & Dowding, L. (2022). *Leadership in health care* (5th ed.). Sage.

Bethea, N. (n.d.). *Overcoming generational divides in nursing.* Health Nurse, Healthy Nation Blog. Retrieved November 27, 2023 from, https://engage.healthynursehealthynation.org/blogs/8/686

Brown, E. N. (2021). *Diversity in the work place.* https://www.amazon.com/Diversity-Work-Place-Inclusive-Unconscious/dp/B09M6ZZRV6

Camelo, G. S., & Lim, F. (2021). When a patient refuses a nurse assignment. *American Nurse Journal, 16*(8), 22–25. https://www.myamericannurse.com/wp-content/uploads/2021/08/an8-Patient-refusal-730.pdf

Cooper Brathwaite, A., Versailles, D., Juüdi-Hope, D., Coppin, M., Jefferies, K. C., Bradley, R., Campbell, R., Garraway, C., Obewu, O., LaRonde-Ogilvie, C., Sinclair, D., Groom, B., & Grinspun, D. (2022). Tackling discrimination and systemic racism in academic and workplace settings. *Nursing Inquiry, 29*(4), e12485. https://doi.org/10.1111/nin.12485

Carson-Neumann University Online. (2022, March 30). *By the numbers: Nursing Statistics 2022.* https://onlinenursing.cn.edu/news/nursing-by-the-numbers

Dinc, L., & Gastmans, C. (2013). Trust in nurse–patient relationships: A literature review. *Nursing Ethics, 20*(5), 501–516. https://doi.org/10.1177/0969733012468463

Duquesne University, School of Nursing. (2020). *Nurse leaders addressing ageism in nursing.* https://onlinenursing.duq.edu/blog/nurse-leaders-addressing-ageism-in-nursing/

Eze, N. (2020). Driving health equity through diversity in health care leadership. *NEJM Catalyst.* https://catalyst.nejm.org/doi/full/10.1056/CAT.20.0521

Garcia, S. E. (2020, June 17). Where did BIPOC come from? *New York Times.* https://www.nytimes.com/article/what-is-bipoc.html

Giger, J. N., & Davidhizar, R. E. (2004). *Transcultural nursing: Assessment and intervention* (4th ed.). Mosby.

Green, C. (2020). The hollow: A theory on workplace bullying. *Nursing Forum, 56,* 433–438. https://doi.org/10.1111/nuf.12539

Harjonto, L., & Batalova, J. (2021). *Vietnamese Immigrants in the United States.* Migration Policy Institute. https://www.migrationpolicy.org/article/vietnamese-immigrants-united-states-2019

Health Stream Resources. (2021). *Benefits of diversity in healthcare leadership.* https://www.healthstream.com/resource/blog/benefits-of-diversity-in-healthcare-leadership

Hendricks, J. M., & Cope, V. C. (2013). Generational diversity: What nurse managers need to know. *Journal of Advanced Nursing, 69*(3), 717–725. https://doi.org/10.1111/j.1365-2648.2012.06079.x

Jean, J. (2022). *6 proven strategies from nurse execs to combat the nursing shortage.* https://nursejournal.org/articles/proven-strategies-to-survive-the-nursing-shortage-2022/

Kennedy, K., Leclerc, L., & Campis, S. (2022). *Human-centered leadership in healthcare: Evolution of a revolution.* Morgan James.

Kile, D., Eaton, M., deValpine, M., & Gilbert, R. (2018). The effectiveness of education and cognitive rehearsal in managing nurse-to-nurse incivility: A pilot study. *Journal of Nursing Management, 27*(3), 543–552. https://doi.org/10.1111/jonm.12709

Kiliç, E., & Altuntaş, S. (2019). The effect of collegial solidarity among nurses on the organizational climate. *International Nursing Review, 66*(3), 356–365. https://doi.org/10.1111/inr.12509

Korn Ferry. (2019). *Women in healthcare: From the ER to the C-Suite.* https://www.kornferry.com/insights/perspectives/perspective-women-in-healthcare

Layne, D. M., Anderson, E., & Henderson, S. (2019). Examining the presence and sources of incivility within nursing. *Journal of Nursing Management, 27*(7), 1505–1511. https://doi.org/10.1111/jonm.12836

Lopez, G., & Wu, A. (2022, September 8). Covid's toll on Native Americans. *New York Times.* https://www.nytimes.com/2022/09/08/briefing/covid-death-toll-native-americans.html

Ma, C., Ghazal, L., Chou, S., Ea, E., & Squires, A. (2020). Unit utilization of internationally educated nurses and collaboration in U.S. hospitals. *Nursing Economics, 38*(1), 33–40, 50. https://www.proquest.com/openview/dd075a21269b32e44289646d0a91ce72/1?pq-origsite=gscholar&cbl=30765

Massachusetts Nurses Association. (2021). *MNA launches effort to combat racism within the association, nursing/health profession, and the health care workplace as tensions rise, and long-standing health disparities for minority communities become glaringly apparent during COVID-19 pandemic.* https://www.massnurses.org/2021/01/18/mna-launches-effort-to-combat-racism-within-the-association-nursing-health-profession-and-the-health-care-workplace-as-tensions-rise-and-long-standing-health-disparities-for-minority-communities-be/

Master Class. (2023). Cross-cultural communication and cultural understanding. https://www.masterclass.com/articles/cross-cultural-communication

McPherson, P., & Buxton, T. (2019). In their own words: Nurses countering workplace incivility. *Nursing Forum, 54*(3), 455–460. https://doi.org/10.1111/nuf.12354

Nowak, T. T. (2003). People of Vietnamese heritage. In L. D. Purnell & B. J. Paulanka (Eds.), *Transcultural health care: A culturally competent approach* (2nd ed., pp. 327–343). F.A. Davis.

Nurse Journal. (2023). *Challenges faced by Black nurses in the profession: Q & A with Jamil Norman.* https://nursejournal.org/articles/challenges-faced-by-black-nurses-in-the-profession-interview

NYU Rory Meyers College of Nursing. (2020). *Hospitals with internationally trained nurses have more stable, educated nursing workforces.* https://nursing.nyu.edu/news/hospitals-internationally-trained-nurses-have-more-stable-educated-nursing-workforces

O'Grady Peyton International (USA) Inc. (2021). *Survey of international nurses.* https://prod.amnhealthcare.com/siteassets/amn-insights/whitepapers/2021-survey-of-international-nursing.pdf

Okougha, M., & Tilki, M. (2010). Experience of overseas nurses: the potential for misunderstanding. *British Journal of Nursing, 19(2),* 102–106. https://doi.org/10.12968/bjon.2010.19.2.46293

Purnell, L. D., & Paulanka, B. J. (Eds.). (2003). *Transcultural health care: A culturally competent approach* (2nd ed.). F.A. Davis

Purnell, L. D., & Paulanka, B. J. (2005). *Guide to culturally competent health care*. F. A. Davis.

Robbins, K. C. (2021). A nurse assignment refused by the patient: What to do. *Nephrology Nursing Journal, 48*(5), 503–504. https://doi.org/10.37526/1526-744x.2021.48.5.503

Saad, L. (2022). *Military brass, Judges among professions at new image lows*. Gallup. https://news.gallup.com/poll/388649/military-brass-judges-among-professions-new-image-lows.aspx

Seo, K., & Kim, M. (2016). Clinical work experience of Korean immigrant nurses in U.S. hospitals. *Journal of Korean Academy of Nursing, 46*(2), 238–248. https://doi.org/10.4040/jkan.2016.46.2.238

Sherman, R. O., & Cohn, T. M. (2023). Assessing unit culture. *American Nurse Journal, 18*(2), 28–32. https://doi.org/10.51256/anj022328

Thomas, S. P. (2022). Finding hope in meaningful steps against racism in nursing. *Issues in Mental Health Nursing, 43*(8), 705. https://doi.org/10.1080/01612840.2022.2104021

The Joint Commission. (2021). Speak up against discrimination. https://www.jointcommission.org/-/media/tjc/documents/resources/speak-up/speak-up-against-discrmination-24x36.pdf

Tropp, L. R., & Barlow, F. K. (2018). Making advantaged racial groups care about inequality: Intergroup contact as a route to psychological investment. *Current Directions in Psychological Science, 27*(3), 194–199. https://doi.org/10.1177/0963721417743282

U.S. Department of Health and Human Services, Health Resources and Services Administration, National Center for Health Workforce Analysis. (2017). *National and regional supply and demand projections of the nursing workforce: 2014-2030*. https://bhw.hrsa.gov/sites/default/files/bureau-health-workforce/data-research/nchwa-hrsa-nursing-report.pdf

Wagner, L. M., Brush, B., Castle, N., Eaton, M., & Capezuti, E. (2015). Examining differences in nurses' accents and comprehensibility in nursing home settings based on birth origin and country of education. *Geriatric Nursing, 36*(1), 47–51. https://doi.org/10.1016/j.gerinurse.2014.10.012

Yoder Stouffer, R. U. (2004). Vietnamese Americans. In J. N. Giger & R. E. Davidhizar. *Transcultural nursing* (4th ed., pp. 455–488). Mosby.

IMPORTANT WEBSITES

For more comprehensive information about Vietnamese people and their cultural heritage.

American Foreign Relations. The Vietnam war and its impact Refugees and "boat people." Retrieved from https://www.americanforeignrelations.com/O-W/The-Vietnam-War-and-Its-Impact-Refugees-and-boat-people.html

Vietnamese Culture. Retrieved from www.vietnam-culture.com/zones-6–1/Vietnamese-Culture-Values.aspx

Vietnamese Embassy of the United States. Retrieved from www.vietnamembassy-usa.org

Vietnamese Touch. Retrieved from www.viettouch.com; web.ebscohost.com/ehost/pdfviewer/pdfviewer?sid = 05133855–3a67–45e8-b257–114ad578dc72%40sessionmgr 114&vid = 4&hid = 123

STEPPING UP TO CULTURAL COMPETENCY

Cultural Considerations When the Patient's Religious or Spiritual Needs Differ From One's Own

Gloria Kersey-Matusiak

Everything in your life is there as a vehicle for transformation. Use it!
—RAM DASS

LEARNING OBJECTIVES

After this chapter, the reader will be able to
1. State a personal definition of spirituality.
2. Explain the difference between spirituality and religion as they relate to the delivery of culturally competent care.
3. Describe the significance of spirituality from both the nurse's and patient's perspective.
4. Recognize clinical indicators of spiritual distress.
5. Identify selected religious groups that are currently practicing in the United States.
6. Identify important religious considerations when delivering culturally competent care.
7. Select appropriate interventions to promote patients' spiritual well-being.

KEY TERMS

Agnosticism	Religion
Atheism	Spirituality
Humanistic	Theistic
Monistic	Unaffiliated

THE PHILOSOPHICAL UNDERPINNINGS OF SPIRITUALITY

Spirituality and/or **religion** are aspects of everyone's culture. Therefore, both the patient and the nurse bring to each nurse–patient encounter their own spiritual values and religious beliefs. When the patient and the nurse come from different backgrounds, the nurse may have little knowledge of the patient's spiritual needs or religious views. For example, in some situations, it may be difficult for the nurse to appreciate the impact that faith and prayer have on healing from the patient's perspective. It may be even more challenging for the nurse to appreciate a patient's spirituality needs when the individual seems to lack religious conviction; for example, if the patient is atheistic (**atheism**) or disbelieves in God, agnostic (**agnosticism**) and neither believes nor disbelieves in God, or believes it is impossible to know of God's existence. Spirituality may be integrated into one's life based on one of three philosophical viewpoints: **monistic**, **humanistic**, or **theistic**. A monistic view holds that there is only one fundamental reality and one source for all things. According to McLeod, someone who practices humanism believes that "it is each person's unique subjective approach to defining reality that's important" (2023, "Psychology") without any belief in a god or deity. Cline (2019) explains that while humanism is often associated with secularism, there is also religious humanism; its basic principles include an overriding concern with humanity, including the needs and desires of human beings and the importance of human experiences. Theism focuses on a belief in at least one or more gods or deities. Most of the world's religions come from a theistic perspective (Cline, 2019).

The Current Religious Landscape in the United States

A significant change in the religious landscape of America has been noted recently by many researchers (Jones, 2021; Neuman, 2021; PBS News Hour, 2019; Pew Research Center, 2022; Public Religion Research Institute [PRRI], 2021). Most notable among researchers' findings is the fact that the percentage of "Americans who describe their religious identity as atheist, agnostic", or "nothing in particular is 26%, in addition, 9% of U.S. adults self-described as atheist or agnostic" (PBS News Hour, 2019). As a National Public Radio (NPR) poll shows, fewer than half of U.S. adults belong to a religious congregation (47%). That number has declined from 50% in 2018 and 70% in 1999. In that study, Catholics were found to have the greatest drop in church membership with an 18% drop, while Protestants showed a 9% decline (Neuman, 2021). According to Jones (2021), among those who do identify with a particular religion, 69% of Americans identify with a Christian religion (in 1971, 90% of Americans identified as Christians). Of those who do identify with a specific religious faith today, 35% identify as Protestant, 22% identify as Catholic, and another 12% identify with another Christian religion. There are significant differences in religious perspectives between Christians who identify with conservative or traditional groups and those who are more liberal in their beliefs. In the same report, 7% identify with a non-Christian religion; this group includes 2% who are Jewish, 1% who are Muslim, and 1% who are Buddhist. In addition, 21% of U.S. adults said they have no religious preference, and 3% did not answer the question (Jones, 2021). The decline in church membership has generally been attributed to the beliefs of younger Americans, with about one in three U.S. younger adults having no religious affiliation. However, the increase in proportion of religiously **unaffiliated** Americans has occurred across all age groups. In 2020, PRRI reported that 23% of Americans identified as religiously unaffiliated.

In any case, irrespective of the nurse's or the patient's religious affiliation, culturally appropriate, evidence-based, and holistic nursing care must include interventions that address the patient's spiritual needs (American College of Cardiology, 2022; Hawthorne & Gordon, 2020; Southard, 2020; Yeşilçinar et al., 2018).

Differentiating Religion From Spirituality

Brady (2020) and Cline (2019), in differentiating religion from spirituality, each describe religion as a set or institutionalized system of attitudes, beliefs, and practices devoted to the service and worship of God or the supernatural. Religion includes public rituals and organized doctrines. It is organized and structured with rules and laws that govern the behavior of its members. The literature reminds us that one does not have to be religious to be spiritual (Table 4.1).

TABLE 4.1 ■ DIFFERENTIATING RELIGION FROM SPIRITUALITY

RELIGION	SPIRITUALITY
1. External; imposed by others, organized, structure 2. Relies on doctrines & rules 3. Is exclusive to followers 4. Belief in God or Higher Being	1. Internal source of strength & direction 2. Seeks personal truth, purpose, & meaning in one's life 3. May or may not have God or Higher Being 4. Seeks balance of mind, body, and spirit

But what, then, is spirituality? Several authors have attempted to define spirituality, but despite these ongoing efforts, there is no clear consensus about its definition (de Brito Sena et al., 2021; Yesilcinar et al., 2018). Most researchers agree that the concept of spirituality is abstract, complex, and most often found in religious and philosophical contexts (Yeşilçinar et al., 2018). In a systematic review of the literature, de Brito Sena and colleagues identified 24 spirituality dimensions that included connection/relation, meaning/purpose, divine/god or higher power, transcendence/immaterial, others/community relationship, and beliefs among the top six dimensions found to refer to spirituality. In this study, the researchers define spirituality as "a complex and multidimensional part of the human experience with cognitive and experiential and behavioral components" (p. 6). Further, they note that the cognitive or philosophic component includes the search for meaning, purpose, and truth and the beliefs and values by which one lives. The behavioral component then becomes the manifestation of one's beliefs. The researchers describe the emotional or experiential component of spirituality as those feelings of hope, love, connection, inner peace, comfort, and support reflected by the "quality of an individual's inner resources" (p. 6). An individual experiencing limited internal spiritual resources, especially at a time when they are facing physical, psychologic, or emotional challenges, may encounter spiritual distress. Spiritual distress is defined as a disruption in a person's belief system. Spiritual distress may be evidenced by such behaviors as crying, apathy, anger, changes in sleep patterns, and/or depression. The spiritual care of patients involves such interventions as contacting a spiritual advisor chosen by the patient, or an on-call chaplain; praying for patients; and praying with patients at their request or with their permission. Cline (2019) argues that spirituality is a personal and private form of religion. This author reminds us that the lines between the two concepts are unclear. Others have described spirituality as "the way individuals seek ultimate meaning, purpose, connection, value, or transcendence" (Harvard T. Chan School of Public Health, 2022). Similarly, the Institute of Medicine, now the National Academy of Medicine (NAM), defines spirituality as "the needs and expectations which humans have to find meaning, purpose, and value in their life" (American College of Cardiology, 2022).

Conducting a Spiritual Assessment

Purnell (2013) defines spirituality as "all behaviors that give meaning to life and provide strength to the individual" (p. 36). Further, Purnell says, "spirituality is a vital human experience shared by all cultures. Spirituality helps bring balance to mind, body, and spirit." "A thorough assessment of spiritual life is essential for the identification of solutions and resources that can support other treatments" (p. 38). He provides a guideline for nurses with suggested spirituality questions. His questions include the identification of the patient's religion, religious practices, the extent to which the person views themself as religious, and those things that the individual views as giving meaning to one's life. The nurse can easily apply these questions in an initial exploration of a patient's spirituality or build on them to conduct a more in-depth exploration of the patient's religious or spiritual beliefs.

Others have also suggested ways to assess an individual's religious or spiritual attitudes and beliefs (Blaber et al., 2015; Hwang, 2022; Zumstein-Shaha et al., 2020). Some writers proposed a narrative approach that simply allowed the patient to tell their story about what gives meaning to their life. As one author notes, most often it is family and their relationships. Some of the available models of religious/spiritual assessments are intended for use by chaplains or other specific health professionals. However, aspects of these models may be used to open up this often challenging conversation.

One very simple model, the HOPE model, may be used by many members of the health-care team. In this model, H stands for Hope. The caregiver can ask the patient what their sources of hope are and what sustains them during difficult times. The O stands for orga-nized religion. The nurse can ask the patient to state their religion and to share how impor-tant it is to that person's life. Culturally competent nurses recognize that people vary in the extent to which they practice their selected religion or consider themselves "spiritual." The P stands for personal spirituality and practices. These include prayer, meditation, reading scripture, attending services, listening to music, or other activities like communing with nature that express an individual's spiritual identity. The E stands for the effect on medi-cal care and end-of-life issues (Hwang, 2022). Asking whether the patient's current clini-cal situation is impacting their relationship with God or the ability to maintain preferred spiritual practices is critical in assessing the patient's spiritual needs. Nurses can then ask the patient what they can do to help them overcome any obstacles that may prohibit them from addressing spiritual needs. By addressing the patient's identified needs, nurses can optimize the spiritual care they can provide and help maintain the integrity of their patients' mind, body, and spirit.

THE SIGNIFICANCE OF SPIRITUALITY IN HEALTHCARE

In a comprehensive analysis of scientific literature, spirituality has been linked to better health outcomes in patient care (Harvard T. Chan School of Public Health, 2022). The researchers in this study encouraged healthcare professionals to ask patients about spirituality as a part of a patient-centered approach to avoid patients feeling "disconnected from the health care system and the clinicians caring for them." The writers also encouraged raising clinicians' awareness of the protective benefits of spiritual community participation. For those who attended religious services, spirituality was associated with healthier lives, greater longevity, less depression and suicide, and less substance use (Balboni et al., 2022; de Brito Sena et al., 2021). Numerous other studies have indicated that spirituality can enhance the quality of life for people with chronic illnesses like heart disease and cancer (Balboni et al., 2022, Harvard T. Chan School of Public Health, 2022; Maciel et al. 2018). One study suggests spirituality can help keep heart failure patients from being readmitted to hospitals. The literature provides much evidence that spirituality can also support caregivers. Therefore, spirituality is a source of coping, managing stress, and empowerment when making difficult health-related deci-sions (Balboni et al., 2022). Research is being done to develop a spirituality screening tool to assess depression and identify heart failure patients who are at risk for spiritual distress. In a study conducted to explore the psychologic benefits of being spiritual without being reli-gious, the researchers found that there were few differences between people who are part of an organized religion and those who practice spirituality on their own than one might think. These authors concluded that, psychologically speaking, nonreligious spiritual and tradition-ally religious participants may be more similar than different.

The literature not only emphasizes the impact that spirituality has on patients' views about their illness, but also on nurses' views of themselves as care providers. While nurses believe strongly that holistic nursing includes assessing and responding to the spiritual needs of patients, many believe they are unprepared to do so. Consequently, some researchers have described spirituality as a central component, essential to human caring, that is often invisible (Southard, 2020). These researchers explain that conceptual confusion about differentiating religion from spirituality and limited education in nursing curricula are factors contributing to this phenomenon. The researchers in this study advocated changes in healthcare systems and nursing education to address this problem. Spirituality, then, is a significant dimension of both the persons giving and receiving care, which ultimately influences patients' health outcomes, as well as nurses' attitudes about the quality of care they provide.

Strategies for Implementing Spiritual Care

To address this issue in nursing, Duquesne University (2022) offers the following tips and reminds us that patient-centered care requires the nurse to take the patient's faith and belief systems into account when providing care, especially during serious illness or at the end of life. They suggest following the *Journal of Palliative Care* and the *Journal of Hospice*'s five key items nurses should bear in mind: Remember, spirituality is not the same as religion; screen for spiritual distress first, then conduct a spiritual history second; a spiritual assessment should be ongoing, not only at admission; there are many ways to conduct a spiritual assessment; and the assessment itself can be therapeutic. Just as nurses are encouraged to assess their own cultural values and beliefs when caring for culturally diverse patients, evaluating one's spiritual well-being is a vital component of a cultural assessment. Nurses who can maintain their own spiritual well-being are better able to provide spiritual care for their patients. At the same time, nurses must be careful not to impose their own religious or spiritual views on their patients.

Many factors influence the nature of one's spiritual well-being, including one's developmental stage of life, family relationships, cultural beliefs, religion, and various life events (Yeşilçinar et al., 2018). Obviously, some life events make more of an impact than others. For example, when individuals are experiencing life-threatening illnesses, they are often compelled to think about the meaning of life in a way most individuals tend to avoid. Loss of loved ones also puts people more in touch with the idea of their own mortality and the value of life as they currently know it. Nurses can maximize the opportunities to enhance these spiritual moments when caring for patients if they themselves are in a place of spiritual well-being that enables them to do so. Alazmani-Noodeh and colleagues (2021) explored nurses' experiences in the ICU when providing perceived futile care. The researchers found that despite not knowing the patient's destiny, having hope of the patient's recovery, a faith in God, and feelings of "self as a useful tool in God's hands" (p. 4, 9) were factors that helped increase nurse's job satisfaction.

Canfield and colleagues (2016) interviewed 30 critical care nurses to determine the nurses' definitions of spirituality. Nurses were asked open-ended questions. The researchers observed that nurses were confused about spirituality and therefore their roles in spiritual care. However, according to Canfield and colleagues (2016), Press Ganey reports indicate that patients place "high importance on spiritual matters and view attention to emotional needs among the top three patient care needs." To meet the nation's end-of-life guidelines, nurse training in spirituality is needed. As the authors state, "the person and the nurse are both unique, but find mutuality upon which to connect . . . [as they] embark upon a mutual search for meaning and wholeness and perhaps for the spiritual transcendence of suffering" (p. 207). The results of this study indicate that while nurse respondents said they generally felt comfortable in providing spiritual care (75%), spiritual care was not usually addressed until end of life. Also, nurses who were unsure of themselves regarding spiritual care called on pastoral care individuals to assist them. Most of the nurses in the study agreed that one does not have to be religious to be spiritual.

Results of this study revealed three patient-centered themes: end-of-life issues, resolutions associated with guilt and hope, and increased need for attention. In addition, "the overarching response was offering . . . [which] was defined as personal presence, praying, touching, holding a hand, or listening" (Canfield et al., 2016, p. 209). One of the respondents mentioned the need for nurses to go beyond the technical aspects of care. Heavy demands of providing physical care were viewed as a barrier by nurses in this study. A few nurses were averse to giving spiritual care.

When caring for culturally diverse groups, Maphosa (2017) explained, patients who are experiencing any physical or emotional illness also encounter spiritual distress; "listening, sympathizing and responding meet the needs of the human spirit for love, understanding, meaning, purpose, and hope" (p. 41). Understanding patients' spirituality requires listening for cues from the patients regarding their religiosity and readiness to discuss their spiritual/religious needs. This writer reminded us that nurses need a working knowledge of major religions—especially their beliefs regarding issues such as health and illness, suffering and death—will be highly relevant to nursing care. Knowledge of customs, ceremonies, cleanliness/ hygiene rules, and food laws will be of practical was paraphrased from page 41. As the author stated, "there are many texts that provide an overview of various religious/spiritual requirements of a number of major faiths" (p. 41).

Based on the various religious groups in the United States that were mentioned at the beginning of this chapter, this section will highlight a few of the groups nurses are likely to encounter as they provide care.

A Growing Muslim Population

Pew Research Center (2021) reported an estimated 3.85 million Muslims of all ages in the United States. The growth of the Muslim population is attributed to the flow of Muslims into the country and the tendency of Muslims to have more children than Americans of other Ethnic groups. However, the Pew Research Center (2021) notes that, since the government does not ask religious affiliation when counting the census, it is difficult to have an accurate count of this population. The Muslim population growth has slowed recently due to the changes in federal immigration policy. Since the terrorist attacks of September 11, 2001, Muslims living in the United States report experiencing much discrimination based on their race or ethnicity (Pew Research Center, 2021). Still, the number of mosques has grown to 2,769, double that of two decades ago. In addition, the number of Muslims continues to gain a larger presence in the public sphere, given the inclusion of four Muslim members in Congress: Rep. Keith Ellison, D. Minn.; Rep. Andre Carson, D. Ind.; Rep. Ilhan Omar, D. Minn; and Rep. Rashida Tlaib, D. Mich. Considering the influx of this relatively new population, nurses need to become familiar with the beliefs and practices that are linked to the Islamic religion (Pew Research Center, 2018). For this reason, a brief discussion follows.

Religious Influences on Care

Swihart and colleagues (2023) and Fowler (2017) offered information that nurses and care providers may use to improve spiritual care given to Muslim patients who practice Islam. Pew Research Center Religious and Public Life (2017) predicted that Muslims will soon replace Jews as the second largest religious group in the United States. For that reason, nurses can benefit by having a working knowledge of this particular religion. First, the term *Moslem* or *Muslim* refers to the people who follow Islam, or the Islamic religion. Because the Middle East is the birthplace of Islam, approximately 90% of Arabs are Muslim, but not all Muslims are Arab. Only 20% of the Muslims in the world are Arab. The rest of the Muslim population can be found throughout the world. About 25% of American Muslims are from South Asia and half are converts to Islam (Pew Research Center, 2018). Like other religious groups, Muslims are diverse culturally, politically, racially, and socioeconomically. Muslims are monotheistic, that is, they believe in one God (Allah) and his prophets, Abraham, David, Jesus, Moses, and Noah. The Islamic holy book is the Qur'an or Koran (Swihart et al., 2023). Followers of Islam believe the book is a compilation of a series of revelations received by the prophet Muhammad, who is considered a messenger from God. The prophet's sayings are found in the Hadith, and Muhammad's words, thoughts, and deeds are found in the Sunnah. The Qur'an and Sunnah provide religious, legal, and ethical guidance for followers of Islam. In the rules or laws that specifically have to do with God, five acts of devotion, or pillars, are described. First is the Islamic profession of faith, saying that there is only one God. Second, Muslims must pray five times a day; third is the duty that Muslims must give to those in need; the fourth is fasting during the holy month of Ramadan, which occurs at different times each year; and the fifth is a religious pilgrimage. Muslims believe in complete submission to God, reward and punishment, judgment day, and life after death. Some Muslim patients may view their illness experience as a means of atonement for their sins (Lawrence & Rozmus, 2001; Swihart et al., 2023).

Fowler (2017) identified several Islamic practices that have nursing implications (a partial list can be found in Table 4.2), including avoidance of pork or any extracts or blood from pork products and any other meat that has not been slaughtered according to "halal" rules. When such avoidance is not possible, Muslims may be offered a vegetarian option. Muslim patients may refuse medications containing gelatin, pork products, or alcohol. The nurse can determine which, if any, medications contain these products and disclose this to their Muslim patients. Patients may be exempted from Ramadan fasting rules, which include liquids, but devout followers may wish to observe the month's daylight hour fast. Pregnant women and children also can be exempt from fasting. Modesty and maintaining privacy is an important concern, so Muslims prefer same-sex caregivers, especially for personal care. The nurse may elicit family members to assist in caring for loved ones. Cleanliness is very important and is a major part of preparation for mandatory prayer, which is performed facing the holy city of Mecca five times a day. Nurses can assist the patient in facing toward Mecca.

TABLE 4.2 ■ CARING FOR MUSLIM PATIENTS

TOPIC	RELIGIOUS PRACTICE	NURSING IMPLICATIONS
Prayer	Muslims are required to pray five times each day; they should face Mecca while doing so. Time of prayer changes with the seasons; accompanied by changes in body positions; floor covered by prayer rug or clean material.	Determine any medical limitations; assist with positioning as needed; patient faces East in North America toward Saudi Arabia; offer clean towel if prayer rug not available; maintain patient's privacy when possible.
Cleanliness	Referred to as "half the faith," strict rules about keeping body clean; essential prior to prayer ritual; must perform ablutions or cleansing of hands, rinsing mouth, nose, ears, and feet with clean water. Body and clothing must be free of urine and stool.	Assist patients with washing, especially if incontinent before prayer. Offer clean water at bedside as much as needed; change clothing as needed.
Dietary restriction	Pork and any extracts or blood products, shellfish, and alcohol are strictly forbidden. All meat must be slaughtered according to halal rules.	Patients may be offered vegetarian options if a halal menu is not available; as appropriate, allow family to bring food from home. Eat with right hand; considered the clean hand.
Fasting	Most Muslims fast, including liquids, during daylight hours during Ramadan. Exemptions for ill health, pregnancy, and breastfeeding; and children may be exempt.	Ask patient about a desire to fast. Determine when food can be offered. Explain necessity of eating during times when medically critical (e.g., for diabetics, wound healing).
Modesty	Modesty is very important to Muslim patients.	Provide same-gender care providers when possible, especially in personal care administration; accept family members' offers to assist when possible.
End-stage care	An imam or family reads from Qur'an, followed by prayers; ritual washing of body by close family; burial as close after death as possible; cremation is not allowed.	Collaborate with imam and family as possible to determine postmortem care needs.

Source: Adapted from Arritt, T. (2014). Caring for...patients of different religions. *Nursing Made Incredibly Easy! 12*(6), 38–45. https://doi.org/10.1097/01.NME.0000454746.87959.46; Fowler, J. (2017). From staff nurse to nurse consultant: Spiritual care. Part 7: Islam. *British Journal of Nursing, 26*(19), 1092. https://doi.org/10.12968/bjon.2017.26.19.1082; Lawrence, P., & Rozmus, C. (2001, July). Culturally sensitive care of the Muslim patient. *Journal of Transcultural Nursing, 12*(3), 228–233. https://doi.org/10.1177/104365960101200307; Swihart, D. L., Yarrarapu, S. N. S., & Martin, R. L. (2023). Cultural religious competence in clinical practice. In: *StatPearls [Internet]*. StatPearls Publishing. https://www.ncbi.nlm.nih.gov/books/NBK493216

Many use a prayer rug if available; nurses can improvise a suitable replacement if necessary. Withdrawing or withholding life-sustaining treatment is discouraged by Muslim tradition and the family may wish to have an imam to assist with end-of-life decision-making. After the patient's death, the family may want to wash the body and point their deceased love one's face toward Mecca. Burial should occur as quickly as possible (Arritt, 2014).

Several other writers have explored the cultural and religious needs of Muslim immigrants. For example, Wolf and colleagues (2016) conducted an ethno-nursing study to explore perceptions of mental illness in Somali immigrants. Among over 35,556 Somali immigrants living in the United States, many had been traumatized by the experiences Somalis encountered in the flight and transition from their war-torn country and had mental health issues like depression. In this study, the researchers interviewed 30 Somali informants living in Minnesota. Among major findings, this study revealed that Somalis believed the Muslim religion significantly influenced their mental health as well as some food choices. Sickness was looked upon as a "test from God and one cannot be healed unless God wills it" (p. 356). Further, the respondents indicated a need to have their Muslim religion incorporated into their care. Specifically, making time for prayer; having access to the Qur'an and same-gender care providers, and time for meditation; recognizing imams, sheiks, and elders, who make community decisions; and other measures would help build trust between Somalis and caregivers. Like other groups, Somalis place a high value on being treated with dignity and respect.

Missal and Kovaleva (2016) interviewed 12 Somali immigrant mothers about their childbirth experiences. Among six themes, these researchers identified the importance of cultural and religious beliefs and practices and concluded that nurses should help facilitate such practices. In another study, Elter and colleagues (2016) investigated the spiritual healing practices of rural Thai women and their families to inform postpartum care. Key informants in this study suggested allowing Somali patients time for praying, meditating, and reading the Qur'an. According to this research, providers of care may need to explain the significance of treatment as a supplement to reading the Qur'an to gain a Somali patient's understanding of the health benefits of treatment measures.

Other practices worth mentioning here are the traditional attitudes toward end-of-life care and organ donation. The Muslim religious leader is an imam. When caring for a Muslim patient, nurses and other health team members should seek collaboration with an imam or the family for advice on spiritual care. At the end of life, the family will want to be with the loved one and may read from the Qur'an and pray. The death ritual includes washing of the body by family members. Prayer for the deceased, led by a male within 72 hours after death, should occur. To facilitate this practice, the death certificate must be signed promptly. Burial should take place as early as possible; an autopsy is only acceptable for legal or medical reasons, cremation is not permitted (Fowler, 2017; Swihart et al., 2023).

In summary, the literature suggests that an individual's spiritual nature serves as an internal resource for experiencing oneself and others while managing life's stressors with some degree of hope. Membership in any of the various religious groups often provides a social support network and sense of belonging for its members. Based on these descriptions of spirituality and religion, nurses can assume that patients they encounter will be influenced by one or both dimensions in their daily lives (Travers, 2021). Therefore, besides having their own sense of what religion and spirituality means to them personally, it is important for nurses to understand the meaning religion and spirituality hold for the patients for whom they are caring. To ensure that each patient receives holistic, culturally competent, and evidence-based care, the nurse must take the spiritual and/or religious nature of the individual into consideration as care is being provided.

All these measures enable the nurse to help patients avoid physical and emotional consequences of spiritual distress or crisis. Often, with serious illness and/or personal losses comes a sense of grieving or loss that may be accompanied by a profound questioning of life's meaning, one's faith, or even one's belief in a higher being. At such times, the nurse provides support to ameliorate the situation so that patients can better cope and accept the clinical circumstances in which they find themselves. Nurses are most effective at providing spiritual care when they themselves are cognizant of their own religious and spiritual attitudes and well-being, but are able to place the patient's spiritual beliefs before their own. Preparing oneself to listen for signs of spiritual distress, to utilize a spiritual assessment tool, and to explore their patients' specific spiritual and/or religious needs are all positive first steps in the process of providing spiritual care.

IMPORTANT POINTS

- There are important differences between spirituality and religion.
- It is important for nurses to be mindful of their own spiritual well-being if they are to be effective in delivering spiritual care to their patients.
- Not all patients are religious, but everyone needs spiritual care, even those who are agnostic or nonbelievers.
- Patients who share the same religion may not all have the same religious perspectives or values.
- When delivering spiritual care, nurses must be careful not to impose their own spiritual and/or religious views on their patients.
- Signs of spiritual distress include crying, apathy, anger, changes in sleep patterns, and/or depression.
- Providing spiritual care involves listening to patients for spiritual clues and assessing for spiritual despair.
- Spiritual care includes seeking a spiritual advisor of the patient's choosing, praying for and with patients, and providing space and time for private prayer.

In the following two case examples, a Jewish patient and a patient who is a Jehovah's Witness, are being presented as prototypes to illustrate situations in which two nurses are caring for someone whose religious or spiritual needs differ from their own. It is not the intent of the author to examine a variety of religious or spiritual belief systems here, but instead to examine ways in which nurses might acquire, through this reading, methods of incorporating spiritual care into their daily nursing practice. Before beginning to address the religious or spiritual needs of patients, nurses must define both terms for themselves, have a general understanding of their own attitudes and beliefs about spirituality and religion, and be open-minded and nonjudgmental about the spiritual beliefs and practices of the patient.

CASE SCENARIO I

A JEWISH PATIENT

Yetta is a 71-year-old Jewish patient. She has been a resident of an upscale Lutheran long-term care facility for the past 2 years. Yetta has been married for 50 years and is quite concerned about her husband, who has recently fallen ill and now rarely visits her. The couple has three children. Two of them, a daughter and a son who is a physician, are married with children. The third child, another son, has a mental disability.

Over the past 15 years, Yetta has suffered from a variety of chronic health problems, including multiple sclerosis and related quadriplegia, diabetes mellitus, hypertension, obesity, decubitus ulcers, and depression. As a result of her multiple clinical problems, she is now totally dependent on the staff for assistance with activities of daily living. Since her admission, Yetta has become progressively more demanding and difficult in her interactions with others. Some of the nurses have commented that this behavior is "typical of Jewish patients." Others have suggested that, perhaps, Yetta is now experiencing a form of dementia.

During a state inspection of the facility, Yetta complained to an official that the staff frequently ignored her. Consequently, the institution established a policy that required all nurses caring for Yetta to visit her at least once each hour. A few of the staff members do so grudgingly and avoid going into her room beyond the designated times. In addition, Yetta's family members visit her infrequently and limit the time of their visits to less than an hour.

Yetta spends much of her time checking her watch and calling for the nurses shortly before her scheduled treatments, meals, medications, and procedures. Karen, one of Yetta's nurses, is frustrated by her patient's behavior. Like many of the other nurses, she dreads going into Yetta's room and caring for her, because the patient constantly criticizes everything she does for her and never seems satisfied. One day, Karen noticed that the only time that Yetta seemed reasonably comfortable was when she was talking to her about her former lifestyle, during which she was much more active in her synagogue. There was a certain twinkle in her eye as she spoke of the many social events that she and her husband participated in through her synagogue. Yetta stated that in the past they had a close relationship with the rabbi. She also described fond memories of her children's Bar and Bat Mitzvahs.

Karen also noticed that although Yetta's conversation with her family is often tense, she seems grateful for the kosher food her family brings during their brief visits. Karen, a Catholic, knew little about the Jewish religion, or Jewish customs and practices. This was her first experience caring for anyone who was of Jewish heritage. She wondered whether Yetta's behavior might be partially a reflection of her separation from her family, cultural traditions, and religious practices. She also wondered if providing Yetta with opportunities to talk more about herself might be helpful in assisting Yetta to better cope with her healthcare problems and relationships with healthcare providers during her stay at this long-term care facility. Karen decided to further investigate Judaism and to learn about the ways to incorporate Yetta's faith and cultural traditions into her care planning.

WHAT NURSES NEED TO KNOW ABOUT THEMSELVES

Application of the Staircase Self-Assessment Model: Self-Reflection Questions

When considering Yetta's case, ask yourself the following questions. If you are the nurse caring for Yetta:

1. What feelings would you have in caring for this patient? On what are these attitudes and feelings based?
2. Where are you on the Cultural Competency Staircase regarding the care of this patient?
3. How will you progress to the next level? (See Chapter 1.)
4. What are your feelings, attitudes, and beliefs about the role spirituality and religion play in coping with illness?
5. Does your religious affiliation differ from the patient's in this case? How might this impact your ability to assist her with spiritual/religious care?
6. How much do you know about the values, traditions, and religious and health beliefs of Jewish patients? What are some ways the nurse might learn?

7. Based on your own religious beliefs and values, what spiritual resources would you seek for yourself if you were hospitalized? Are those kinds of resources applicable in this case?
8. Do you have any underlying assumptions or biases (barriers) that may interfere with positive intercultural communication with a patient who behaves like Yetta?
9. How easily would you be able to communicate with the patient and her family to assess the patient's cultural/spiritual needs?
10. What spiritual assessment tool would you use to collect data about this patient's spiritual needs?

Responses to Self-Reflection Questions 4, 5, 6, 8, 9, and 10

Response: What are your feelings, attitudes, and beliefs about the role spirituality and religion play in coping with illness?

One of the most important ways to address this question is to ask yourself whether or not you are a believer in a being or power higher than yourself. Whether you call that power God or Allah is not as important as determining how much your relationship with that being influences your life, especially during times of illness or stress. If your answer is no, on what systems do you rely during these times as a means of comfort and support? Second, if you practice a formal religion, to what extent does it influence your attitudes and beliefs about health, illness, life, and death? Answering these questions enables you to discover commonalities and differences between your patient's values and beliefs and your own. Most importantly, acknowledging these differences nonjudgmentally affords the nurse a place from which to build a helping relationship with the patient, while utilizing the patient's own internal and external resources for coping with their health issues.

Response: Does your religious affiliation differ from the patient's in this case? How might this impact your ability to assist her with spiritual/religious care?

The patient in one scenario is of the Jewish faith, and the other is a Jehovah's Witness. Are these religions ones with which you are familiar? When caring for a patient of a religion that is unfamiliar, the nurse can use each encounter with the patient to demonstrate interests and seek information about the ways to respect the principles and practices of the religion during the hospitalization to promote adherence to dietary, prayer, and other traditional practices. One example is assisting Muslims in fasting during Ramadan.

Response: How much do you know about the values, traditions, and religious and health beliefs of Jewish patients? What are some ways the nurse might learn?

Asking the patient and family members is a place to start, but in seeking information about any spiritual needs that Yetta might have, the nurse might reach out to a rabbi for suggestions about how best to meet Yetta's dietary concerns and health needs in general within the guidelines of the Jewish tradition.

Response: Do you have any underlying assumptions or biases (barriers) that may interfere with positive intercultural communication with a patient who behaves like Yetta?

Nurses may be frustrated when caring for Yetta based on her behaviors, but those who made remarks about Yetta's religion/ethnicity are making assumptions that are biased and prejudicial. There are many factors that help explain Yetta's behavior, including personality, separation anxiety, dementia, and so on. For this reason, nurses should strive to prevent these feelings from interfering with the provision of quality care.

Response: How easily would you be able to communicate with the patient and her family to assess the patient's cultural/spiritual needs?

The nurse's ability to communicate with this patient and others much depends on the motivation and desire of the nurse to bridge any interpersonal barriers to communication and gain the patient's confidence and trust. Demonstrating concern, interest, patience, and understanding during initial interactions will facilitate the establishment of a positive working relationship with the patient.

Response: What spiritual assessment tool would you use to collect data about this patient's spiritual needs?

The LEARN model is a good choice when caring for patients with whom the nurse might be having communication problems. Using this model, the acronym LEARN stands for listening, explaining, acknowledging, recommending, and negotiating (www.heartland alliance.org/wp-content/uploads/sites/20/2016/07/learn_model.pdf). The nurse begins by actively listening to the patient, explaining what the nurse believes the patient is saying, acknowledging, recommending, and finally negotiating. In this case, the nurse works collaboratively with Yetta to determine her preferred needs. The nurse might also use the HOPE model, previously discussed in this chapter, to assess Yetta's spiritual needs.

WHAT THE NURSE NEEDS TO KNOW ABOUT THE PATIENT

Selecting a Cultural Assessment Model

Purnell's Model for Cultural Competence

Purnell's model identifies 12 domains for assessing the ethnocultural attributes of an individual.

These attributes include a spirituality assessment (see Table 4.3). When using this model, the nurse may select one or more areas that are relevant to this patient's situation.

A Rationale for Care

There is evidence in the information provided that several factors are having a direct impact on the patient's quality of life while living in this extended care facility. It may be helpful to identify physiologic reasons that might explain the patient's anxiety and related behavior (patient's blood sugar, blood pressure, level of clinical depression, and specific medications) as these add to our understanding of both her physiologic and psychologic

TABLE 4.3 ▪ APPLYING PURNELL'S MODEL FOR CULTURAL COMPETENCE

DOMAIN	APPLICATION
• Overview, inhabited localities	• Jewish ethnicity; Yetta is living in Lutheran home
• Communication	• In this case, poor communications between patient and staff
• Family roles and organizations	• Family is very significant in Jewish culture. Yetta has a strained
• Workforce issues	relationship with her family.
• Biocultural ecology	• Does patient prefer kosher food?
• High-risk behaviors	• Jewish religion: Need to determine what role religion plays in
• Nutrition	Yetta's life. Is she Orthodox or Reform?
• Pregnancy/childbirth practices	• Is Yetta restricted in any way by cultural values?
• Death rituals	• Patient is age 71 (late adulthood). Developmental task
• Spirituality	(integrity vs. despair)
• Healthcare practices	• Does Yetta hold traditional health beliefs or share those of
• Healthcare providers	Western medicine?

Source: Purnell, L. D., & Fenkl, E. A. (2021). *Textbook for transcultural health care: A population approach* (5th ed.). Springer.

needs. Even though the medical care that Yetta requires is probably being provided, it is obvious that the patient is unhappy with her care and that many other psychosocial needs are going unmet. This aspect of Yetta's care is the primary focus of this discussion.

According to the standards of professional nursing practice, it is the responsibility of the nurses to carry out nursing actions that promote patients' psychological as well as physiological well-being, involve the family in the planning of care, and evaluate the quality of the care provided on an ongoing basis (American Nurses Association [ANA], 2021). Further, based on Culturally and Linguistically Appropriate Services (CLAS) standards developed by the Department of Health and Human Services (DHHS), and those established by The Joint Commission (TJC), nurses also have a responsibility to "ensure that patients receive from all staff members effective, understandable, and respectful care that is compatible with their cultural health beliefs and practices."

Implications of the Patient's Religion and Culture

According to the Pew Research Center (2021), Jews made up about 2.4% of the U.S. adult population in 2020. In 2022, there were approximately 7,387,992 people of Jewish ancestry (Jewish Virtual Library, n.d.). However, not all individuals who identify as Jewish by ethnic background or culture identify as being religiously Jewish. Today, around one third of the total population identifies as being Jewish by culture only. In 2020, 0.6% of adults who are classified as Jews reported being of no religion, while others identified with another religion such as Christianity.

In Yetta's case, the fact that she happens to be of Jewish heritage and has, for reasons unknown, been placed in a religious facility that is different from the religion she practices may be complicating an already challenging situation. Some staff members have implied having some assumptions about Jewish patients and find it difficult to relate to her. Yetta's estrangement from her husband due to his illness, her limited contact and somewhat strained relationship with her family, and multiple chronic health problems provide many sources of stress and frustration for her.

Like all patients hospitalized, or in tertiary care facilities for chronic illnesses, there are several physiologic and psychologic care needs to be addressed. More specifically, in this case it is important that nurses caring for Yetta understand her healthcare beliefs, spirituality needs, family relationships and support systems, patterns of communication, and dietary preferences in order to provide her with culturally competent nursing care.

Planning Culturally Competent Care: Staircase Self-Assessment

If Yetta is to receive culturally competent care, the nurses must begin with a self-assessment. During this assessment, nurses acknowledge their own personal feelings and attitudes when caring for this patient and recognize the impact these have on the quality of care they are able to provide. Culturally sensitive nurses will also reflect on their personal attitudes and beliefs about the role spirituality plays in the promotion, maintenance, and restoration of health and how these attitudes may differ from those of the patient. Recognizing anxieties, biases, and frustrations is the first step in preventing barriers to communication between the patient and the nurse. Those nurses who express feelings that Yetta's behavior reflects a cultural or ethnic norm must consider this a personal bias that is probably based on limited information about patients who are Jewish. Caring for even 25 Jewish patients does not afford nurses enough exposure to generalize about all of them.

Considering Jewish Traditions

There is evidence in this case scenario that suggests there are reasons other than cultural heritage that may explain Yetta's behavior. The roles spirituality and religion may be playing cannot be overlooked. If dementia does exist, this is a medical diagnosis that must become a factor when planning the patient's care. There are ethical considerations when caring for all patients with dementia, but there are specific implications for care of a patient with dementia who happens to be Jewish (Quinn & Grossman, 2020).

A wide variation exists between members of the Jewish religion and cultural group based on their denomination and adherence to Jewish law and traditions. Additionally, all people have unique characteristics based on their personality. Since one of the nurses has already established that "Yetta seems happier" when discussing her religion, further conversation should be encouraged to determine how much Yetta's religion means to her. Would she benefit by having a rabbi or members of her own or a neighboring synagogue called in to see her?

The Jewish Culture: A Brief Overview as a Reference for This Case Scenario

It is important that nurses caring for Yetta attempt to understand what being Jewish means to her. Equally important is for nurses to have some basic knowledge about the important aspects of Judaism. This knowledge should incorporate information about Yetta's cultural values and healthcare beliefs. What does Yetta believe about her illness and its consequences and her ability to lead a normal life? What are her expectations of the staff nurses and physicians? Nurses can assess Yetta's knowledge level, feelings, and attitudes using a variety of assessment measures and begin to develop a plan that is more congruent with the patient's goals.

As is the case in every cultural group, there is no monolithic group of Jewish patients. Individual members of the same cultural group differ in ways that are specific to their own personality traits and circumstances. Therefore, there is no standard culturally sensitive way to manage the care of patients who happen to be Jewish, especially when they are experiencing complex medical problems like Yetta's. Nurses can benefit from knowing some important aspects of Jewish culture that may be applicable in providing care to patients of Jewish heritage. However, it is equally important to keep in mind the aspects of Yetta's or other Jewish patients' situations that make them unique. Jewish patients may belong to one of three main branches of the Jewish religion, *Orthodox* (highly traditional), *Conservative* (less strict), or *Reform* denomination (considered liberal or progressive). While *Ultra-Orthodox* Jews, like Hasidics, adhere strictly to all religious laws and practices of Judaism, Conservative Judaism places emphasis on obeying most of the Jewish laws with some degree of compromise with modern times (Purnell, 2013). Reform Jews modify traditional practices to incorporate contemporary social and cultural norms, which include being flexible regarding the use of Hebrew for religious services and dietary practices. There are many converts to Judaism and many of these become more conservative in their adherence to Jewish law than some of those who are born Jewish. Given this range of participation in the Jewish faith, it is helpful for the nurse to know to which group the patient belongs.

For all practicing Jews, religion is based on the Torah, which is the first five books of the Hebrew Bible or the Old Testament of the Christian Bible. The Talmud is the body of scholarly teaching about early Jewish civil and religious law. Prominent Jewish scholars provide a third source of Jewish legal authority in the Responsa literature, which provides an interpretation of the Bible and Talmud while keeping it relevant to contemporary times (History. com, 2020; Selekman, 2013). In Judaism, the spiritual leader is the *rabbi*, who is often consulted regarding questions having to do with Jewish religious law. Jews are permitted to question or challenge tenets of the religion as a means of enhancing their understanding. Jews celebrate the Sabbath on Saturday, beginning at sundown Friday evening and ending sundown on Saturday evening. This time is considered a holy day of rest for observant Jews.

The language spoken for religious services is *Hebrew*. Major faith beliefs lie in the sanctity and preservation of life and living up to one's potential. According to Jewish tradition, all life is God-given and the value of one's life is determined by the good deeds, or

informed her that he was a Jehovah's Witness and would not accept blood as it was "against his religion." Susan explained to the patient that without the transfusion, Mr. Jackmon's hemoglobin was likely to drop even more. Still, Mr. Jackmon refused. Susan felt strongly that the patient should change his mind about accepting the transfusion, since his hemoglobin was so low. Susan decided to discuss the matter with Rachel, another staff nurse on the unit. Rachel explained to Susan that there were alternatives to being transfused with packed cells when the patient objected to having a blood transfusion. Rachel added that she believed it was important to respect the patient's religious values. Susan called the physician so that he might meet with the patient to discuss the dilemma and determine the next course of action. Both nurses were anxious to stabilize Mr. Jackmon medically and recognized that the patient was becoming anxious about his medical situation. Despite his anxiety, Mr. Jackmon remained alert and oriented, and steadfast in his religious commitment. Later, that afternoon, a second laboratory report revealed a hemoglobin of 3 g/dL. Susan feared that time might be running out for Mr. Jackmon and something needed to be done soon. Perhaps it was the morphine he was receiving for pain that was clouding his judgment, one of the nurses remarked. "I don't understand some of these patients, how can you help them when they won't try to help themselves?"

WHAT NURSES NEED TO KNOW ABOUT THEMSELVES

Application of the Staircase Self-Assessment Model: Self-Reflection Questions

In attempting to address Mr. Jackmon's case, ask yourself the following questions if you are the nurse caring for Mr. Jackmon:

1. Where am I on the staircase in relation to this patient? How can I move to the next level?
2. How familiar am I and the nursing and medical staff with the religious beliefs, values, and attitudes of people who are Jehovah's Witnesses?
3. What major differences exist in health beliefs of followers of this religion and other Christian traditions? How different is this religion from my own?
4. What feelings and attitudes do I have about Mr. Jackmon's beliefs about receiving blood?
5. How helpful are these attitudes toward the development of cooperative interaction between myself and the patient?
6. Are there alternative ways of treating this patient's hemoglobinemia?
7. On what religious beliefs does Mr. Jackmon base his refusal of blood, despite his need for it?
8. From whom could the nursing staff gain more insight about the patient's healthcare beliefs?
9. What strategies might be useful in meeting the physiologic and psychologic needs of this patient?
10. What resources might the nursing staff utilize to assist them in meeting the needs of this patient?

WHAT NURSES NEED TO KNOW ABOUT THE PATIENT

Selecting a Patient-Focused Cultural Assessment Model

An assessment model that may be useful in this case example was developed by Berlin and Fowkes (1982) and can be found at www.ncbi.nlm.nih.gov/pmc/articles/PMC1011028/?page=5. In this model, the authors use the mnemonic LEARN and identify five steps in the cultural assessment process. The framework was developed by the authors to enhance physician–patient communication and promote better compliance with treatment plans. The model has since been used by all healthcare providers as a tool in improving cross-cultural communication. In Step 1, the nurse *listens* to the client to determine their understanding of the patient's illness and related problems. At Step 2, the nurse *explains* their perception of the problem. At Step 3, the nurse *acknowledges* similarities and differences in perception between the patient and the nurse. At Step 4, the nurse makes *recommendations* in collaboration with the patient, and in Step 5, the pair *negotiates* a mutually agreed on plan of treatment.

Some hospitals are beginning to utilize cultural assessment tools in obtaining patient admission histories. Collecting these kinds of data early on enhances the nurse's understanding of the patient's needs and provides a foundation from which nurses can build an arsenal of knowledge about future patients who share the same cultural backgrounds or faith traditions. It is important for nurses to recognize that while many commonalities exist among members of the same ethnic, cultural, or religious groups, there are often individual differences in attitudes and beliefs. For example, not all patients who identify themselves as Jehovah's Witness agree with the blood policy (Arritt, 2014; DeLoughery, 2020). Many parents will agree to permit blood transfusions in an emergency involving their children. Generally, Jehovah's Witnesses' refusal of blood based on religious beliefs applies to red blood cells, granulocytes, platelets, plasma, and whole blood. The decision to use minor derivatives of blood products like cryoprecipitate and immunoglobulins is left up to the individual (DeLougherty, 2020).

Listen

The nurse caring for this patient must focus attention on the patient's health-related beliefs, religious orientation and values, and treatment efficacy. Obviously, this is a critical time in this patient's hospitalization. Mr. Jackmon's immediate clinical problem is not only anxiety producing, but also life threatening. Nevertheless, the patient's perspective on his illness and preferred treatment approach must be heard.

Explain

It is equally important that the patient fully understands the consequences of his healthcare decisions, but that he also be given adequate information about alternative methods of treating his hemoglobinemia. Today there are many strategies for replacing blood loss in patients who do not wish to be transfused. These methods include a toolkit of various interventions: iron replacement in anemia and blood loss, erythropoiesis-stimulating agents (ESAs), tranexamic acid, recombinant factor VIIa, prothrombin complex concentrate (PCC), fibrinogen concentrate, thrombopoietin agonists, interventional radiology, and artificial blood or artificial oxygen carriers (Deloughery, 2020).

Many Jehovah's Witnesses, but not all, will submit to autologous blood transfusions. Acceptance of this approach will depend on the method in which the blood is retrieved (DeLoughery, 2020). It is important for nurses to recall that for Jehovah's Witnesses, the determination to abstain from blood is based on references to scripture (Jehovah's Witness JW.org, 2021). Since many Jehovah's Witnesses are strong believers in the Bible, it may be useful to provide time and privacy for scripture reading as a means of offering emotional and spiritual support.

Acknowledge

Nurses can act as advocate for this patient by making his values and beliefs known to other members of the healthcare staff.

During the initial assessment, the nurses caring for Mr. Jackmon must fully determine the patient's level of understanding about the nature of his illness, its cause, possible consequences, and methods of treatment. It is equally important for the nurse to be knowledgeable about the value that this patient places on his religious and spiritual beliefs. Several authors provide information about caring for clients who are Jehovah's Witnesses that can aid nurses in providing care for members of this religious group (American College of Surgeons [ACS], 2018; Arritt, 2014; Deloughery, 2020). With this knowledge, nurses will be able to conduct a thoughtful and comprehensive evaluation of the patient's cultural background and healthcare attitudes and beliefs to plan an effective treatment approach.

Spirituality and Jehovah's Witnesses

According to the JW.Org (2023), there are 8,699,048 Jehovah's Witnesses around the world. The world headquarters for the Jehovah's Witnesses is in Brooklyn, New York, and there are more than 100 branch offices around the world. The King James version of the Christian Bible serves as the basis of Jehovah's Witnesses' religious beliefs.

Members believe in the value of a strict interpretation of the scriptures as the word of God and a guide for life. Jehovah, the Hebrew name for God, is believed to be the source of all human life and that all life is sacred and precious to him. Among other values shared by members of this religion are loving their fellow man, teaching others about God's kingdom, and avoiding political and social controversies. Many Jehovah's Witnesses are conscientious objectors, as they do not support any acts of war or aggression against their fellow human beings. Other taboos of religion include a disdain for gambling, lying, stealing, taking revenge, fornication, premarital sexual relations, incest, and homosexuality.

Members hold meetings for bible study in Kingdom Hall, the Witnesses' place of worship. Jehovah's Witnesses recognize Jesus as the son of God, but do not celebrate traditional Christian holidays such as Christmas and Easter. They do observe the night of the Last Supper as a memorial of Christ's death on a day that corresponds to Nisa 14 of the Jewish calendar, which occurs sometime in March or April (Jehovah's Witness JW.org, 2021). Members of the Jehovah's Witnesses congregation do not believe in magical spells or practice faith or spiritual healing, nor do they celebrate birthdays, as they believe that this practice is derived from ancient false religions. Within the congregations, volunteer "elders" or "overseers" serve as leaders and provide spiritual comfort and guidance, without pay or special status, to the congregants. All members and elders willingly visit the sick and pray with them, so this is an excellent resource for nurses seeking psychologic support for patients who are members of this religion. Naturally, a better place to start, in this case, is with the patient's own family.

Family Roles and Traditions

Based on the biblical beliefs, Jehovah's Witnesses consider the husband the head of the household and he is expected to honor and respect his wife; serve as spiritual leader for the family; and provide food, clothing, and shelter for the family. The wife is expected to assist her husband in caring for the children and teaching them the tenets of the religion. Children are required to obey their parents and to study the Bible with them. Within the marriage, partners are encouraged to be forgiving through marital difficulties and to use the Bible in confronting these issues. Divorce is frowned on, and adultery is the only acceptable grounds for divorce for a Jehovah's Witness.

Considering this background information about Jehovah's Witnesses, one realizes that there are many facets of this patient's situation that represent either a real or perceived threat to his personal integrity. As breadwinner and head of household, he may worry about his family's ability to sustain itself through what is potentially a long-term illness with loss of employment days. Once the patient's health situation is stabilized, culturally sensitive nurses in cooperation with social workers and the patient's family can work together to find methods of support.

Healthcare Beliefs and Values

All life is deeply valued and respected by Jehovah's Witnesses; therefore, abortion, suicide, euthanasia, and violence against others are all unacceptable practices. Unhealthful practices that do not support a healthy life, such as smoking, taking drugs, and excessive drinking, are also forbidden by practicing members of this group.

Blood is also considered sacred and Jehovah's Witnesses consider it wrong to eat the meat of an animal that has not been appropriately bled (Jehovah's Witness JW.org, 2021). Some members of this religious group also consider it wrong to accept a blood transfusion even when the patient's own blood is the source. They believe that this is a serious sin against God. At times, children have been made wards of the court when physicians, seeking authorization for transfusions, have believed that a medical condition necessitated a blood transfusion. Nonblood volume expanders, surgical procedures without accompanying blood transfusions, surgical procedures, and biopsies are accepted by Jehovah's Witnesses, but adherence to God's laws is valued over sustaining one's life.

Applying Principles of Cultural Competency

Nurses caring for Mr. Jackmon will need to recognize that the ability to provide culturally sensitive and congruent healthcare is jeopardized when the desire to impose one's own values (in this case, regarding adherence to Western medical practices) conflicts with the desire to do what is in the best interest of the patient (from the patient's own perspective). The inability to respect Mr. Jackmon's right to decide what medical interventions are acceptable based on his religious convictions is a critical factor interfering with positive cross-cultural communication between some of the nurses and this patient. Nurses who can accept the patient's perspective, even as it conflicts with their own personal views, are in a much better position to establish a trusting relationship based on mutual respect, and to act most effectively in this patient's behalf.

Culturally sensitive nurses and other healthcare providers will utilize cultural assessment measures that explore the patient's level of understanding about his health risks, clinical status, and alternative methods of treatment for his hemoglobinemia. Measures will be taken to utilize the family and community supports to provide spiritual and emotional support during this time of crisis.

Role of Spirituality

In caring for this patient, the nurse will need to determine what role religion and spirituality play in Mr. Jackmon's and his family's life and incorporate this in his plan of care. A meeting with his wife to further assess Mr. Jackmon's level of anxiety about his hospitalization and other stresses is necessary. As patient advocate, the culturally competent nurse can collaborate with the physician and other health professionals to determine appropriate treatment options for him.

CONSIDERATIONS WHEN PROVIDING CULTURALLY COMPETENT CARE TO JEHOVAH'S WITNESSES

- Jehovah's Witnesses do not celebrate birthdays or Christian holidays like Christmas and Easter.
- Jehovah's Witnesses place much emphasis on physical, mental, moral, and spiritual cleanliness, and will not eat meat that has not been bled properly or accept blood transfusions.
- Jehovah's Witnesses will accept blood substitutes or plasma expanders.
- Witnesses believe that we live in an unclean world and that Witnesses must strive daily to overcome threats to their moral integrity and, indirectly, their relationship with God. Truth telling, keeping a clean house, and avoiding people who do not adhere to God's laws is a way of life for Jehovah's Witnesses.
- Members are encouraged to teach God's word at least 10 hours each month.

NCLEX®-TYPE QUESTIONS

1. Which of the following statements is accurate about the difference between spirituality and religion? *Select all that apply.*
   A. Religion is internal and spirituality is external and exclusive.
   B. Spirituality relies on doctrines and rules.
   C. Religion is focused on specific values, beliefs, and a framework for ethical behavior.
   D. Spirituality is internal and inclusive.

2. Which statement/s are true about the major religious groups in the United States? *Select all that apply.*
   A. There are significant within group differences in religious perspectives.
   B. Most groups are strongly traditional in their religious thinking.
   C. Most Protestants are conservative.
   D. Most Catholics are liberal.

3. During a cultural assessment, when asked about his religion, the patient tells the nurse that he is an agnostic. The nurse acknowledges that this term means:
   A. The patient believes in the oneness of the human family
   B. The patient does not believe in God
   C. The patient is uncertain about the existence of God
   D. The patient believes that there are many deities

4. The primary reason that the culturally competent nurse questions patients to learn about the value they place on God and religion in their lives is because:
   A. Attitudes about God and religion vary among individuals
   B. Some patients will not require spiritual care
   C. Most patients are religious
   D. This is a sign of a patient's coping capacity

5. Which of these statements provides a rationale for the nurse to assist patients in maintaining their spiritual well-being? *Select all that apply.*
   A. Spirituality gives patients a sense of purpose.
   B. Spirituality provides a means for coping with stress.
   C. Spirituality positively influences the nurse–patient relationship.
   D. Spirituality strengthens patients' religious beliefs.

6. According to research, most Americans belong to which of the following religious groups?
   A. Catholic
   B. Protestants
   C. Muslims
   D. Christians

7. The percentage of Americans in 2019 who considered themselves agnostics or nonbelievers is:
   A. 2%
   B. 5%
   C. 9%
   D. 22.8%

8. When defining spirituality, a common theme seems to be that spirituality is an expression of one's views about which of the following? *Select all that apply.*
   A. Life's direction
   B. Meaning and purpose
   C. Cultural attitudes
   D. God

9. When culturally competent nurses administer spiritual care to diverse patients, they recognize that it is important to focus their attention on the spiritual well-being of which individuals? *Select all that apply.*
   A. The patient only
   B. The patient and his family
   C. The patient and the nurse
   D. The nurse only

10. Which of the following are some important aspects of spiritual care? *Select all that apply.*
    A. Listening for spiritual clues
    B. Remaining nonjudgmental
    C. Consulting with other healthcare professionals as needed
    D. Incorporating one's own religious and moral views in patient care decision-making

11. The culturally competent nurse observes patients for indications of spiritual distress. These include which of the following? *Select all that apply.*
    A. Depression
    B. Crying
    C. Apathy
    D. Insomnia
    E. Moodiness

12. The nurse's selection of a spiritual advisor for the patient is based on:
    A. The nurse's knowledge of the patient's religion
    B. The patient's expressed desire
    C. The availability of a spiritual advisor within the healthcare system
    D. The family's wishes

13. When caring for the patient who is Muslim, which statement indicates an important cultural nursing consideration? *Select all that apply.*
    A. The nurse assists the patient with ambulation after surgery.
    B. The nurse frequently offers clean water to ensure the patient's cleanliness.
    C. The nurse reheats the patient's food to ensure that it stays warm.
    D. The nurse provides quiet and private time for meditation and prayer.

14. During Ramadan, the Muslim patient is most likely to express the need to:
    A. Sleep longer through the night
    B. Fast during daylight hours
    C. Request more frequent visitors
    D. Read the Qur'an

ANSWERS TO NCLEX-TYPE QUESTIONS

1. C and D
2. A
3. C
4. A
5. A and B

6. D
7. C
8. A and B
9. C
10. A, B, and C

11. A, B, C, D, and E
12. B
13. B and D
14. B

AMERICAN ASSOCIATION OF COLLEGES OF NURSING COMPETENCIES ADDRESSED IN THIS CHAPTER

1. Apply knowledge of social and cultural factors that affect nursing and healthcare across multiple contexts.
2. Promote achievement of safe and quality outcomes of care for diverse populations.
3. Participate in continuous cultural competence development.

 A robust set of instructor resources designed to supplement this text is located at http://connect.springerpub.com/content/book/978-0-8261-8302-6. Qualifying instructors may request access by emailing textbook@springerpub.com.

REFERENCES

Alazmani-Noodeh, F., Abdi, K., & Ranjbar, H. (2021). The moderating effect of spiritual beliefs on job dissatisfaction related to the futile care. *BMC Nursing, 20*(1), Article 64. https://doi.org/10.1186/s12912-021-00582-7

American College of Cardiology. (2022, March 28). *Spirituality can improve quality of life for heart failure patients, study finds.* Science Daily. https://www.sciencedaily.com/releases/2022/03/220328141002.htm

American College of Surgeons. (2018). *Statement on recommendations for surgeons caring for patients who are Jehovah's Witnesses.* https://bulletin.facs.org/2018/09/statement-on-recommendations-for-surgeons-caring-for-patients-who-are-jehovahs-witnesse

American Nurses Association. (2021). *Scope of practice.* nursingworld.org

Arritt, T. (2014). Caring for patients of different religions. *Nursing Made Incredibly Easy! 12*(6), 38–45. https://doi.org/10.1097/01.NME.0000454746.87959.46

Balboni, T. A., VanderWeele, T. J., Doan-Soares, S. D., Long, K. N. G., Ferrell, B. R., Fitchett, G., Koenig, H. G., Bain, P. A., Puchalski, C., Steinhauser, K. E., Sulmasy, D. P., & Koh, H. K. (2022). Spirituality in serious illness and health. *JAMA, 328*(2), 184–197. https://doi.org/10.1001/jama.2022.11086

Berlin, E. A., & Fowkes, W. C., Jr (1983). A teaching framework for cross-cultural health care. Application in family practice. *The Western Journal of Medicine, 139*(6), 934–938. https://www.ncbi.nlm.nih.gov/pmc/articles/PMC1011028/

Blaber, M., Jone, J., & Willis, D. (2015). Spiritual care: which is the best assessment tool for palliative settings?. *International Journal of Palliative Nursing, 21*(9), 430–438. https://doi.org/10.12968/ijpn.2015.21.9.430

Brady, A. (2020). Religion versus spirituality: The difference between them. *Chopra.* https://chopra.com/articles/religion-vs-spirituality-the-difference-between-them

Canfield, C., Taylor, D., Nagy, K., Strauser, C., Vankerkhove, K., Wills, S., Sawicki, P., & Sorrell, J. (2016). Critical care nurses' perceived need for guidance in addressing spirituality in critically ill patients. *American Journal of Critical Care, 25*(3), 206–211. https://doi.org/10.4037/ajcc2016276

Cline, A. (2019, March 16). *What is religious humanism?* Learn Religions. https://www.learnreligions.com/what-is-religious-humanism-248118

de Brito Sena, M. A., Damiano, R. F., Lucchetti, G., & Peres, M. F. P. (2021). Defining spirituality in healthcare: A systematic review and conceptual framework. *Frontiers in Psychology, 18*(12), 756080. https://doi.org/10.3389/fpsyg.2021.756080

DeLoughery, T. G. (2020). Transfusion replacement strategies in Jehovah's Witnesses and other who decline blood products. *Clinical Advances in Hematology & Oncology, 18*(12), 826–836. https://www.hematologyandoncology.net/files/2020/12/ho1220DeLoughery.pdf

Duquesne University. (2022). *Spiritual care in nursing: Guidelines and tips.* https://onlinenursing.duq.edu/blog/spiritual-care-in-nursing

Elter, P. T., Kennedy, H. P., & Chesla, C. A. (2016). Spiritual healing practices among rural postpartum Thai women. *Journal of Transcultural Nursing, 27*(3), 249–255. https://doi.org/10.1177/1043659614553515

Fowler, J. (2017). From staff nurse to nurse consultant: Spiritual care. Part 7: Islam. *British Journal of Nursing, 26*(19), 1092. https://doi.org/10.12968/bjon.2017.26.19.1082

Harvard T. H. Chan School of Public Health. (2022). *Spirituality linked with better health outcomes, patient care.* Chan School of Public Health. https://www.hsph.harvard.edu/news/press-releases/spirituality-better-health-outcomes-patient-care/

Hawthorne, D. M., & Gordon, S. C. (2020). The invisibility of spiritual nursing care in clinical practice. *Journal of Holistic Nursing: Official Journal of the American Holistic Nurses' Association, 38*(1), 147–155. https://doi.org/10.1177/0898010119889704

History.com. (2020). *Judaism.* https://www.history.com/topics/religion/judaism

Hwang, J. (2022). *Spirituality for the contemporary world: Hope: A spiritual assessment tool.* https://scholarblogs.emory.edu/spirituality/2022/04/22/hope-a-spiritual-assessment-tool/

Jehovah's Witness JW.org. (2021). *The watchtower study edition.* https://www.jw.org/en/library/magazines/watchtower-study-august-2021

Jewish Virtual Library. (n.d.). Jewish population in the United States by state.(1899–present). Retrieved October 10, 2023, from https://www.jewishvirtuallibrary.org/jewish-population-in-the-united-states-by-state

Jones, J. M. (2021). *How religious are Americans?* Gallup. https://news.gallup.com/poll/358364/religious-americans.aspx

JW.Org. (2023). *Jehovah's Witnesses around the world.* https://www.jw.org/en/jehovahs-witnesses/worldwide/

Lawrence, P., & Rozmus, C. (2001). Culturally sensitive care of the Muslim patient. *Journal of Transcultural Nursing, 12*(3), 228–233. https://doi.org/10.1177/104365960101200307

Maciel, A. M. S. B., Alexandre, A. C. S., Ferreira, D. M. B., & Silva, F. C. (2018). The condition of spirituality in oncological nursing care. *Journal of Nursing UFPE On Line, 12*(11), 3024–3029. https://doi.org/10.5205/1981-8963-v12i11a234609p3024-3029-2018

Maphosa, S. (2017). The role of spirituality in nursing: Part 2. *Nursing Update, March/April*, 40–42. Retrieved from https://web-p-ebscohost-com.ezproxy.sju.edu/ehost/pdfviewer/pdfviewer?vid=4&sid=e83ede7d-2e67-4da5-b65f-7907329229b7%40redis

McLeod, S. (2023, February 16). *Mind-body relationship in psychology: Dualism vs monism*. Simply Psychology. https://www.simplypsychology.org/mindbodydebate.html

Missal, B., & Kovaleva, M. (2016). Somali immigrant new mothers, childbirth experiences in Minnesota. *Journal of Transcultural Nursing, 27*(4), 359–367. https://doi.org/10.1177/1043659614565248

Neuman, S. (2021). *Fewer than half of U.S. adults belong to a religious congregation, new poll shows NPR*. https://news.gallup.com/poll/358364/religious-americans.aspx

PBS News Hour. (2019). *Number of Americans with no religious affiliation growing*. https://www.pbs.org/newshour/nation/number-of-americans-with-no-religious-affiliation-growing

Pew Research Center. (2018). *New estimates show U.S. Muslim population continues to grow*. https://www.pewresearch.org/short-reads/2018/01/03/new-estimates-show-u-s-muslim-population-continues-to-grow

Pew Research Center. (2021, May 11). *Jewish Americans in 2020*. https://www.pewresearch.org/religion/wp-content/uploads/sites/7/2021/05/PF_05.11.21_Jewish.Americans.pdf

Pew Research Center. (2022). *How U.S. religious composition has changed in recent decades*. https://www.pewresearch.org/religion/2022/09/13/how-u-s-religious-composition-has-changed-in-recent-decades/

Pew Research Center Religious and Public Life. (2017, April). *The changing global religious landscape*. http://www.pewforum.org/2017/04/05/the-changing-global-religious-landscape

Public Religion Research Institute. (2021). *The 2020 census of American religion: The American religious landscape 2020*. https://www.prri.org/research/2020-census-of-american-religion

Purnell, L. (2013). *Transcultural health care: A culturally competent approach* (4th ed). F. A. Davis.

Quinn, K. L., & Grossman, D. L. (2020). At the crossroads of religion and palliative care in patients with dementia. *Israel Journal of Health Policy Research, 9*, 43. https://doi.org/10.1186/s13584-020-00401-5

Selekman, J. (2013). People of Jewish heritage. In L. Purnell (Ed.), *Transcultural health care: A culturally competent approach* (4th ed., pp. 339–356). F. A. Davis.

Southard, M. E. (2020). Spirituality: The missing link for holistic health care. *Journal of Holistic Nursing, 38*(1), 4–7. https://doi.org/10.1177/0898010119880361

Swihart, D. L., Yarrarapu, S. N. S., & Martin, R. L. (2023). Cultural religious competence in clinical practice. In: *StatPearls [Internet]*. StatPearls Publishing. https://www.ncbi.nlm.nih.gov/books/NBK493216

Travers, M. (2021). Is it better to be spiritual or religious? *Psychology Today*. https://www.psychologytoday.com/us/blog/social-instincts/202112/is-it-better-be-spiritual-or-religious*

Wolf, K. M., Zoucha, R., Mcfarland, M., Salman, K., & Dagne, A. (2016). Somali immigrant perceptions of mental health and illness: An ethnonursing study. *Journal of Transcultural Nursing, 27*(4), 349–358. https://doi.org/10.1177/1043659614550487

Yeşilçinar, I., Acavut, G., Iyigun, E., & Tastan, S. (2018). Eight-step concept analysis: Spirituality in nursing. *International Journal for Human Caring, 22*(2), 34–42. https://doi.org/10.20467/1091-5710.22.2.34

Zumstein-Shaha, M., Ferrell, B., & Economou, D. (2020). Nurses' response to spiritual needs of cancer patients. *European Journal of Oncology Nursing, 48*, 101792. https://doi.org/10.1016/j.ejon.2020.101792

IMPORTANT WEBSITES

Institute for Jewish Medical Ethics. Retrieved from www.icjme.com
Islamic Institute of America. Retrieved from www.iiofa.org
Jehovah's Witnesses Official Webpage. Retrieved from www.jw.org/en
Jewish Community Online Internet Resources (Family/Health and Bioethics). Retrieved from www.ourjewishcommunity.org
Judaism 101. Retrieved from www.jewfaq.org

5

Cultural Considerations When Caring for Patients With Physical, Psychologic, or Intellectual Disabilities

Gloria Kersey-Matusiak

Just because a man lacks the use of his eyes doesn't mean he lacks vision.
—STEVIE WONDER

LEARNING OBJECTIVES

After this chapter, the reader will be able to
1. Describe the various types of disabilities found in American society.
2. Discuss the impact of discrimination or bias on persons with disabilities.
3. Examine the demographics found among persons with disabilities.
4. Identify groups and organizations that may be used as resources when caring for persons with disabilities.
5. Explore common attitudes of healthcare providers toward persons with disabilities.
6. Recognize the implications for nurses when caring for persons with disabilities.
7. Determine strategies and interventions to enhance the quality of care for persons with disabilities.

KEY TERMS

Americans With Disabilities Act	Disability
Arc	Healthcare disparities
Barriers	Social determinants of health

INTRODUCTION

According to the United Nations (UN) in 2022, roughly 15% of the world's population, over 1.3 billion people (or 1 in 6 people), live with a significant disability. In fact, 80% of people with disabilities live in developing countries, an estimated 46% of older people aged 60 years and older have disabilities, and one in every 10 children is a child with a disability. In the United States, 26% or one in four members of the adult population (61 million people) lived with a disability (Centers for Disease Control and Prevention [CDC], n.d.-a, n.d.-b). Among children in the United States in 2019, 4.3% had a disability. The most common types among children 5 and older were cognitive difficulties (Young, 2021).

A report by the World Health Organization (WHO) in 2022 showed evidence of a higher risk of premature death and illness among persons with disabilities than among persons without disabilities. Health disparities among people who live with disabilities are attributed to unfair factors within the healthcare system including negative attitudes of health providers, health information in formats that are not understandable, and difficulties accessing a health center due to the physical environment, lack of transport, or financial barriers (UN, 2022).

For this reason, in 2018 the UN developed a plan to include consideration of people with disabilities in all its work. For example, included among the 17 UN Sustainable Development Goals is #10 regarding reducing inequalities (United Nations, Sustainable Development Goals, 2023). In its facts and figures related to this goal, it states that one third of persons with disabilities experience discrimination and women with disabilities are at highest risk. Women are particularly vulnerable to discrimination and sexual violence, especially with intersecting identities (United Nations, Department of Economic and Social Affairs, 2023).

DEFINING DISABILITIES

The CDC defines "**disability** as any condition of the body or mind (impairment) that makes it more difficult for the person with the condition to do certain activities and interact with the world around them." The term *people with disabilities* sounds like a description of a homogeneous population, a collective of individuals sharing the same characteristics. However, like many other groups in society, it is very diverse, crossing all racial, ethnic, and age groups, and refers to people who differ in the nature and type of impairment they live with temporarily or permanently. In addition, even when two different individuals have the same type of disability, depending on many factors their experiences can be vastly different. A disability can be present at birth, like Down syndrome, and affect functioning in later life; be discovered in childhood, like attention deficit hyperactivity disorder (ADHD), and be considered developmental; be related to an injury, like a traumatic brain injury (TBI); or be acquired in adulthood and associated with a longstanding condition, like loss of vision due to diabetes mellitus (CDC, n.d.-c).

The WHO describes three disability dimensions: impairment, activity limitation, and participation restrictions. An impairment can occur in one's body structure or function, like loss of a limb, or mental impairment, like loss of memory. An example of an activity limitation would include restrictions on one's ability to walk. A participation restriction limits one's ability to work or engage in social and recreational activities. In addition, ADA.gov reminds us that some disabilities are visible, and others are not (ADA.gov, n.d.). See Box 5.1 illustrating some common examples of disabilities of various types including cancer; cerebral palsy; deafness or blindness; epilepsy; mobility disabilities that require the use of a wheelchair, walker, or cane; intellectual disabilities; major depressive disorders; and TBI. Of course, these lists are not all inclusive of all the various disabilities in the world, or even the United States.

A comprehensive discussion of the topic of disabilities is beyond the scope of this text. Rather, it is the goal of the author to highlight some of the common types of disabilities found in the United States; to discuss some of the major challenges people living with disabilities encounter; examine the impact of implicit bias and discrimination on the health and general well-being of people living with disabilities; and determine ways to combat implicit bias to ensure the provision of equitable, quality nursing and healthcare for all people living with disabilities.

BOX 5.1   Various Types of Disabilities

Autism	HIV
Blindness	Intellectual disabilities
Cancer	Low vision
Cerebral palsy	Major depressive disorders
Deafness	Mobility disabilities (use of a wheelchair, walker,
Diabetes	or cane)
Epilepsy	Traumatic brain injury
Hearing loss	

Source: ADA.gov

Intellectual and Development Disabilities

The National Institutes of Health (NIH) defines *intellectual and developmental disabilities* (IDDs) as differences that are usually present at birth and that uniquely affect the trajectory of the individual's physical, intellectual, and/or emotional development. Many conditions affect multiple body systems.

Intellectual disabilities start at any time before age 18 and are characterized by differences with both intellectual functioning and adaptive behavior including social and life skills. Developmental disabilities often refer to lifelong challenges that can be intellectual, physical, or both. The signs of IDDs vary for conditions. More severe IDDs may occur early, and signs may include delayed mobility in children, delayed or difficulty in speaking, difficulty remembering things, difficulty understanding the rules of social behavior, understanding the outcome of actions, or having trouble problem-solving (NIH, n.d.).

Cooper (2022) described the role of a breast care nurse in the United Kingdom (UK) who provided support to a newly diagnosed breast cancer patient with a learning disability. Because of the learning disability, the nurse recognized the need for close communication with the patient's next of kin, to communicate each step of the treatment process in a manner that was understandable to the patient or in a way that would facilitate the patient's family member passing the information on to the patient. The nurse needed to support the patient through all the different treatment modalities including surgery, chemotherapy, radiotherapy, and endocrine therapy. "We explained the findings to both the patient and her relative, not ignoring any questions, or comments, and trying to find ways to explain the diagnosis at a level she understood" (p. 1151). When explaining the diagnosis, the nurse allowed the patient more time to process the information and provided an easy-read booklet for her to read at home. The nurse coordinated the patient's care and arranged for two best interest meetings with the GP, learning disability liaison nurses, the community with the family and disabilities team, the surgeon, and the patient's family. The patient displayed some behavioral issues, becoming very aggressive and uncooperative with washing, dressing, and taking medications. These behaviors manifested at a time when one of the patient's wounds became infected. Since there were COVID-19 hospital visitation restrictions, the family was not allowed to visit. During this time, the nurse was able to keep a clear communication pathway between the team, the patient, and her family. The author credits the team in providing the intensive care this patient needed and ensuring that she received all treatments that any patient with a similar diagnosis would receive, despite her IDD.

In another study of nurses caring for patients with IDDs, Cashin and colleagues (2022) surveyed 69 registered nurses across contexts of practice: primary care and community, intensive care, acute hospital, emergency department, pediatrics, and intellectual disabilities/autism spectrum disorder (ID/ASD) to explore their preparedness and comfort to care for people with IDs and ASD. Age, years of experience, educational content and exposure, comfort, and confidence were dependent variables. The authors observed that while all nurses encounter people with IDD and/or ASD, there are noticeable differences, by context in their confidence, comfort, and knowledge. The researchers also noted that nurses have been identified in studies in multiple countries to feel unprepared to care for patients with ID and/or ASD. Results of this study indicate that nurses' level of comfort and feelings of preparedness to care for patients with IDs or ASD was dependent on the context in which they worked. In this study, nurses working in the public, mainstream care environment reported low levels of knowledge and confidence to care for ID/ASD patients as compared to nurses occupying roles in ID/ASD settings with reported higher levels of educational preparedness, professional development, and postgraduate education relevant to caring for patients with ID/ASD. Findings indicate a need for the inclusion of information about caring for patients with ID/ASD at all levels of nurse preparation for all practice areas and continuing professional development to enhance confidence and comfort when working with this patient population. Today, the care of persons with learning disabilities has moved away from long-term care facilities toward more frequent use of general health services. Therefore, it is more likely that nurses may see persons with learning disabilities during their professional careers. Many organizations are available as resources to support people with disabilities and their caregivers.

The Arc is one of several organizations of and for people with IDDs. This organization provides information, resources, and services for millions of individuals and their families who struggle with IDDs. Members of this and other organizations that support persons with disabilities seek their inclusion in society and in the workplace. The Arc's philosophy and mission are rooted in several key beliefs and principles: "Society in general and the Arc in particular benefits from the contributions of people with diverse personal characteristics (including but not limited to race, ethnicity, religion, age, geographic location, sexual orientation, gender and type of disability); people with intellectual and developmental disabilities are entitled to the respect, dignity, equality, safety and security accorded to other members of society, and are equal before the law" (The Arc, 2017). The Arc represents, supports, and acts on behalf of individuals and their families regardless of level of disability or membership in the organization. The organization empowers people with disabilities by providing needed resources to assist them in making informed decisions and choices.

The Americans With Disabilities Act

Before the enactment of the **Americans With Disabilities Act (ADA)**, there was widespread discrimination of people with disabilities in employment, education, housing, and healthcare (ADA.gov, n.d.). In July of 2022, America celebrated 32 years of the ADA, a federal law that promotes inclusion and protects the civil rights of people living with disabilities. The law guarantees that people with disabilities have the same rights as everyone else to enjoy employment, purchase goods and services, and participate in state and local government programs. The ADA also prohibits discrimination based on disability. The ADA requirements are stated in five sections, Title I to V, with each title designating requirements for a specific group. Title I is for employers, Title II is for all service programs of state and local government, Title III is for businesses and nonprofits serving the public, Title IV is for telecommunications, and Title V provides miscellaneous provisions. Since the passage of the ADA, much has happened to eliminate discrimination and other injustices against people living with disabilities, but much work still needs to be done.

DISABILITIES, DIVERSITY, AND DISPARITIES

According to the CDC, persons with disabilities from diverse racial and ethnic groups vary in their incidence of disabilities. Among Native Americans and Alaskan Natives, three in 10 have a disability. Among Blacks, one in four has a disability. Among Whites, one in five has a disability. Among Native Hawaiian/Pacific Islanders, one in six has a disability. Among Hispanics, one in six has a disability. And among Asians, one in 10 has a disability.

Smoking and obesity among people with disabilities were also found to vary based on race and ethnicity. Among American Indians/Alaskan Natives, 40.6% are obese and 41.2% smoke; among Blacks, 47.3% are obese and 28.1% smoke; among Whites, 35.5% are obese and 28.7% smoke; among Native Hawaiians/Pacific Islanders, 31.8% are obese and 28.2% smoke; among Hispanics, 39.9% are obese and 20.6% smoke; and among Asians, 20.3% are obese and 12.8% smoke (CDC, n.d.-d).

During the beginning months of the COVID-19 pandemic, the United States learned harsh lessons about the impact of racism and healthcare disparities on Black and Indigenous People of Color (BIPOC) as the disproportionate number of deaths from COVID-19 occurred and the disease relentlessly struck members of those groups, initially killing loved ones, especially older adults, and separating families at rates higher than those seen in the general population. According to data gathered by the National Disability Institute (NDI) in 2020, individuals with disabilities were also overrepresented among lives lost during the COVID-19 pandemic. During the pandemic, amid tragic losses, all families were forced to isolate themselves from one another out of fear of contracting the disease themselves, as COVID-19 raged on. At one point in 2020, the COVID-related hospitalization rates for non-Hispanic Black and indigenous people was five times that of non-Hispanic Whites, followed by the Latinx community at four times that of Whites (NDI, 2020).

According to the CDC, adults with disabilities are three times more likely to have heart disease, strokes, diabetes, or cancers than adults without disabilities. In addition, on many of the measures of the **social determinants of health** like education, jobs, poverty levels, and housing, researchers found disparities between families in which there are people with disabilities when comparing these families to the larger population. These disparities are further differentiated by race and ethnicity. For example, among BIPOC Americans with disabilities, 35% lost their jobs, especially between January of 2020 and May of that year. Based on a 2019 community survey by the Census Bureau, across all racial groups 35% of people without disabilities have a bachelor's degree or higher, while 15% of people with disabilities have attained that level of education (NDI, 2020).

Across all racial groups, 26% of individuals with disabilities are living below the poverty line compared with 11% of individuals without disabilities. The rate of BIPOC families with disabilities is higher than the rate of White communities regardless of disability status (NDI, 2020).

Across all racial groups, households with a disabled, working householder were worth an average of $14,180 compared to other households which were worth $83,985. Notable here is that non-Hispanic White householders' net worth at $27,100 in households with a disability is higher than that of Black and Hispanic families without a disability. The lowest net worth was at $1,282 for Black householders with a disability (NDI, 2020).

Households that spend more than 30% of their income on housing are considered cost burdened. In addition, 44% of households with one or more members with a disability are cost-burdened as compared to 34% of households without a member with a disability. Being cost-burdened places a household at risk for foreclosure or eviction. Because the COVID-19 pandemic caused loss of jobs, especially for those families with a member with a disability, families in this group are even more cost burdened and at risk of losing their homes (www.census.gov/programs-surveys/ahs).

The Challenges of Living With Disabilities

Implicit Bias and Discrimination

Despite the long-standing existence of the ADA, healthcare literature tells us that people with disabilities in the United States and elsewhere still encounter implicit bias and discrimination along with other challenges based on their disability (Acheampong et al., 2022; Foreman, 2023; Iezzoni, 2022; Lagu et al., 2022).

The WHO (2023) reported on perceptions of healthcare workers toward people with disabilities. The researchers noted that as the world population ages, so do the numbers of people with disabilities. Findings reveal that people with disabilities globally receive negative publicity, face discrimination, are stigmatized, and are considered deviant. Sakairi (2020) discussed the societal view that adults with disabilities are asexual and their sexuality needs are often neglected. Also, many people with disabilities are met with pity, anxiety, and avoidance. Further, the authors observe that service providers' perceptions of service users are an important aspect of human service. Negative healthcare attitudes or misperspectives significantly influence the likelihood of delivering quality care. The way a disabled person is treated can be a barrier or facilitator. Past negative experiences by healthcare professionals discourage future service. According to the WHO, the findings of several studies reveal healthcare professionals show negative attitudes toward people with disabilities, use derogatory language, have difficulty establishing a rapport, and cited physical and mental abuse. Having preconceived stereotypes leads to devaluation of people with disabilities. At times, the stigma associated with people with disabilities leads to passing moral and psychologic judgment, leading to total social rejection.

Mark and Sisirak (2022) discussed the implicit bias directed toward people with disabilities and the ableist view of them as being less than whole. The researcher also noted the results of a previous study in which healthcare professionals stated they preferred working with people without disabilities. Lagu and colleagues (2022) conducted three focus groups of physicians and identified physical, communication, and attitudinal barriers to care for people with disabilities. In this study, physicians reported feeling overwhelmed by the demands of practicing medicine in general, and the requirements of the ADA of 1990 caused them to feel inadequately reimbursed for accommodations. Some stated for this reason that they attempted to discharge people with disabilities from their practice. The findings of this study suggest that physicians' bias and general reluctance to care for patients with disabilities plays a role in perpetuating healthcare disparities.

Acheampong and colleagues (2022) explored attitudes and perceptions held by persons with disabilities in a peri-urban district of Ghana regarding healthcare providers and access to healthcare. In low and middle-income countries in Africa, it is estimated that 76% and 99% of people with severe disabilities, respectively, do not have access to treatments they need. In this study, the researchers conducted 28 face-to-face interviews of 28 healthcare providers. The authors explained that many Sub-Saharan Africans link having a disability to sin or punishment for violations or a wrong committed by the individual with the disability or a family member. In healthcare settings, healthcare professionals including nurses participate in this stigma. In this study, researchers conclude that healthcare professionals generally hold negative perceptions about people who are disabled and interactions between them are likely to be hostile. The authors conclude that these perceptions will have negative implications for the care patients with disabilities will receive by the healthcare professionals in these settings.

As the WHO (2023) observes, most human beings will be subject to a temporary or permanent disability during their lifetime. In this article, a nurse/nurse educator who sustained a broken right foot injury describes her experience living with a temporary disability, the surprising treatment she received from others, and the impact it had on her life. Foreman (2023) discussed the challenges of negotiating her physical environment with a temporary disability that restricted her walking due to a fractured right fourth metatarsal that required wearing a stabilizing orthopedic boot. After several falls, she began using a metal walker. Since she maintained her employment as a full-time nursing instructor, she received support from her family to transport her back and forth to work. As the author states, "students and colleagues were tolerant of her new physiological challenges, but people outside the university were not" (Foreman, 2023, p. 13). The author described several incidents of intolerance directed at her because of her disability. She was surprised by the lack of compassion and the disrespect she encountered while experiencing this temporary disability. Drivers shouted at her to move faster, she was cursed at in parking lots, shoppers told her to get out of the way in supermarkets, and people cursed or grumbled as they passed or went around her on public sidewalks. One man kicked the front of her walker and shouted, "if you can't walk stay home." The author, who has recovered from her injuries, encourages her students to complete values clarification (self-assessment about their attitudes and thoughts regarding people with disabilities). She compares the treatment she received from the public with that which she should receive from nurses. This author also encourages compassion and respect from her students for all people with disabilities. Unfortunately, the stories shared by the author of this article and others support healthcare literature on society's perceptions of people with disabilities.

One remedy to this problem of misperceptions and misunderstandings about people with disabilities is offered by Marks and Sisirak (2020), who discuss the fact that nursing students with disabilities and nurses with disabilities are excluded from employment opportunities, thereby limiting nurses' opportunities to utilize this invaluable human resource. The authors remind us that nurses with disabilities themselves can assist other nurses in various ways. "Nurses with disabilities can offer patient-provider concordance, which is a shared identity based on demographic variables, which have been linked to establishing trust, patient satisfaction, and enhanced understanding between provider and patient" … in this case, between patients who are disabled and the nurse. Having a nurse who has a disability promotes role modeling by that individual and helps foster an enhanced understanding of issues and challenges confronting patients with disabilities, thereby enabling nurses to address healthcare disparities more fully. The authors suggest that as nurses with disabilities become more visible and supported by proponents of diversity and cultural competence, they can collaboratively support equitable care for patients with disabilities. This patient–provider concordance would mirror the same concordance nursing continues to seek in other realms of diversity like gender, race, and ethnicity, and create an environment in which people with disabilities are valued.

Even though much of the literature depicting healthcare professionals' attitudes toward caring for people with disabilities seems negative, not all stories reflect a total lack of caring for people living with disabilities. Some indicate true concern about their health and well-being, and a sincere desire to provide support. However, at times this desire to be supportive can lean toward paternalism and a disregard for the feelings and attitudes of the patient living with the disability.

Appelgren and colleagues (2022), in a study of homecare nurses working with patients with IDDs in a home-care setting, interviewed RNs to determine Swedish nurses' perceptions of caring for patients with IDDs. Nurses in this study believed they had too little time to establish a meaningful relationship with patients to determine their needs and had to rely too much on auxiliary personnel to provide them with information about the patients. The nurses felt most of their time was "putting out fires" and not enough time was spent in building trust and long-term relationships between themselves and patients. The nurses considered these critical elements of care, but the work structure was counteracting these efforts. The RNs also believed that support staff did not have adequate knowledge in care or know how to express themselves in a way the RNs could understand. Sometimes the support staff were helpful in that patients felt supported when support staff were present, since they had established a relationship with them. The analysis of this study revealed three categories: nursing held hostage in the context of care, care that was dependent on intuition and proven experience, and situations of contending for the patients' rights to adequate care. The findings show that the home care context and organization were not adjusted to the needs of the patients, so nurses felt unable to provide the care according to their values regarding how they believed patients should receive care. Nurses also believed they overused supportive staff to interpret the needs of patients and had not mastered the available augmentative and alternative communication tool. Nurses in this study viewed these patients as stigmatized, marginalized, and overlooked, and they advocated for the patients' right to receive the right care at the right time and by the right person.

The findings in this study reveal the RNs felt they could not give the care that was needed by their patients and that they wanted to give to their patients. One suggestion from the authors was the development of an IDD specialist RN to improve care and outcomes for IDD patients. There is an urgent need for professional development within the IDD field to ensure all nurses caring for IDD patients have adequate knowledge and communication skills that are needed to care for IDD patients. Further, the author notes, there is an absence of a broad base of evidence about what works best for this group of patients in a home-care setting.

Safety, Autonomy, and Quality of Life

Barkan (2021) begins the story of his "beautiful life" as a young, happily married person, with two children, newly diagnosed with amyotrophic lateral sclerosis (ALS), and given 3 to 4 years to live. Now nearly 5 years later, the author is living with ALS with a "skilled, reliable, stable, and well-paid healthcare team and 24-hour home care," with the support of his private insurance and supplemented by "wealthy friends." He lives at home with his family and the necessary accommodations that he believes is "keeping him alive," while "millions of children, seniors and adults with disabilities are on waiting lists for Medicaid's home- and community- based plan in danger of being removed from their homes and placed in institutions" (p. 22). Most people want to stay in their homes, but they can't afford it, since neither Medicare nor most private insurance companies will pay for home care. Barkan advocates fully funding homecare so older adults and those with disabilities can have a choice to live at home. The author reminds us that despite our nation's wealth and the country's ability to spend on a variety of other costs, during the COVID-19 pandemic 134,000 nursing home residents died from the disease. He offers this fact as evidence that "America's misplaced national choices are depriving millions of disabled people and our loved ones of invaluable years and priceless days." There is an urgent need, he says, "to fully fund a plan that ensures everyone has basic health care" and can chose to stay at home with a chronic condition if they wish.

Iezzoni (2022) also discussed the fact that most people with significant disabilities, even when told by their healthcare professionals that it is unsafe to stay at home, despite having numerous care needs, want to remain at home in their community. However, few have adequate financial resources to afford personal assistance services (PAS), and there are long waiting lists for Medicaid's home- and community-based services (HCBS), the major public payor for PAS. These waiting lists and the difficulties of getting Medicaid prevent many beneficiaries from obtaining these supports. For example, in 2017, more than 707,000 Medicaid beneficiaries were on waiting lists across 40 states; about two thirds were individuals with IDD, and 28% were older persons or people with significant physical disabilities.

In addition, the author notes that being forced into a nursing home diminishes one's quality of life. This is a complex problem from both sides of the argument as health professionals have an ethical responsibility to advocate for the safety of their patients, while also maintaining patient's autonomy. On the other hand, nursing homes, while addressing some needs of patients, are often understaffed and not fully capable of meeting patients' needs for ongoing support of activities of daily living (ADLs). The author shares a story of a friend who has complete quadriplegia, due to primary progressive multiple sclerosis (MS), and lives alone. He was able to avoid involuntary placement into a nursing home, but requires the care of a primary care physician, a neurologist, a physiatrist, and a urologist. The patient also requires nursing visits to manage his skin care and supra-pubic tube; he has no family to support him in instrumental ADLs, like shopping, meal preparation, and laundry. As this patient's needs increased over time, he could no longer pay agency fees for PAS and was encouraged to join PACE (Program of All-Inclusive Care for the Elderly), a program that supports Medicare and Medicaid beneficiaries over 55 years old with severe disabilities or extensive chronic health problems to stay in their homes and communities. PACE transports typical participants to day care during the day and brings them home at night, but the patient refused the day care experience. During his enrollment in PACE, the patient encountered a series of events that landed him in the hospital, development of severe neurogenic pain, skin breakdown, wound infection with a need for medication twice a day (which required a home visiting nurse) and wound care, then forced admission to a nursing home by PACE, and a strong reluctance on the part of the hospitalists to discharge the patient back to his home. From the patient's account, the nursing home stay was miserable. The patient was ultimately able to find a new primary care physician and geriatrician, who was able to return him to his home. According to the author, this doctor provided meticulous care, empathy, and made all decisions collaboratively with the patient, who now enjoyed his home and had a better quality of life.

Considering the previous two cases, for patients with complex disabilities and care needs, there are pros and cons to both living at home and in nursing home situations. Neither can probably meet all patients' needs when there are extensive disabilities and care needs. However, the conversation raises several important questions. First, when both nursing home stays and the cost of living at home are costly but equivalent and the patient wishes to remain at home, who should decide? Second, should public funds be utilized to support those wanting to stay at home? Third, when potential safety risks exist when caring for patients with disabilities, how should ethical principles be prioritized, especially in terminal illness where autonomy and quality of life are at stake?

Mental Distress

Considering the previous discussions about the many challenges people living with disabilities face, the following information seems a foregone conclusion. A 2018 study conducted by the CDC that annually screens patients 18 years of age and older for mental health concerns found that adults with disabilities reported mental distress 4.5 times more often than those without disabilities. More than half of all adults with both mobility and cognitive disabilities reported mental distress.

Characteristics that indicated higher risk for mental distress among people with disabilities included cigarette smoking, depressive disorders, insufficient sleep, obesity, physical inactivity, or unmet health needs due to cost. Individuals who had disabilities and these characteristics reported more mental distress.

Barriers for People Living With Disabilities

The WHO defines **barriers** as factors in a person's environment that, through their absence or presence, limit functioning and create disability. These factors include attitudinal, communication, physical, policy, programmatic, social, and transportation issues (CDC, n.d.-c). See Table 5.1.

Stigma, implicit bias, prejudice, and discrimination were included in the previous discussion about the challenges of living with disabilities. However, people living with disabilities face some, if not all, these barriers each day of their lives. Understanding how these barriers work to impede quality healthcare access and/or to reduce the quality of one's life is essential for nurses and other healthcare professionals who wish to provide quality care for patients living with disabilities (Liebel et al., 2018).

TABLE 5.1 ■ BARRIERS AND EXAMPLES FOR PEOPLE LIVING WITH DISABILITIES

ATTITUDINAL	COMMUNI-CATION	PHYSICAL	POLICY	PROGRAM	SOCIAL	TRANS-PORTATION
• Stereotypes • Stigma • Implicit bias • Discrimination	• Signage with health promotion • Messages in small print • Technical language • For people with cognitive impairment	• Steps and curbs that block a person's ability to move	• Denying qualified individual access • Denying reasonable accommo-dations	• Provider's attitudes or lack of understand-ing about people with disabilities	• Employment • Education • Income	• Lack of access to accessible transpor-tation

IMPLICATIONS FOR NURSES

Many nurses have special opportunities to interact with people who have disabilities. The problem is that many others have limited opportunities and exposures to people with disabilities and operate from stereotypes and misperceptions. In any case, the context in which nursing occurs plays a role in determining the type of nursing care, the quality of resources, and the services that are made available to patients with disabilities. For example, in rehabilitation nursing, nurses in close collaboration with other rehabilitation team members are prepared to provide care that more specifically addresses the needs of patients with disabilities.

In these settings, a multidisciplinary planned approach that focuses on potential and actual problems that may be related to the client's cultural background is already in place. By acting as patient advocate, the nurse sets the tone for other members of the health team. In recognizing the specific needs of individuals with disabilities, nurses can make a tremendous positive difference in ensuring that care is appropriate and culturally sensitive. From the patient's perspective, much depends on how recently the disability was acquired, the severity of the disability, whether the disability is permanent, and the extent to which there are adequate family or other support systems. Certainly, patients who have recently become disabled due to trauma, stroke, or other unanticipated events will experience psychologic effects that will need to be considered when planning care. Patients with long-standing disabilities may have adapted to the inconveniences of the disability itself and may not consider it a "problem" at all. Nurses and others should always use people-first language that acknowledges personhood before the disability (New York State Department of Health, 2009).

To effectively care for patients with disabilities, it is important for nurses and all healthcare professionals to remember two major principles embedded in the ADA law. First, people living with disabilities have the same rights as everyone else to enjoy employment, purchase goods and services, and participate in state and local government programs. This means that people with disabilities are entitled to the same quality of healthcare services as everyone else. Second, the ADA prohibits discrimination based on disability. For these two reasons, nurses as healthcare professionals are compelled to ensure that these ADA goals are met when caring for patients from this population. Understanding how the social determinants of health are impacting a patient's health and well-being, and being able to recognize challenges and barriers blocking their access to quality care, are important strategies for helping to dismantle them. As the largest group of health professionals, nurses are positioned well to assess their patients' risk factors, limitations, strengths, and the resources they may or may not have to overcome their health issues. Living with a disability is a chronic condition that affects each person differently, so there is no recipe, nor one size fits all approach to care.

However, what is always needed is kindness and compassion when caring for any patient. As Larsen (2023) wrote, "Chronic illness is the lived experience of the individual and family diagnosed with the condition or disease. The individual's and family's values impact their perceptions and beliefs about the condition or disease and thus their illness and wellness behaviour" (Larsen, p. 75). The culturally competent nurse will discover the information needed to develop an appropriate, individualized plan of care through the establishment of a trusting and collaborative relationship with the patient that is respectful of the client's perspectives and identified needs, regardless of the nature of the disability.

IMPORTANT POINTS

Strategies for Delivering Culturally Competent Care

1. Treat adults as adults. Address people with disabilities by their first name only after they have given permission. Never patronize them by patting them on the head or shoulders, regardless of their age.
2. Be aware of and sensitive to factors influencing the patient's experience of illness, such as the nature of the disability, the realistic problems it creates, the person's attitude, the person's material resources, and the attitude of the patient's family and/or social group.
3. Avoid looking down, either figuratively or literally, on patients who utilize wheelchairs. Be seated for face-to-face encounters that allow you to make direct eye contact with patients.
4. Listen attentively when you are talking to people who have difficulty speaking. Be patient! Do not interrupt them, correct them, or speak for them. Do not pretend to understand. Repeat what you understand and allow them to elaborate.
5. Avoid leaning or hanging onto a person's wheelchair. The chair is part of their personal space.
6. Avoid negative language; for example, use of terms like *afflicted, handicapped, stricken, deaf and dumb, retarded, victim, confined to wheelchair, unfortunate,* and so on. Refer to a person with a disability as a person first who has a particular disability.
7. Remember that issues of sexuality are important. Although these issues are frequently ignored by the nurse and other health professionals, they are often of great concern for young and older persons experiencing new onset or permanent disabilities (Sakairi, 2020).
8. Seek appropriate resources to assist in addressing the patient's concerns.
9. Consider issues of mobility from the patient's perspective to ensure that patients are permitted to move freely and to have the most autonomy that the clinical situation permits. This may require collaboration with the physical or occupational therapy staff.
10. Be flexible in allowing adequate time for the patient to perform ADLs at a pace that is appropriate given the nature of the disability.
11. Provide privacy and assistance with physical or body requirements such as catheterizations, toileting, or wound care according to the patient's specific needs.
12. Teach patients with disabilities new skills to assist them in adapting to their environment.

Utilize available resources (see References) to address home care needs of patients with disabilities when planning for the patients' discharge. For example, the Individuals With Disabilities Education Act (IDEA) provides transitional services for children age 16 years or younger, including transportation, rehabilitation counseling, social work assistance, and other services.

A more complete list of do's and don'ts when communicating with people with disabilities can be found at People First Language (www.disabilityisnatural.com) and at Person-First and Destigmatizing Language (https://www.nih.gov/nih-style-guide/person-first-destigmatizing-language)

In short, nurses caring for patients with disabilities must have an awareness of their own attitudes, values, and beliefs; have cultural knowledge about patients for whom they care; be skilled at optimizing each nurse–patient encounter; and most importantly, be highly motivated to provide care that is congruent with what the patient needs and desires.

Source: Adapted from Delaware County Board of Developmental Disabilities. (2018). *People first language style guide.* https://www.dcbdd.org/wp-content/uploads/2018/01/People-First-Language-Style-Guide-1.pdf

CASE SCENARIO 1

Jimmy Watson is a 28-year-old White male patient with paraplegia caused by falling two stories from a ladder while doing construction work. This event occurred 4 months ago, and Jimmy has had extensive previous hospitalizations for multiple trauma injuries during the acute and subacute phase of his injury. Jimmy was transported from the very rural area in which he lives to a rehabilitation hospital in an urban area, which is several hundred miles from his hometown. This occurred because there was no facility of this kind in the area where he lived. Jimmy's father and younger brother live several hundred miles away and are unable to visit.

During the first weeks of his admission to the unit, Jimmy was pleasant and cooperative in his interactions with the hospital staff. All the nurses enjoyed working with him. Jimmy worked very hard to cooperate with the rehabilitation team in following his treatment regimen. After several weeks of hospitalization and several setbacks, including wound infections, high fevers, and several discharge postponements, Jimmy became despondent. At times, he became hostile when interacting with the staff. He frequently apologized for his discourteous behavior but became increasingly unhappy with his care. The nurses were perplexed. Bob, one of the nurses, comments, "I know he doesn't like the food here and wants to go home, but I don't understand why he seems to have given up. We are doing the best we can for him."

CASE SCENARIO 2

Milton Thomas, a 26-year-old Black male patient with quadraplegia, is admitted to a medical–surgical unit. Four years ago, he was a victim of a gunshot wound to his spine. He has since been living at home with his wife. He was admitted to a medical–surgical unit with a urinary tract infection, large sacral decubitus ulcer, and a fever of 103°F. He arrived at the unit on a stretcher accompanied by his wife. Milton and his wife were escorted to a room that was occupied by an older adult male patient with dementia. Kate, a young White female nurse, came into the room to perform the nursing history and initial assessment and discovers the patient is angry, hostile, and requesting a room change. The nurse explains that presently there are no other beds available, but they will consider moving him when possible. In assessing Milton, the nurse determines that because of his quadriplegia, need for extensive wound care, and problem with urinary retention, he will need much assistance with his personal care. Over the next several days, Milton's condition slowly improves but his attitude toward the hospital personnel becomes increasingly strained. He has several altercations with different members of the staff. One nurse commented, "I actually felt sorry for him at first, but I am fed up with his abusive behavior." Nurses assigned to work with Milton complain that he is uncooperative and at times rude toward them. Others are intimidated by his behavior and avoid going into his room at all. Another nurse refuses to answer Milton's call bell at night because, she says, he deliberately puts on the light as soon as the nurse leaves the room. A psychologist and social worker have been consulted. It is determined that Milton is having some marital difficulties and he anticipates possibly being placed in a nursing home following his discharge. His wife feels that she is no longer able to care for him because she has to work, and Milton is unable to care for himself at home.

CASE SCENARIO 3

Carlotta, a 38-year-old, Spanish-speaking, married mother of three is admitted to a medical unit after several weeks of neurologic changes that involved progressive weakness of her lower extremities. Prior to this, Carlotta and her family had recently moved to Philadelphia, Pennsylvania, from Puerto Rico, where she had a full-time job as a secretary. She has been active in her church and community. She and her husband also enjoyed swimming, but she has not felt up to doing any of these activities for the past several weeks. She was brought to the unit in a wheelchair. When Steve, Carlotta's nurse, attempts to assist Carlotta to bed, the patient waves him away. "I'm okay," she says. "I can do it." The admitting nurse learns that Carlotta is being evaluated to determine if she has MS or some other neurologic disease.

During the interview, the nurse learns that Carlotta speaks only a little English. She learned that Carlotta has three teenage children. The patient denies any complaints beyond the general muscle weakness that she is currently experiencing in her lower extremities. The nurse tries to explain that over the next 2 days testing has been planned to determine the nature of Carlotta's illness. That afternoon, Carlotta interacts pleasantly with the nursing staff and enjoys a visit with her husband and several other members of her family. While giving a report, the nurse states, "She is a nice lady, but a real puzzle. I don't understand why, despite her growing weakness, she does not really let you do anything for her. She wants to do it all by herself." Later that evening, on making her rounds, the evening nurse discovers Carlotta sobbing in her room.

WHAT NURSES NEED TO KNOW ABOUT THEMSELVES

Application of the Staircase Self-Assessment Model: Self-Reflection Questions

The patients in these cases are experiencing various stages in their encounter with disabilities, and each has unique circumstances that influence their ability to cope with their disability and to participate in their care. In attempting to address these cases, ask yourself the following questions. If you were the nurse caring for these patients, how would you respond?

1. Where are you on the staircase in working with patients with disabilities? How will you prepare to progress to the next level?
2. Which case would be the most challenging for you and why?
3. What attitudes and feelings would you have toward the patients in each of these scenarios? How might these attitudes influence care?
4. What skills or resources would be useful to you and the other nurses when caring for these patients?
5. What information would you need to provide these patients with culturally sensitive and competent care?
6. During each patient–nurse encounter, what strategies would strengthen the nurse–patient relationship?

RESPONSES TO SELF-REFLECTION QUESTIONS 3, 4, 5, AND 6

Response: What attitudes and feelings would you have toward the patients in each of these scenarios? How might these attitudes influence care?

In all the cases, the nurses' attitudes toward the patient seem directly related to the attitude and/or behavior of the patient. In Case 1, Bob, Jimmy's nurse, indicates his frustration with Jimmy's depression and is somewhat defensive in stating, "We're doing all we can for him." In Case 2, the nurses express a range of emotions that include anger, feeling intimidated, and "feeling sorry for the patient." Again, each of these emotions is a direct reflection of the patient's behavior toward the nurses. In Case 3, the nurses again expressed "feeling sorry for the patient" in the wheelchair and confusion about the patient's insistence on remaining independent.

As a human being, it is difficult when you believe that you are doing the best that you can on someone's behalf and feel that it is unappreciated by that person. However, none of these attitudes or feelings expressed by the nurses, including "feeling sorry for the patient," really helps meet the patient's needs. Acknowledging rather than denying frustration, anger, intimidation, or even sympathy toward the patient during peer group discussions may help alleviate some of the related stress that is associated with these feelings. This acknowledgment enables nurses to focus their energy on identifying and responding to the specific needs of the patient rather than focusing on their own personal feelings. By doing so, nurses become better able to confront patient care issues more objectively, while providing support for one another.

Response: What skills or resources would be useful to you and the other nurses when caring for these patients?

Regardless of the nature and type of the disability, it will be helpful for the nurse to gain specific knowledge about the patient's health-related beliefs and practices and cultural values, disease incidence and prevalence, and treatment efficacy. This includes learning from patients how they view the world; what they value or really care about; and what they believe about their illness, disease, or clinical situation. It also involves gaining information about any predispositions to disease or health risks that may be attributed to ethnicity or race and determining the effectiveness of the treatment plan being utilized. Another consideration is the preferred style of interaction or communication that the patient utilizes. This style is usually dependent on whether the patient is "culturally immersed" in his own culture or acculturated to another. Many American patients will use a "traditional style" that neither rejects nor accepts their cultural identity. In this case, patients will frequently say, "I'm just an American." Members of culturally diverse groups may be more likely to be acculturated, bicultural, or culturally immersed, rejecting all values except those held by their own cultural group.

In any case, nurses must recognize that there are also intracultural differences. For example, Americans from rural, suburban, and urban areas may choose different styles of interacting when placed in an environment that is new to them. Besides learning that is acquired through textbooks and conferences, healthcare professionals must gain cultural knowledge directly through interactions with the patient. Cultural knowledge comes through asking questions, seeking clarification, and sharing cultural information about differences and commonalities between the patient and the nurse.

Response: What information would you need to provide these patients with culturally sensitive and competent care?

In these three cases, it would be helpful for the nurses to first select and utilize a cultural assessment model that will enable them to develop a profile of the patient, identify pertinent healthcare needs, and plan care that is culturally congruent with the patients' values and beliefs. Because patients who are disabled are a heterogeneous population, they will have a wide variation in background factors that will contribute to both their responses to illness and their specific needs for care. In addition, the developmental stage and age of the patient will also have an impact on the type of care they will require. In culturally assessing the patient, the nurse can gain information about the patient's family support systems; values, religion, and spirituality needs; food preferences and health beliefs; and attitudes.

One approach the nurse can utilize is the assessment model first proposed by Purnell and Paulanka (2013). This model focuses on 14 interconnected domains that may be applied in assessing individuals' families and groups within various cultures: overview, inhabited localities and topography, communication, family roles and organizations, workforce issues, biocultural ecology, high-risk health behaviors, nutrition, pregnancy, childbearing practices, death rituals, spirituality, healthcare practices, and healthcare practitioners. Obviously, the nurse will need to decide which of the domains is relevant in the care of a particular patient or selected population. When applying any assessment model, nurses will also need to utilize good communication skills. It is particularly critical that the nurse has the ability to actively and objectively listen to patients without making judgments about their statements or attributing negative connotations to issues about which the patient and the nurse disagree. Human resources to assist the nurse when needed in planning culturally sensitive care include the family, clergy, social service personnel, interpreters, and other members of the health team.

Response: During each patient–nurse encounter, what strategies would strengthen the nurse–patient relationship?

Each patient-care encounter affords the nurses opportunities to learn more about the patient and to apply that information to patient-care planning. For example, in Case 1, during interactions with Jimmy, nurses can attempt to learn more about the differences between the rural lifestyle and hospital experiences that the patient is accustomed to and his experience in this urban hospital outside of his local region. In what ways can nurses assist the patient in coping with those differences? It is especially helpful to determine how significant the absence of family members is to this patient. Are there extended family members nearby? Could the nurse facilitate periodic phone conversations or video conversations between the patient and the family? If interaction between the patient and his family is not possible, what kinds of social support or activities can be arranged for this patient? What are some food preferences or substitutes that may be acquired through consultation with dietary services? In resolving some of these issues, the nurse may be better able to assist the patient in coping with his medical situation.

Clearly the nurse–patient encounters in Case 2 have not been positive ones. The nurses are angered and frustrated by the interactions they are having with this "hostile patient." However, psychologic consultations have revealed some underlying reasons for the patient's angry behavior. Are there also race and gender issues influencing the nurse–patient interaction in this situation? Can these issues be explored by assigning a male nurse or nursing assistants from the patient's ethnic background to assist the other nurses with his care? If this is not possible, perhaps the nurses can collaborate with the psychologist, clinical nurse specialist in psychology, or other members of the healthcare team to identify effective strategies for interacting with the patient.

In encounters with patients like the patient in Case 3, who speaks little English, the nurse can use the LEARN model (see Chapter 2 to review)

The acronym LEARN represents listen, explain, acknowledge, recommend, and negotiate. Nurses using this model will acknowledge and discuss the similarities and differences between the patient's explanation and the clinical or medical explanation of that patient's illness. However, use of an interpreter will facilitate interactions with this patient. The nurses will need to determine the following:

- What role the interpreter will play
- How advocacy and support for the patient and family will occur
- How a nonjudgmental attitude will be maintained
- The appropriate setting for the encounter between the patient and the interpreter
- How linguistic competence will be evaluated
- How the patient will be provided with thorough and accurate information
- How time will be managed
- How confidentiality and other ethical issues will be handled during patient encounters

Despite the nurse's best intentions and best efforts, it is sometimes difficult for the nurse and the patient to like one another. Nevertheless, the culturally competent nurse must be willing to respect differences while remaining flexible in adapting care so that it is culturally congruent with the patient's values and needs. Additionally, regardless of the patient's behavior, the nurse remains accepting of the patient as partner in the development of an appropriate plan of care. Without sincere cultural humility and motivation to provide culturally sensitive care to patients, it is impossible to do so.

In caring for patients with physical disabilities, in addition to the considerations mentioned previously there are some general guidelines that may be helpful to include when planning care. All of these are because people who are physically disabled do not want to be viewed as handicapped, but rather as individuals with a disability who, like everyone else, can benefit by understanding and receiving respectful help in meeting any problems.

NCLEX®-TYPE QUESTIONS

1. When planning care for persons with disabilities, the nurse recognizes that according to the Centers for Disease Control and Prevention (CDC) a disability is defined as:
   A. A physical limitation or bodily impairment that disallows freedom of mobility
   B. An emotional or psychologic illness that interferes with learning
   C. A psychologic impairment that hinders a person's normal development
   D. Any condition of the body or mind (impairment) that makes it more difficult for the person with the condition to do certain activities and interact with the world around them

2. According to the Centers for Disease Control and Prevention (CDC), what percent of the U.S. population has a disability?
   A. 10%
   B. 26%
   C. 30%
   D. 40%

3. The abbreviation IDDs applies to which of these conditions? *Select all that apply.*
   A. Autism
   B. Intellectual disabilities
   C. Mobility disabilities
   D. Developmental disabilities

4. The nurse cares for a person who uses a wheelchair who questions why able-bodied people are sometimes so insensitive to the needs of persons with disabilities. The nurse explains that according to some researchers:
   A. Most able-bodied people have had little prior exposure to persons with disabilities and are unaware of the problems they face in society

    B. Persons who are insensitive are those who usually lack social skills or compassion

    C. Most able-bodied people try hard to demonstrate compassion when meeting people with disabilities

    D. Persons who have disabilities are often given considerations that able-bodied persons are denied

5. For nurses caring for persons who have disabilities, it is important to remember that issues of sexuality:

    A. Have little or no significance after diagnosis of a physical disability

    B. Are of great concern to persons with disabilities but are often ignored by nurses

    C. Are meaningless when learning or cognitive disabilities exist

    D. Affect only persons who are able bodied

6. The nurse considers the care needs of a person who uses a wheelchair. When planning a meeting with the patient, the nurse recognizes that the best approach is to:

    A. Maintain eye contact when speaking with the patient to monitor nonverbal clues

    B. Stand facing the patient's chair when speaking with them

    C. Stand beside the patient's chair to promote safety

    D. Sit facing the patient to maintain eye-to-eye contact

7. The nurse is teaching a community class about the incidence of disabilities in the United States. According to the World Health Organization (WHO), what factors account for the increasing number of persons with disabilities in the United States?

    A. Aging

    B. The emergence of chronic diseases

    C. Injuries caused by road crashes

    D. HIV/AIDS

    E. All of these

8. Two organizations that primarily provide support for persons with intellectual and developmental disabilities are:

    A. American Disability Association (ADA) and International Council of Nurses (ICN)

    B. The World Health Organization (WHO) and ADA

    C. The Arc and Learning Disabilities Association of America (LDA)

    D. National Center for Health Statistics (NCHS) and WHO

9. The nurse caring for persons with disabilities recognizes that the concept of "people first" refers to the belief that:

    A. All persons with disabilities have strengths, abilities, and inherent value, and are equal in the law

    B. Persons with disabilities should be given first priority in clinical settings

    C. Persons with disabilities must first overcome them before actively participating in society

    D. Persons with disabilities should be first to receive healthcare benefits

10. What situation describes the problem of disability disparities among persons with disabilities?

    A. Low-income, working-age adults with physical disabilities experience problems with transportation accessibility and privacy barriers.

    B. A person is born with a learning disability.

    C. Children who have cerebral palsy experience problems with mobility.

    D. There is a high percentage of physically disabled among the young.

11. The nurse is interviewing a patient with a disability who has a problem speaking clearly. The patient is struggling to explain the situation. The best initial action by the nurse is to:

    A. Correct the patient's mispronunciations and unclear statements

    B. Listen patiently without interrupting, then answer the question to clarify

    C. Speak directly instead to a family member who can interpret the patient's meaning

    D. Pretend to follow the conversation to minimize the patient's embarrassment

12. The culturally competent nurse recognizes that the use of certain language can be demoralizing to persons with disabilities. Which of these statements suggest that the nurse is using culturally appropriate language when caring for clients with disabilities?
    A. The nurse giving a report at change of shift mentions that the patient is afflicted with mobility problems and has recently been stricken with multiple sclerosis (MS).
    B. The ED triage nurse explains that "since you are handicapped, I'll place you in a larger cubicle for your assessment."
    C. The nurse explains to the doctor, "I believe this young lady may have a hearing impairment."
    D. A nurse exclaims, "I was just assigned to a mentally retarded patient!"

13. The nurse is caring for a patient who is paralyzed from the waist down due to a gunshot wound to the spine. To encourage the patient's participation in his care, the nurse offers the patient a basin with hot soapy water. On the nurse's return a half hour later, the patient is still washing himself. The best initial response by the nurse is to:
    A. Take over for the patient and complete the bath
    B. Ask if he needs any assistance or wants the nurse to return later
    C. Take the wash basin away, as this is taking too long
    D. Ask a nursing assistant to work with the patient to complete his bath

14. When admitting a 73-year-old patient with dementia to their unit, what approach by the nurse is most appropriate?
    A. Calling the patient by their first name to establish an informal and relaxed rapport with them
    B. Asking the patient by which name they wish to be called
    C. Stating their own name but referring to the patient as "sweetie"
    D. Avoiding the use of names in relating to the patient

ANSWERS TO NCLEX-TYPE QUESTIONS

1. A
2. C
3. B
4. A
5. B

6. B and D
7. E
8. C
9. A
10. A

11. B
12. C
13. B
14. B

AMERICAN ASSOCIATION OF COLLEGES OF NURSING COMPETENCIES ADDRESSED IN THIS CHAPTER

1. Apply knowledge of social and cultural factors that affect nursing and healthcare across multiple contexts.
2. Use relevant data sources and best evidence in providing culturally competent care.
3. Promote achievement of safe and quality outcomes of care for diverse populations.
4. Advocate for social justice, including commitment to the health of vulnerable populations and the elimination of health disparities.
5. Participate in continuous cultural competence development.

 A robust set of instructor resources designed to supplement this text is located at http://connect.springerpub.com/content/book/978-0-8261-8302-6. Qualifying instructors may request access by emailing textbook@springerpub.com.

REFERENCES

Acheampong, E., Nadutey, A., Anokye, R., Agyei-Baffour, P., & Edusei, A. K. (2022). The perception of healthcare workers of people with disabilities presenting for care at peri-urban health facilities in Ghana. *Health & Social Care in the Community*, 30(4), e944–e952. https://doi.org/10.1111/hsc.13496

ADA.gov. U.S. Department of Justice Civil Rights Division. (n.d.). *Introduction to the Americans With Disabilities Act.* https://www.ada.gov/topics/intro-to-ada

Appelgren, M., Persson, K., Bahtsevani, C., & Borglin, G. (2022). Swedish registered nurses' perceptions of caring for patients with intellectual and developmental disability: A qualitative descriptive study. *Health & Social Care in the Community, 30*(3), 1064–1076. https://doi.org/10.1111/hsc.13307

The Arc. (2017). *Diversity annual report: A new beginning.* https://thearc.org/wp-content/uploads/2019/08/2017-Diversity-Annual-Report-1.pdf

Barkan, A. (2021, September 8). Home care keeps me alive. It should be fully funded. *The New York Times.* https://www.nytimes.com/2021/09/08/opinion/als-home-health-care.html

Cashin, A., Pracilio, A., Buckley, T., Morphet, J., Kersten, M., Trollor, J. N., Griffin, K., Bryce, J., & Wilson, N. J. (2022). A cross-practice context exploration of nursing preparedness and comfort to care for people with intellectual disability and autism. *Journal of Clinical Nursing, 31*(19/20), 2971–2980. https://doi.org10.1111/jocn.16131

Centers for Disease Control and Prevention. (n.d.-a). *Disability and health overview.* https://www.cdc.gov/ncbddd/disabilityandhealth/disability.html

Centers for Disease Control and Prevention. (n.d.-b). *Disability and health promotion: Many adults with disabilities report frequent mental distress.* https://www.cdc.gov/ncbddd/disabilityandhealth/features/adults-with-disabilities-mental-distress.html

Centers for Disease Control and Prevention. (n.d.-c). *Common barriers to participation experienced by people with disabilities.* https://www.cdc.gov/ncbddd/disabilityandhealth/disability-barriers.html

Centers for Disease Control and Prevention. (n.d.-d). *Disability impacts all of us infographic.* https://www.cdc.gov/ncbddd/disabilityandhealth/infographic-disability-impacts-all.htm

Cooper, D. (2022). Supporting a patient with learning disabilities through screening and treatment for primary breast cancer. *British Journal of Nursing, 31*(22), 1150–1153. https://doi.org10.12968/bjon.2022.31.22.1150

Foreman, R. A. (2023). A nurse's disability experience: Seeking compassion and respect. *Missouri Nursing News, 3*(3), 9. https://www.healthecareers.com/nurse-resources/missouri-nursing-news-april-2023/a-nurses-disability-experience-seeking-compassion-and-respect

Iezzoni, L. I. (2022). Project Muse: Dignity of risk and living at home despite severe disability. *Perspectives in Biology and Medicine, 65*(2), 252–261. https://doi.org/10.1353/pbm.2022.0021

Lagu, T., Haywood, C., Reimold, K., DeJong, C., Sterling, R. W., & Ienoni, L. I. (2022). "I am not the doctor for you": Physicians' attitudes about caring for people with disabilities. *Health Affairs, 41*(10), 1387–1395. https://doi.org/10.1377/hlthaff.2022.00475

Larsen, P. D. (2023). Advancing the care of persons with chronic illness and disability. *Rehabilitation Nursing, 48*(3), 75–76. https://doi.org/10.1097/RNJ.0000000000000415

Liebel, D. V., Powers, B., Salo, J., & Burgen, D. (2018). Managing the elephant in the room: What home health care nurses do and don't do to support productive interaction. *International Journal of Integrated Care, 18*, 1–2. https://doi.org/10.5334/ijic.s2358

Marks, B., & Sisirak, J. (2022). Nurses with disability: Transforming healthcare for all. *Online Journal of Issues in Nursing, 27*(3), 10. https://doi.org/10.3912/OJIN.Vol27No03Man04

National Disability Institute. (2020). *Race ethnicity, and disabilities: The financial impact of systemic inequality and intersectionality.* https://www.nationaldisabilityinstitute.org/reports/research-brief-race-ethnicity-and-disability

National Institutes of Health. (n.d.). *Eunice Kennedy Shriver National Institute of Child Health and Human Development (NICHD).* https://www.nih.gov/about-nih/what-we-do/nih-almanac/eunice-kennedy-shriver-national-institute-child-health-human-development-nichd

New York State Department of Health. (2009). *People first language: Communicating with and about people with disabilities.* https://www.health.ny.gov/publications/0951.pdf

Purnell, L., & Paulanka, B. J. (2013). *Transcultural health care: A culturally competent approach* (3rd ed.). F. A. Davis.

Sakairi, E. (2020). Medicalized pleasure and silenced desire: Sexuality of people with disabilities. *Sexuality and Desirability, 38*, 41–56. https://doi.org/10.1007/s11195-020-09618-3

United Nations, (2022). *Transformative solutions for inclusive development: The role of innovation in fueling an accessible and equitable world.* https://www.un.org/en/observances/day-of-persons-with-disabilities

United Nations, Department of Economic and Social Affairs. (2023). *5 things you should know about persons with disabilities.* https://www.un.org/en/desa/5-things-you-should-know-about-persons-disabilities

United Nations, Sustainable Development Goals. (2023). *Goal 10: Reduce inequality within and among countries.* https://www.un.org/sustainabledevelopment/inequality

World Health Organization. (2023). *Fact sheet: Disability.* https://www.who.int/news-room/fact-sheets/detail/disability-and-health

Young, N. A. E. (2021). *Childhood disability in the United States: 2019.* https://www.census.gov/library/publications/2021/acs/acsbr-006.html

IMPORTANT WEBSITES

American Association of People With Disabilities. Retrieved from https://www.aapd.com

California Nonprofit Organization for Children with Special Needs. Retrieved from https://americandisabilityassociation.org/

The Arc. Retrieved from https://thearc.org/

People First Language: Retrieved from https://www.nih.gov/nih-style-guide/person-first-destigmatizing-language

Project Empowerment: Improving Minority Disability. Retrieved from http://www.worksupport.com/NewSite0513/projects/index.html

6

Cultural Considerations When the Patient Speaks a Different Language

Gloria Kersey-Matusiak

The language of the lips is easily taught, but who can teach the language of the heart?

—MAHATMA GANDHI

LEARNING OBJECTIVES

After this chapter, the reader will be able to
1. Describe the impact of language barriers on patients' access to quality healthcare.
2. Recognize the various types of language diversity and their impact on nurse–patient interactions.
3. Explain some myths related to language diversity.
4. Discuss the influence of linguistic style and nonverbal communication on nurse–patient communication.
5. Develop strategies for overcoming language barriers when working with culturally diverse groups.

KEY TERMS

Culturally and Linguistically Appropriate
    Services (CLAS) Standards in Healthcare
In-person face-to-face
Language barriers
Limited English proficiency (LEP)
Linguistic style

Literacy
Nonverbal communication
Telephonic approach
Video remote interpretation
Web-based translation applications

UNDERSTANDING THE NEED FOR CULTURALLY LINGUISTIC CARE

According to the U.S. Census (Dietrich & Hernandez, 2022), nearly 68 million people living in the United States spoke a language other than English in the home in 2019. Among the top languages spoken were Spanish, Chinese (including Mandarin and Cantonese), French (including Cajun and Creole), Tagalog, and Arabic. In addition, several African languages, such as Amharic, Igbo, Swahili, and Yoruba, were spoken. Among these groups, many individuals do not speak English very well or at all and are considered **limited English**

proficient (LEP). In 2018, 47% of immigrants ages 5 years or older were classified as LEP (Betancur et al., 2020). A designation of LEP indicates that an individual whose primary language is not English has a low proficiency in reading, speaking, writing, or understanding English. Pew Research Center (Bialik et al., 2018) reported that the term *English language learners* (ELLs) refers to a diverse group from many different states and native language backgrounds. Nearly 5 million ELLs were enrolled in U.S. schools in 2015, or 9.5% of the U.S. public school enrollees. ELLs represent a growing part of the student population in the United States.

For patients who are LEPs, this means having a need for support in understanding the medical system, their diagnosis, and the related plan of care. While U.S individuals who are unauthorized immigrants are more proficient in English than a decade ago, individuals who are unauthorized immigrants are much less likely to be proficient in English than lawful entrants (Passel & Cohn, 2019). The literature also links being considered LEP to education. For example, 64% of Asian immigrants with college degrees also had higher levels of English proficiency that increased with time in the United States. However, there are also high percentages of LEPs among some other Asian groups, such as Chinese (33%), Koreans (32%), and Vietnamese (31%). Unauthorized immigrants from Mexico and the Northern Triangle (El Salvador, Guatemala, and Honduras) were among the largest groups with less than a high school diploma and high numbers of LEP. Although more people are coming to the United States today from countries with high English proficiency, limited English skills have increased among immigrants to California, Texas, New York, Florida, Illinois, and New Jersey (Passel & Cohn, 2019). Given these facts, as nurses increasingly interact with culturally diverse patients, they can be certain to encounter **language barriers** at some point during their careers. Communicating effectively with patients requires nurses to be able to listen, observe, and understand the beliefs and needs of their patients and to use culturally relevant concepts when communicating with them (Campo et al., 2015; Montie et al., 2016; Sobel & Metzler Sawin, 2016).

The National Standards for **Culturally and Linguistically Appropriate Services (CLAS) Standards** in Health and Health Care have challenged nurses and healthcare institutions to provide services that address the linguistic needs of patients (U.S. Department of Health and Human Services [DHHS], 2013). More specifically, in the revised CLAS standards under the category Communication and Language Assistance in Standard 5, healthcare agencies are mandated to "offer language assistance to individuals who have limited English proficiency and/or other communication needs, at no cost to them, to facilitate timely access to all health care and services" (DHHS, 2013, p. 72). (See Important Websites at the end of this chapter for a link to the CLAS standards Fact Sheet.) Language enables us to establish a rapport with our patients, communicate our ideas, and negotiate our plan of care.

Impact of Limited English Proficiency on Patient Care

The healthcare literature identifies numerous problems for patients who are LEP, such as not being able to access and navigate the healthcare system and communicate with physicians, nurses, and other health team members effectively to provide an accurate account of their chief complaint and medical history (Betancur et al., 2020; Lopez-Bushnell et al., 2020; Hu, 2018; Pew Research Center, 2022). Patients who are LEP also have difficulty understanding their diagnosis, medical instructions, the recommended treatment plans, and their own role in clinical decision-making.

Obviously, when the patient and the nurse speak different languages or have only minimal understanding of one another's primary language, this greatly inhibits the establishment of a culturally sensitive and ethically appropriate nurse–patient relationship (Alpern et al., 2016). The literature tells us that "linguistic barriers between nurses and patients can threaten quality nursing care by perpetuating stereotypes and fostering the delivery of care based on misinformation and assumptions" (Hunter-Adams & Rother, 2017; Meuter et al., 2015).

In addition, DeWilde and Burton (2017) discussed the consequence to patients who did not receive culturally competent care, labeling it cultural distress. These writers proposed a theoretical framework that is based on the Leininger culture care diversity and universality theory. This theory describes the experience of illness, which they say is accompanied by a baseline level of stress. According to this theory, the level of stress is increased as patients feel alienated or marginalized because of cultural differences based on skin color, language, physical ability, gender, and/or when their cultural beliefs and attitudes are not considered. This process is referred to by the authors as "othering." Further, they stated that although the process may be unintentional, othering can "create and reinforce positions of dominance and subordination, and exclusion by the recipient" (p. 336). These authors cited reports of such adverse outcomes in African Americans as shorter life expectancy, increased infant mortality, and hypertension as examples of the "othering" effect on health. "The process of othering itself creates barriers to access and to care, because patients feel unwelcome and are less inclined to seek care" (p. 337). The writers noted that as globalization increases, so too will the likelihood of increased cultural distress among culturally diverse patients. The authors acknowledged that nurses cannot be all things to all cultural groups. However, when caring for patients from diverse backgrounds, nurses can recognize the significance of culture in patient–nurse relationships and provide care that strives to be culturally congruent with the patients' cultural values and beliefs.

At the same time, physicians and nurses struggle with their own inability to communicate important health information to patients who are LEP when they cannot speak the patient's primary language. They express concerns that their time might be better served in addressing the needs of those patients with whom they are better able to communicate. Many health professionals are also frustrated by the additional time it takes to care for patients with language barriers when language resources to assist them are limited, unavailable, or when they are untrained in the use of such resources. Squires and colleagues (2019) explored home healthcare professionals' perspectives about how workload changes from managing language barriers influence quality and safety in home healthcare. These researchers concluded that having non-English speaking, LEP patients in their caseload increased visits and working days, and may pose a threat to the quality of care patients receive, adding to workload stress and job dissatisfaction. Based on their findings, the researchers in this study suggested that when home health agencies have large populations of LEP patients they should consider making policies about patient assignments based on language preferences when possible.

The Impact of Limited English Proficiency on Patient Safety

Besides the impact language barriers have on communication between patients and healthcare professionals, the literature also stressed the potential health consequences that result from the language barriers LEP patients encounter. Many researchers cite extended length of stay (LOS), risks of delayed diagnosis, surgical delays, readmission within 30 days, failure to recognize symptoms, or risk of adverse effects of treatment and other safety risks caused by language barriers (Hu, 2018; Lopez-Bushnell et al., 2020; Trube & Yeo, 2023). Hu (2018) warned of the unintentional and often greater harm LEP patients encounter caused by acts of omission and commission. In this study, researchers conducted a 7-month analysis of adverse incident reports in six hospitals and found 49.1% of patients who were LEP experienced higher levels of detectable physical harm compared to 29.5% who spoke English. Higher levels of physical harm ranged from moderate temporary harm (46.8%) to death (24.4%). The authors defined "moderate temporary harm as that which is not severe or did not cause permanent injury" (p. 409). Trube and Yeo (2023) examined published government documents from 2017 to 2022 and discussed issues faced by individuals with LEP who are anticipated to be diagnosed with a new cancer diagnosis. Based on their findings, these authors predict that 145,000 individuals with LEP will be diagnosed with a new cancer annually. Even though federal law prohibits discrimination based on immigration status, people with LEP with limited understanding of the healthcare system often experience delayed cancer diagnosis and often receive inadequate treatment.

The Impact of Language Diversity

Besides differences between users of diverse languages, sometimes problems in communication are encountered when patients have some knowledge of English but lack the confidence in their ability to speak it with native speakers. Because a lack of English-speaking skills is often stigmatized in America, foreign speakers of English sometimes fear ridicule or negative judgments about their intelligence. At the same time, while Americans insist on immigrants learning English, they are unmotivated to learn a second language themselves. Only 18% of Americans as compared to 53% of Europeans speak a second language. This lack of motivation is attributed to a variety of factors including nativism among some and a belief that speaking only English is a sign of Americans' national pride. Two myths about language diversity may also influence nurses' judgment about linguistically diverse patients. First, some believe that emphasizing the importance of Americans gaining knowledge of a second language other than English may minimize the importance of English as the primary language of the United States. Yet, English remains the dominant language. Second, there are those who believe that minority members, especially recent immigrants, are not eager to learn English. However, experience in local communities tells us that there are many groups throughout the country that provide English-learning programs. For example, the author of this chapter recently worked with a group of very committed and diligent Spanish-speaking English-language learners who viewed learning English as a way of gaining employment and successfully completing tests for naturalization. These programs are highly sought out and attended by recent and older immigrants who strive to prepare themselves for living and working in the United States. There is also the belief that English is widespread globally; however, 75% of people in the world do not speak it. Americans also generally learn other languages starting at the high school level, whereas Europeans start language programs much earlier in elementary school. It has been documented that children are more likely to learn new language skills rapidly. *The New York Times* (Engle, 2019) reported 20% of K–12 students in the United States study a foreign language compared with 92% in Europe, and only 10 states and the District of Columbia make foreign language learning a high school graduation requirement. In addition, from 2013 to 2016 enrollment in college modern language courses dropped 9.2%, and language options are limited in many colleges (Friedman, 2015). All of these factors place America behind in competing in the global economy. As one writer observed, "to prosper economically and to improve relations with other countries, Americans need to read, speak, and understand other languages" (Primavera, 2017, para. 10).

Besides being able to manage the issue of English as a second language (ESL), nurses must also learn to bridge the communication gap that is created by differences in patients' **linguistic style**, dialect, **literacy**, and **nonverbal communication** patterns. For each of these aspects, communication can significantly influence cross-cultural interactions between the patient and the nurse.

Another important nursing consideration during cross-linguistic communication is the cultural context in which the language is spoken. When speaking in their language, some cultural groups rely on the use of many words to convey a particular message. Such groups are considered "low context." The English, German, and French fall under this category. High-context languages use fewer words and meaning is found between the lines as more attention is paid to the nonverbal or cultural cues transmitted through body language. High-context languages include Native American languages and Chinese (Milincic, 2020).

Linguistic style refers to the way in which words are used to send messages. This includes tone of voice, rate of speed, and degree of loudness (Britannica, 2023) and reflects the speaker's vocabulary, pace, pitch, and intonation choices. Linguistic style also relates to an individual's tendency to be direct or indirect when communicating (Milincic, 2020). Linguistic style is influenced by a variety of cultural factors, such as ethnic background, geographical origin, and gender. It is useful for nurses to recognize that linguistic style and dialect variations are reflections of a cultural group's shared patterns of communicating, usually due to geographical norms: Consider a speaker who comes from Rhode Island and another from the rural South, for example. One way of speaking is not superior to another, nor is linguistic style an indication of one's intelligence or ability. However, language-related conflicts occur due to feelings and attitudes of fear and mistrust of "otherness" as reflected by a difference in one's style of communicating. These attitudes emerge from long-held assumptions about differences that may be inaccurate.

There are also variations in patients' levels of literacy, or their ability to read and write the spoken word, whether it be in English or in the patient's native language. The term *health literacy* refers to the ability of patients to find, understand, and use their health information and services to inform health-related decisions (American Academy of Pediatrics, 2021).

Therefore, the nurse cannot assume that patients understand medical forms or documents even when distributed in the patient's language. Just as in America some persons who speak their own language at a conversational level of fluency are unable to read it, so nurses must assess reading capacity of patients from both English-speaking and linguistically diverse backgrounds. To members of some cultural groups, nonverbal communication is even more important than the spoken word. Often by our gestures, facial expressions, eye contact, stance, or hand movements, we communicate to others messages we do not intend. When communicating cross-culturally, it is especially important for nurses to pay attention to differences in patterns of nonverbal communication between themselves and the patient. When differences in linguistic style and nonverbal behavior coexist with the inability to share a common language, either the patient or the nurse may become frustrated and abandon the efforts to communicate at all. This is evidenced by the tendency by some nurses to avoid the room of a patient who may have a different way of communicating that is offensive or intimidating to the nurse. However, an attitude of unwillingness to seek new ways to overcome language barriers is the greatest barrier of all. Failure of the nurse to communicate effectively with the patient can lead to serious consequences for the patient. (Specifically, barriers to communication can adversely affect patients' access to healthcare, ability to give informed consent and to understand medical and nursing diagnoses, health education, and healthcare outcomes). To overcome the barriers created by differences in language and communication style between the patient and the nurse, nurses must first be aware of their own patterns and styles of communication. By acknowledging differences that exist between themselves and their patients and the potential problems these differences create, they can identify appropriate strategies to overcome them.

STRATEGIES TO ADDRESS LINGUISTIC BARRIERS

In efforts to overcome the impact of language barriers and miscommunication, most researchers suggest the use of professionally trained healthcare interpreters when caring for patients designated LEP (Betancur et al., 2020; Lopez-Bushnell et al., 2020; Papadis et al., 2022). In addition, Title VI of the federal Civil Rights Act requires all health agencies to provide interpreters for all LEP patients and those with disabilities that affect their ability to communicate (Hu, 2018). In addition to recommendations to provide trained healthcare interpreters, the literature provides information about various other strategies to enhance communication between providers and patients who are LEP. For example, the Agency for Healthcare Research and Quality (AHRQ) created the Team Strategies and Tools to Enhance Performance and Patient Safety for individuals with LEP (see webpage at the end of the chapter). The AHRQ also offers tips for working with in-person interpreters. See Chart 6.1.

CHART 6.1 ■ BEST PRACTICE TIPS WHEN WORKING WITH AN IN-PERSON INTERPRETER IN CLINICAL PRACTICE.

General Principles	• Avoid the use of family members and friends as interpreters. • Document the use of trained professional interpreters in the patient's medical record. • Recognize that interpreted encounters take longer, but save time in the long run.
Specific Skills	• Position yourself to maximize interaction with the patient. • Address the patient directly. • Watch the patient carefully; don't miss valuable clues (especially nonverbal). • Avoid medical jargon. • Speak in short units, keep a comfortable pace, and allow time for interpreter. • Check in with the patient to determine accuracy. • Use return demonstrations to make sure the patient is understanding you via the interpreter.

Source: Agency for Healthcare Research and Quality, & Larliner, L. S. (2018). *When patients and providers speak different languages.* https://psnet.ahrq.gov/web-mm/when-patients-and-providers-speak-different-languages

In addition, legal and regulatory obligations posed by the Office of Civil Rights, the U.S. DHHS, and The Joint Commission to provide language access services for patients with LEP are found in the healthcare literature (Karliner, 2018). Karliner weighs the advantages and disadvantages of in-person interpretation and remote interpretation (either telephonic or videoconferencing) and offers the reader best practice tips when using an in-person interpreter. The literature suggests the best modality for accessing professional interpreter services depends on the needs and resources of a particular agency. However, in-person professional interpretation has proven to be effective in increasing patient satisfaction, ensuring a better understanding of patients' social and cultural backgrounds, facilitating an easy patient rapport, and improving care outcomes (Karlinger, 2018). Nevertheless, in-person interpretation is not without its faults because the use of in-person interpreters requires that the hospital can provide staff to offer assistance with many languages and that staff will be available on an on-call basis and travel from place to place whenever needed. Therefore, since this modality creates time constraints and limited availability when there are many LEP patients requiring services, the authors recommend the use of multiple modalities, including telephonic or videoconferences, to increase access and efficiency, especially in a large health system.

Modes of Interpretation

Several modes of interpretation have been described in the literature (Chart 6.2). For example, there is **in-person face-to face,** during which the interpreter is present with the provider and patient. This approach lends itself to viewing nonverbal aspects of the interaction and enhances communication. The **telephonic approach** is used when patient and provider connect with one another through an audio device. This approach facilitates communication to remote areas or for use when a language is not commonly spoken. However, this approach limits access to nonverbal cues that the patient may express. **Video remote interpretation** is increasingly being used and can include advanced technology that employs features such as having the spoken word as text appearing on the screen. This approach is especially useful for patients with hearing impairments without a sign-language interpreter. **Web-based translation applications** enable voice-to-voice and text-to-text communications. This approach is considered best when used in simple, low-risk

CHART 6.2 ■ SUMMARY OF TEXT DESCRIPTION MODES OF INTERPRETATION.

1. In person face-to-face
2. Telephonic approach
3. Remote interpretation
4. Web-based translation

healthcare encounters because of patient safety concerns in more complex healthcare situations (Habib et al., 2023).

Hu (2018), in a review of the literature, discussed Lindholm and colleagues' (2012) investigation of the LOS and 30-day readmission rates associated with LEP patients receiving interpretation at admission or discharge. This study found that those who did not use an interpreter during either time had a significantly longer stay in the hospital, but readmission rates were not found to be statistically significant. However, these results conflict with others in the literature that suggest use of interpreters during a hospital stay increases the LOS compared with English-speaking patients. The current study does indicate that use of interpreters affords LEP patients opportunities for better communication between themselves and care providers, enhanced history taking, quicker diagnosis, and greater understanding of their diagnosis and treatment.

Sonoda and colleagues (2022) discussed a study in which they surveyed Japanese adult patients in an ambulatory, family healthcare setting with two Japanese-speaking physicians. The study explored the effectiveness of using the Japanese–English communication (JEC) sheet, a communication sheet intended to facilitate communication between patients and non–Japanese-speaking clinical staff. More than half of the study's participants found this tool to be useful in facilitating communication with the staff and reducing inequities based on linguistic and cultural barriers. In this study, researchers also found that using a communication sheet like this in other settings and with different languages can advance quality and safety of patient care at the individual and institutional level.

When the nurse communicates with patients who speak ESL, there are three important strategies the nurse can use. First, the nurse must listen *actively* while paying particular attention to the patient's use of silence throughout the conversation. Listening actively means asking for clarification when the patient uses unfamiliar terms or the nurse is unclear about the patient's use of English terms. Second, the nurse should seek to clarify nonverbal communication to avoid misinterpretation. Third, regardless of the type of language barrier, the nurse should remember to strive to convey patience and caring through nonverbal measures. These actions by the nurse include moving about in a nonhurried manner, facing the patient when communicating, touching when culturally acceptable, and smiling. In this way, the nurse acknowledges an appreciation of how stressful cross-cultural interactions may be for the patient. This approach also signals to patients the nurse's desire to minimize their anxiety and ultimately bridge the cultural gap that exists in these situations.

Using an Interpreter

When a nurse recognizes that the patient is unable to speak English, the nurse should attempt to recruit someone who can address the patient in their native language. Many texts outline the best approach when utilizing an interpreter (Andrews & Boyle, 2013; Habib et al., 2023; Purnell & Fenkl, 2021). To maintain patients' privacy and confidentiality, children and family members should be avoided as interpreters or translators when possible. Purnell (2013) offers several recommendations for working with an interpreter, including using dialect-specific interpreters whenever possible who also understand the culture and who are age- and gender-appropriate when sensitive or personal issues are discussed. Habib and colleagues (2023) suggest the nurse schedule the interview, allowing for extra time to meet with the interpreter before the encounter to build a rapport and share information about the patient's background and expectations during the interview. During the consultation, the nurse should introduce and identify everyone present and position the interpreter and provider side-by side in an inpatient setting so the patient can see both easily. The nurse should make the patient the focus of attention; demonstrate interest in the conversation; maintain eye contact with them throughout the interaction; speak clearly and slowly; avoid slang, medical jargon, or acronyms; and speak directly to the patient. When relating to the interpreter, insist on sentence-by-sentence interpretation and allow adequate time for a response to your question. During any periods of silence, observe the patient for nonverbal clues while formulating your next question. Check and reinforce the patient's understanding through techniques like return demonstrations, then summarize key points of the conversation. After the consultation, the nurse should thank the interpreter and discuss or clarify medical, social, cultural, or ethical concerns; plan follow-up appointments or referrals; and document the use of the interpreter in the patient's clinical record (Habib et al., 2023).

Finally, should there be no immediate availability of an interpreter and the nurse is unable to speak the patient's language, remember to demonstrate warmth and compassion by smiling, introducing oneself as the nurse that will be caring for the patient, and using any known appropriate words in that patient's language that convey caring and understanding of the patient's situation. Phrase books, picture cards displaying common words, or communication sheets are also helpful supports during these encounters. Seek help from age-, gender-, and culturally appropriate individuals who speak the patient's language. Remember, the goal is to enhance understanding between the patient and the nurse and to ensure the patient's safety from any harm that may result from ineffective communication.

IMPORTANT POINTS

- Nearly 68 million, or 21.5%, of the U.S. population speaks a language other than English as a primary language.
- In 2018, 47% of immigrants aged 5 years and older were classified as LEP.
- Only 18% of Americans speak a second language.
- Among the top non-English languages spoken in the United States are Spanish, Chinese, French, Tagalog, and Arabic.
- CLAS standards are national guidelines and mandates that compel hospitals and healthcare providers to provide culturally linguistic care.
- Language diversity includes ESL issues as well as linguistic style, dialect, literacy, and non-verbal communication patterns.
- Literacy refers to the ability to read, write, and understand in English or one's own language.
- Linguistic style refers to the way in which words are exchanged. This includes tone of voice, rate of speed, and degree of loudness.
- Linguistic style does not reflect an individual's intelligence or ability.
- Language barriers can adversely affect patients' access to healthcare, ability to give informed consent, medical and nursing diagnosis, health education, patient safety, and healthcare outcomes.
- Some myths about language diversity influence nurses' attitudes about caring for linguistically diverse patients.
- The person selected to assist the nurse by translating and interpreting for the patient should ideally be a trained medical interpreter who understands both the patient's language and culture.
- Using family members, especially children, may violate patients' confidentiality and privacy rights.
- Strategies for caring for linguistically diverse patients include actively listening, seeking clarification, using an appropriate interpreter, and paying attention to nonverbal communication.
- Modes of interpretation include in-person face-to-face, telephonic, video remote, and web-based applications.
- It is important to document the session and its outcome with the interpreter.

When there is no interpreter:

- Greet patient by identifying oneself as the nurse, and shaking hands or touching only if it is culturally (gender) appropriate.
- Smile; speak slowly, using simple words; and demonstrate warmth and caring.
- Attempt to use any words you know in the patient's language.
- Obtain phrase books, picture cards, or communication sheets.
- Seek age- and gender-appropriate individuals who speak the patient's language and dialect to assist you.

CASE SCENARIO

Mrs. Garcia is a 67-year-old woman who is visiting her daughter from Puerto Rico. She suddenly experiences an episode of severe chest pain. Her daughter, who recently delivered a healthy 8-pound newborn, calls for an ambulance but is unable to accompany her mother to the hospital. Although the daughter speaks English fluently, Mrs. Garcia speaks only Spanish and can understand only a little English. She is rushed to the nearest hospital, where the staff struggles to communicate with her as best they can. In the ED, Mrs. Garcia holds her hand over her chest and grimaces as the pain seems to grow more severe.

One of the ED nurses grabs Mr. Rodriguez, a staff member in environmental services, and asks him to assist by translating for the nurses and doctors caring for Mrs. Garcia because it is 8 a.m. and the only Spanish-speaking medical interpreter, Mr. Sanchez, is not due in until 10 a.m. Based on the ECG findings and first lab results, the staff believes that Mrs. Garcia is experiencing a myocardial infarction (MI). They ask that Mr. Rodriguez explain to her that they are awaiting the results of other laboratory studies to confirm the medical diagnosis but believe that she probably had a heart attack and will need further testing to confirm the medical staff's suspicion. Mrs. Garcia becomes extremely anxious and begins to cry. The staff is baffled about what to do next.

WHAT NURSES NEED TO KNOW ABOUT THEMSELVES

Application of the Staircase Self-Assessment Model: Self-Reflection Questions

1. Where are you on the Cultural Competency Staircase regarding this patient's language and culture? How will you progress to the next level? (Review Chapter 1 and the Staircase Model.)
2. What knowledge do you need to have about this patient, including cultural/language needs, to provide this patient with culturally sensitive care?
3. What would you personally do to address the needs of this patient?
4. What resources do you need and how would you obtain them?
5. What cultural assessment model would you plan to use to assess this patient?

Responses to Self-Reflection Questions

Response: Where are you on the Cultural Competency Staircase regarding this patient's language and culture? How will you progress to the next level?

Finding your place on the Cultural Competency Staircase enables you to determine your readiness for caring for this patient. Wherever you find yourself, it is important to think of ways to progress up the staircase. Is it knowledge of the culture you lack, or the ability to communicate in the language? In this chapter, we examined strategies for communicating with individuals who speak languages other than English. Which of these strategies can you apply here? Do you need an interpreter?

Response: What knowledge do you need to have about this patient, including cultural/ language needs, to provide this patient with culturally sensitive care?

A good question to ask yourself in this situation is, "What do I know about the specific Hispanic culture represented in this case scenario?" Although many texts offer information generally about Latinos/Hispanics, you really want to identify relevant information about

Puerto Ricans and provide specific information about this cultural group. Texts by Purnell and Fenkl (2021), among others, reminds us that there is diversity among members of this group. For example, many Puerto Ricans are Catholic, but there are also many Protestants among the group. Puerto Ricans vary in their level of education and socioeconomic status. Some are highly educated, while some others may be illiterate both in English and in Spanish. Through the patient, her family, and an interpreter, you can gain insight into the patient's cultural attitudes and beliefs, dietary preferences, spirituality needs, and health beliefs.

Response: What would you personally do to address the needs of this patient?

Because of the emergent medical problem, it is important for the nurse to have some general medical information about this patient immediately. Calling the family and attempting to speak with someone who can give information about the onset of Mrs. Garcia's symptoms and precipitating factors is important. We know that Mrs. Garcia's daughter is an adult and can speak English fluently. Whether you are able to speak Spanish or not, there are some verbal and nonverbal ways to communicate with this patient. Emphasis should be placed on reducing this patient's anxiety through the nurse's verbal and nonverbal communication of support. Using phrase cards or other visual devices that enable the nurse to communicate caring to the patient is important.

Response: What resources do you need and how would you obtain them?

If the daughter is available, she may be an age-appropriate alternative when the interpreter is not available. Because the patient is experiencing a medical crisis, it is critical to contact either the daughter or the interpreter at home to provide this service for the patient. The environmental services person is of least effectiveness in this situation, because of the medical knowledge limitations and potential for breaching the patient's confidentiality and privacy rights.

Response: What cultural assessment model would you plan to use to assess this patient?

It is important to select a model that can be quickly applied in this situation. The LEARN model is one of several that seems appropriate here. Remember, the acronym stands for *listen, explain, acknowledge, recommend,* and *negotiate.*

The nurses *listen* with sympathetic ears to the patient and the interpreter and then *explain* their perceptions of what the patient is saying, in this case through an interpreter, while always facing and addressing the patient. This process is also referred to as reflective or active listening. During interviews with Mrs. Garcia, the nurse restates and/or clarifies information, always responding with acceptance and empathy to what Mrs. Garcia says. (See Chapter 2 for the discussion on the LEARN model and more information about active listening at www.analytictech.com/mb119/reflecti.htm.) The nurses in this case should attempt to identify the differences and similarities in perceptions between the patient and her family and the medical staff, as they *recommend* appropriate treatment. After the nurse and the other healthcare providers finally *negotiate* the treatment plan with the patient, they should offer her clinical options based on the patient's values and goals for care.

NCLEX®-TYPE QUESTIONS

1. The culturally competent nurse recognizes that the consequences of misunderstandings between the nurse and linguistically diverse patients are most likely to result in which of the following? *Select all that apply.*
    A. Misdiagnosis
    B. Suboptimal pain management

C. Reduction in the cost of care
D. Poor patient satisfaction
E. Enhanced treatment of chronic care

2. When delivering cross-linguistic nursing (CLN), to ensure evidence-based practice, the nurse reviews the literature on cultural competency and finds which of the following statements is accurate about language differences between nurses and their patients? Language differences between patients and nurses often:
A. Perpetuate discrimination and compromise care
B. Impact doctors and nurses equally
C. Impact doctors more than nurses
D. Enhance nurse–patient interactions

3. What may be a potential outcome when the nurse uses informal or ad hoc translators such as family members or untrained hospital staff? *Select all that apply.*
A. It breaches patient confidentiality.
B. It ensures compliance with the Office of Minority Health.
C. It meets ethical standards.
D. It is intrusive of patient privacy rights.

4. The nurse admits Mr. Smith, a member of the Cherokee Tribe, to the unit. When preparing to conduct the initial nursing interview and assessment, the nurse considers that Mr. Smith's cultural heritage suggests that his language is most likely to be:
A. Low context
B. High context
C. Nonverbal
D. Mid-context

5. The nurse complains to his charge nurse that one of his patients is threatening and intimidating because of his loud and forceful tone of voice. The culturally competent charge nurse recognizes that this behavior most likely reflects this patient's:
A. Cultural beliefs
B. Linguistic style
C. Language context
D. Cultural language

6. When the nurse plans cross-linguistic care for her newly admitted patient, she is most concerned by patient behaviors that suggest differences in:
A. Linguistic style
B. Language context
C. Literacy
D. Cultural attitudes

7. When language diversity is first suspected, the initial response by the nurse should be to:
A. Provide an interpreter
B. Notify the physician of this concern
C. Determine the patient's primary language and their ability to speak and read it
D. Conduct a full cultural assessment

8. A female patient who is unable to speak English is discovered by the nurse crying alone in her room. What *initial* action by the nurse is most appropriate?
A. The nurse goes to contact the family before entering the room.
B. The nurse approaches the patient smiling and offers the patient tissues.
C. The nurse contacts an interpreter.
D. The nurse speaks in English and tells the patient that everything will be all right.

9. The nurses on a medical–surgical unit are offered an opportunity to take a night course in Spanish for healthcare personnel. One nurse refuses to take the course because she believes that this action by the nurses would discourage Spanish-speaking patients from appreciating the importance of learning and speaking English. This way of thinking is based on:
   A. Myths about language diversity
   B. Evidence-based practice
   C. Cultural sensitivity
   D. Linguistic diversity

10. The interpreter arrives on the unit to see Mr. Nam, a Vietnamese patient. The nurse's initial action before beginning the interpreting session is to:
    A. Discuss the clinical situation and goals of the interview with the interpreter
    B. Introduce the patient and interpreter
    C. Provide a list of questions to ask the patient
    D. Allow the interpreter an opportunity to determine how the interview should be conducted

ANSWERS TO NCLEX-TYPE QUESTIONS

1. A, B, and D
2. A
3. A and D
4. B

5. B
6. C
7. C
8. B

9. A
10. A

AMERICAN ASSOCIATION OF COLLEGES OF NURSING COMPETENCIES ADDRESSED IN THIS CHAPTER

1. Apply knowledge of social and cultural factors that affect nursing and healthcare across multiple contexts.
2. Use relevant data sources and best evidence in providing culturally competent care.
3. Promote achievement of safe and quality outcomes of care for diverse populations.
4. Advocate for social justice, including commitment to the health of vulnerable populations and the elimination of healthcare disparities (based on the application of nursing ethics as it relates to culturally linguistic nursing care).
5. Participate in continuous cultural competence development.

A robust set of instructor resources designed to supplement this text is located at http://connect.springerpub.com/content/book/978-0-8261-8302-6. Qualifying instructors may request access by emailing textbook@springerpub.com.

REFERENCES

Alpern, J., Davey, C. S., & Song, J. (2016). Perceived barriers to success for resident physicians interested in migrant and refugee health. *Bio-medical Central Health Services Research, 16,* 178. https://doi.org/10.1186/s12909-016-0696-z

American Academy of Pediatrics. (2021, May 3). *Addressing low health literacy and limited English proficiency.* https://www.aap.org/en/practice-management/providing-patient--and-family-centered-care/addressing-low-health-literacy-and-limited-english-proficiency

Andrews, M. M., & Boyle, J. S. (2012). *Transcultural concepts in nursing care* (6th ed.). Lippincott Williams & Wilkins.

Betancur, S., Walton, A. L., Smith-Miller, C., Wiesen, C., & Bryant, A. L. (2020). Cultural awareness: Ensuring high quality for limited English proficient patients. *Clinical Journal of Oncology Nursing, 24*(5), 530–537. https://doi.org/10.1188/20.CJON.530-537

Bialik, K., Scheller, A., & Walker, K. (2018, October 25). *6 Facts about English language learners in U.S. public schools.* Pew Research Center. https://www.pewresearch.org/short-reads/2018/10/25/6-facts-about-english-language-learners-in-u-s-public-schools

Britannica. (2023). *Language: Meaning and style.* https://www.britannica.com/topic/language/Meaning-and-style-in-language

Campo, S., Kohler, C., Askelson, N. M., Ortiz, C., & Losch, M. (2015). It isn't all about language: Communication barriers for Latinas using contraceptives. *Journal of Transcultural Nursing, 26*(5), 466–472. https://doi.org/10.1177/1043659614524784

DeWilde, C., & Burton, W. (2017). Cultural distress: An emerging paradigm. *Journal of Transcultural Nursing, 28*(4), 334–341. https://doi.org/10.1177/1043659616682594

Dietrich, S., & Hernandez, E. (2022, December 6). *Nearly 68 million people spoke a language other than English at home in 2019.* U.S. Census Bureau. https://www.census.gov/library/stories/2022/12/languages-we-speak-in-united-states.html

Engle, J. (2019, March 29). How important is knowing a foreign language? *The New York Times.* https://www.nytimes.com/2019/03/29/learning/how-important-is-knowing-a-foreign-language.html

Friedman, A. (2015). America's lacking language skills. *The Atlantic.* https://www.theatlantic.com/education/archive/2015/05/filling-americas-language-education-potholes/392876

Habib, T., Nair, A., Von Pressentin, K., Kaswa, R., & Saeed, H. (2023). Do not lose your patient in translation: Using interpreters effectively in primary care. *South African Family Practice, 65*(1), e1–e5. https://doi.org/10.4102/safp.v65i1.5655

Hu, P. (2018). Language barriers: How professional interpreters can enhance patient care. *Radiologic Technology, 89*(4), 409–412.

Hunter-Adams, J., & Rother, H. A. (2017). A qualitative study of language barriers between South African health care providers and cross-border migrants. *Bio-Med Central Health Services Research, 17*(1), 1–9. https://doi.org/10.1186/s12913-017-2042-5

Karliner, L. S. (2018). *When patients and providers speak different languages.* Agency for Healthcare Research and Quality (AHRQ). https://psnet.ahrq.gov/web-mm/when-patients-and-providers-speak-different-languages

Lindholm, M., Hargraves, J. L., Ferguson, W. J., & Reed, G. (2012). Professional language interpretation and inpatient length of stay and readmission rates. *Journal of General Internal Medicine, 27*(10), 1294–1299. https://doi.org/10.1007/s11606-012-2041-5

Lopez-Bushnell, F. K., Guerra-Sandoval, G., Schutzman, E. Z., Langsjoen, J., & Villalobos, N. E. (2020). Increasing communication with healthcare providers for patients with limited English proficiency through interpreter language services education. *MedSurg Nursing, 29*(2), 89–95. https://www.thefreelibrary.com/Increasing+Communication+with+Healthcare+Providers+for+Patients+with...-a0641362810

Meuter, R. F., Gallois, C., Segalowitz, N. S., Ryder, A. G., & Hocking, J. (2015). Overcoming language barriers in healthcare: A protocol for investigating safe and effective communication when patients or clinicians use a second language. *Bio-Med Central Health Services Research, 15,* 371. https://doi.org/10.1186/s12913-015-1024-8

Milincic, A. (2020). Differences in high context and low context communication style. *LinkedIn.* Accessed at https://www.linkedin.com/pulse/differences-high-context-low-context-communication-styles-milincic

Montie, M., Galinato, G., Patak, L., & Titler, M. (2016). Spanish-speaking limited English proficiency patients and call light use. . *Hispanic Health Care International, 14*(2), 65–72. https://doi.org/10.1177/1540415316645919

Papadis, M., Sander, A. M., Struchen, M. A., & Kurtz, D. M. (2022). Soy differente: A qualitative study on the perception of recovery following traumatic brain injury among Spanish-speaking U.S. immigrants. *Disability and Rehabilitation, 44*(11), 2400–2409. https://doi.org10.1080/09638288.2020.1836045

Passel, J. S., & Cohn, D. (2019, May 23). *U.S. unauthorized immigrants are more proficient in English, more educated than decades ago.* Pew Research Center. https://www.pewresearch.org/short-reads/2019/05/23/u-s-undocumented-immigrants-are-more-proficient-in-english-more-educated-than-a-decade-ago

Primavera, J. (2017, April 5). Americans need to learn another language. *Massachusetts Daily Collegian.* https://dailycollegian.com/2017/04/americans-need-to-learn-foreign-languages

Pew Research Center (2022). *How Asian immigrants receive help while navigating language barriers.* https://www.pewresearch.org/race-ethnicity/2022/12/19/how-asian-immigrants-receive-help-while-navigating-language-barriers/

Purnell, L. (2013). *Transcultural health care: A culturally competent approach* (4th ed.). F. A. Davis.

Purnell, L., & Fenkl, E. A. (2021). *Textbook for transcultural health care: A population approach. Cultural competence concepts in nursing care* (5th ed.). Springer Publishing Company. https://doi.org/10.1007/978-3-030-51399-3

Sobel, L. L., & Metzler Sawin, E. (2016). Guiding the process of culturally competent care with Hispanic patients: A grounded theory study. *Journal of Transcultural Nursing, 27*(3), 226–232. https://doi.org/10.1177/1043659614558452

Sonoda, K., Takedai, T., & Salter, C. (2022). Communication sheet eases barriers for Japanese patients and health professionals. *BMC Health Services Research, 22,* 976. https://doi.org/10.1186/s12913-022-08371-x

Squires, A., Milner, S., Liang, E., Lor, M., Ma, C., & Witkoski Stimpfel, A. (2019). How language barriers influence provider workload for home health care professionals: A secondary analysis of interview data. *International Journal of Nursing Studies, 99,* 103394. https://doi.org/10.1016/j.ijnurstu.2019.103394

Trube, C. L., & Yeo, T. P. (2023). Patients with limited English proficiency: A challenge for oncology nursing providers. *Clinical Journal of Oncology Nursing, 27*(2), 147–153. https://doi.org/10.1188/23.CJON.147-153

U.S. Department of Health and Human Services: Office of Minority Health. (2013). *National Standards for Culturally and Linguistically Appropriate Services in Health and Health Care: A blueprint for advancing and sustaining CLAS policy and practice.* https://thinkculturalhealth.hhs.gov/assets/pdfs/enhancedclasstandardsblueprint.pdf

IMPORTANT WEBSITES

Agency for Healthcare Leadership (AHRQ): Retrieved from www.ahrq.gov/sites/
default/files/wysiwyg/professionals/systems/hospital/lepguide/lepguide.pdf

Do You Speak American? Retrieved from www.pbs.org/speak/education/curriculum/
college/style

Guide to Developing a Language Access Plan: Retrieved from https://www.cms.gov/
About-CMS/Agency-Information/OMH/Downloads/Language-Access-Plan-508.pdf

LEP.gov: Retrieved from https://www.lep.gov/faq/faqs-rights-lep-individuals/
commonly-asked-questions-and-answers-regarding-limited-english

The National CLAS Standards. Fact Sheet. Retrieved from https://health.wyo.gov/
wp-content/uploads/2016/02/43-17343_NationalCLASStandardsFactSheet.pdf

Practicing Medical Spanish: Retrieved from www.practicingspanish.com

7

Culturally Competent Care for the Older Adult

Gloria Kersey-Matusiak

I've learned from experience that the greater part of our happiness or misery depends on our disposition, not our circumstances.

—MARTHA WASHINGTON

LEARNING OBJECTIVES

After this chapter, the reader will be able to

1. Explain the rationale behind considering older adults in the United States as members of a vulnerable population in society.
2. State the age categories used to describe the older adult in the United States.
3. Explore the process of aging as it relates to the Erikson stages of psychosocial development.
4. Describe the cultural, geographical, and socioeconomic profile of American older adults.
5. Examine the various U.S. perspectives on aging and their impact on older adults.
6. Discuss the common health problems associated with aging in the United States.
7. Identify issues of death and dying as they relate to older adults.
8. State the factors impacting health and quality of life in the older adult.
9. Determine strategies for providing culturally competent care to older adults.

KEY TERMS

Black, Indigenous, People of Color (BIPOC)

Erikson's stages of psychosocial development

Integrity versus despair

Frail older adult

INTRODUCTION

Older adults over age 65 represent 16.8% of the U.S. population or 55.8 million people (Caplan, 2023). It is also the one group to which all Americans and citizens of the world, if fortunate, may one day belong. Yet, this collective of diverse individuals is often looked upon as monolithic, maligned and depicted in negative ways, frequently targeted by social media, victimized by ageism in the workplace, and must endure a variety of myths about the impact of aging. As Bergeron and Lagace (2021) observed, reactions to ageism and discrimination by the older adult may also be culturally dependent. Additionally, findings from the 2021 International Health

Policy Survey of Older Adults revealed that "more older adults in the United States have suffered from economic hardship during the COVID-19 pandemic compared with their counterparts in other high-income countries" and those with chronic conditions were more likely to have appointments cancelled or postponed (Williams et al., 2021, "Toplines"). Consequently, older adults more than other age categories had a higher morbidity or succumbed to COVID-19. These facts were especially true for **Black, Indigenous, and People of Color (BIPOC)**. For these reasons, the older adult is included here in this edition of the text to place them rightfully among the other most vulnerable in our society, to separate truth from fiction, and to discover ways to ensure equitable and culturally competent care to our most senior Americans.

Profile of the Older Adult

Like other groups described in this text, there is much diversity between and within categories of individuals we call "older adults." These individuals can be classified as young-older adults (age 55–74) or old-older adults (75 and older). In 2022 in the United States, there were 97,104 people who were over 100 years of age (Fitzgerald, 2022). As people are living longer, some categorize older adults as being young-old adults (65–74), middle older adults (75–84), and oldest older adults (85 and older). Since these age categories do not consider one's level of functioning, older adults vary in their physical, emotional, and cognitive health.

In 2020, individuals who reached age 65 had an average life expectancy of an additional 18.5 years (19 years for women and 17 for men; Administration for Community Living [ACL], 2020).

Older adults include individuals from all races, socioeconomic classes, and genders. Among the 55.6 million people living in the United States who are over age 65, 30.8 million are women and 24.8 are men. Of those over age 65, 60% lived with a spouse, while 27% lived alone. In 2020, 51% of Americans age 65 lived in nine U.S. states: California, Florida, Texas, New York, Pennsylvania, Ohio, Illinois, North Carolina, and Michigan (ACL, 2022; see Chart 7.1).

The median income for older persons in that age 65 group in 2020 was $26,668 ($35,808 for men and $21,245 for women). The median household income for homeowners age 75 and older was $36,200 in 2019. In 2020, about 1.1 million people aged 60 or older were responsible for the basic needs of at least one grandchild under 18 who was living with them. In 2021, 10.6 million Americans age 65+ were actively working or seeking employment while 16% of those in that age group lived below poverty (ACL, 2022).

In 2020, 24% of persons age 65 and older were members of racial or ethnic minority populations—9% were African American (not Hispanic), 5% were Asian American (not Hispanic), 0.6% were American Indian and Alaska Native (not Hispanic), 0.1% were Native Hawaiian/Pacific Islander (not Hispanic), and 0.8% of persons age 65 and older identified

CHART 7.1 ■ GEOGRAPHIC DISTRIBUTION OF OLDER ADULTS IN THE UNITED STATES

STATE	NUMBER OF OLDER ADULTS
California	6 million
Florida	4.6 million
Texas	3.9 million
New York	3.4 million
Pennsylvania	2.4 million
Ohio	2.1 million
Illinois	2.1 million
North Carolina	1.8 million
Michigan	1.8 million

Source: The Administration for Community Living. (2020). *2020 profile of Hispanic Americans age 65 and older.* https://acl.gov/sites/default/files/Profile%20of%20OA/HispanicProfileReport2021.pdf

themselves as being of two or more races. Persons of Hispanic origin represented 9% of the older adult population (ACL, 2022).

Health Among Older Americans: Integrity Versus Despair

Psychologists, counselors, and nurses today use the Erikson stage theory of psychosocial development when planning care for older adults; therefore, it is helpful to review his theory and its application to the older adult (Cherry, 2023). According to Erikson, the eighth and final stage of human development that occurs between ages 65 and death involves resolving the conflict or crisis he describes as **integrity versus despair**. The primary conflict or dilemma at this stage is answering the question of whether one has led a meaningful, satisfying life. Erikson believed that most people experience a balance between integrity and despair rather than completely accept one belief versus the other about themselves. One's decision to feel integrity versus despair is based on many factors, such as feeling a sense of accomplishment in one's life's work and/or achievements, having a supportive network of family and friends, and feeling that one has contributed to society through their work or children. On the other hand, individuals feeling a lack of these things and/or feelings of regret over past mistakes, decreased life satisfaction, increased depressive mood, sadness, and bitterness can ultimately lead to despair (Cherry, 2023). According to Erikson, individuals who are able to successfully resolve this crisis of integrity versus despair gain ego integrity, wisdom, peace and fulfillment, a general satisfaction, and even an acceptance when confronting death.

Several studies have examined factors contributing to health and quality of life among older adults (Emiliussen et al., 2023; Kurnat-Thoma et al., 2022; Luo et al., 2020, 2021). There is no question that people who reach age 65 and beyond often face a variety of health challenges that include cognitive, visual, and mobility problems that threaten their ability to perform activities of daily living (ADLs) in a way that they were used to at younger ages. However, many older adults have been able to overcome these challenges through good medical care, exercise, and a healthy diet. For example, Clark and colleagues (2018) in a study of community-dwelling older women aged 70 to 80 years at baseline found that higher levels of physical exercise modified risks of incident impairment in executive function over a 9-year period. Therefore, in this study, greater levels of caloric expenditure were associated with better executive function. The researchers in this study cited an earlier study of older men who completed 150 minutes of vigorous physical activity per week and were more likely to remain free of mood, cognitive, or functional impairments after 10 to 13 years compared with those who did not complete as much physical activity.

According to Allison and colleagues (2021, p. 219), "frailty is a state of increased vulnerability across multiple health domains that leads to adverse health outcomes." It is a geriatric syndrome, not a normal aspect of aging, affecting 5% to 17% of older adults and placing them at risk for falls, disabilities, hospitalizations, and death. Symptoms of frailty include generalized weakness, exhaustion, slow gait, poor balance, decreased physical activity, cognitive impairment, and weight loss. Researchers in this study note that there are a variety of validated assessment tools to screen for this syndrome in older adults, who are then diagnosed as not-frail, prefrail, or frail. Frail patients are at higher risk for poor health outcomes (Verghese et al., 2021).

Kurnat-Thoma and colleagues (2022), in a study of 5,553 older adults older than 60 years of age in a cross-sectional National Health and Nutrition Examination Survey (NHANES) study, found 482 participants (9%) were frail, and 2,432 (44%) were prefrail. In this study, the four factors highly associated with frailty were difficulty with one or more ADLs (77%), having two or more hospitalizations in the previous year (17%), having two comorbidities (27%), and polypharmacy (66%). The researchers recommended that nurses utilize a rapid assessment of frailty in low resource settings to streamline nursing care coordination and facilitate targeted frailty interventions to support healthy aging in vulnerable populations (Kurnat-Thoma et al., 2022). The findings in this study affirm past research, and as the researchers stated, frailty and prefrailty in North America in community dwelling adults older than age 65 is estimated at 15% and 45%, respectively. The authors also identified a higher prevalence of frailty in female participants, which was attributed to decreased lean muscle mass and muscle strength compared to men. Study results also revealed significant differences in frailty and prefrailty by race and ethnicity. Frailty rates were as follows: Whites (9.9%), non-Hispanic Blacks (9.1%), non-Black Hispanics (7.3%), and Asians (4.2%). Prefrailty rates were highest in non-Hispanic Blacks (47.9%).

Perceptions on Aging and Quality of Life in the United States

The literature reveals various perspectives on aging in the United States, however, many take a negative posture toward growing older (Makita et al., 2021). In a study of college students' perceptions of "old people" compared to "grandparents," Newsham and colleagues (2021) acknowledged that college students frequently hold negative or ambivalent views of aging and older adults. However, these attitudes toward older adults in general differed from their perceptions of grandparents, who were viewed more positively. Reasons cited for the negative perceptions of older adults reflected limited time spent with older adults and inaccurate portrayals of older adults in TV shows, commercials, magazines, and other media forms. There is also much negativity about aging and older people on social media. The researchers in this study suggest that the lack of time with older adults leads to "othering," or viewing aging "as foreign and only happening to other people" (p. 64). The combined impact of having limited exposure to older adults and inaccurate media portrayals leads to ageism, a bias against people who are older. Having positive interactions with older adults early in life can help mitigate the effects of ageism and stereotyping of older adults. Findings from this study indicate that college students more "frequently associate emotional (typically positive) and personality-related terms with grandparents, while associating medical and physical descriptors with older people in general" (p. 67).

Lu and colleagues (2020) explored the relationship between concepts of self-perceptions of aging (SPA) and control of life (COL) over a 9-year period in a health and retirement study. In this study, researchers found that older adults' SPA are associated with aging outcomes such as physical functioning, cognitive performance, psychologic well-being, and health behavior. The more negatively older adults viewed aging predicted decreases in their attitudes about their COL 4 years later. Another study examined how SPA affected one's spouse's self-perception and its influence on the health of husbands and wives. In this study, researchers found that intimate relationships influence the health of each partner. Specifically, "wife's SPA have an evident influence on her husband's physical health, and husband's SPA have a clear influence on his wife's mental health" (Luo et al., 2020, p. 163).

Emiliussen and colleagues compared life quality perceptions among residents, care workers, relatives, and managers in care homes. They found differences in perceptions about life quality between these four groups that may lead to disagreements and potential conflicts. They also warned against considering older adults as one homogeneous group, since older adults hold diverse and sometimes conflicting ideas on quality of life. In this study, residents found it difficult to say what life quality and a good life are indicating, and that present life quality partly relies on past and present experiences and interpretations of the past. "Being satisfied, expressing 'I can't complain,' were viewed as indications of having had a "good life" (Emiliussen et al., 2023, p. 34). The researchers concluded that "a good life" has to do with autonomy (or agency), the ability to move, and having something to do (tasks). In this study, all four groups focused on activity as a reflection of quality of life.

The researchers also observed that older people living in nursing homes score higher on depression, hopelessness, and suicidal ideation than those living in the community. To address this phenomenon, the researchers encourage nursing care actions based on establishing close relationships with residents regarding their integrity and enabling "at-homeness" as a way of mediating their well-being. Care workers are encouraged to balance their own values on good health and healthcare while incorporating residents' and relatives' values in the provision of individualized care to residents.

Perceptions of Death and Dying Among Older Adults

Older adults vary in their attitudes about death and dying. Stibich (2022), Tjernberg and Bökberg (2020), Sjöberg and colleagues (2018), and Österlind and colleagues (2017) examined older adults' experiences in nursing home facilities and their attitudes toward death and dying. Although there are some shared feelings about death and dying among human beings, the way one feels about the process when it is happening to a loved one or to oneself is unique and informed by one's values, beliefs, and experiences over a lifetime. Also, the stages of grief identified by Kubler Ross in 1969 (denial, anger, bargaining, depression, and acceptance) are not always followed in the same order, intensity, or duration. These emotions may also be revisited, but are generally thought of as those that someone contemplating death will usually experience (Stibich, 2022).

The older adult who is anticipating an imminent death may fear the potential for pain and suffering. Tjernberg and Bökberg interviewed 36 older persons living in a nursing home about their thoughts about death, dying, and the future. Their analysis revealed three main themes: the *unavoidable and unknown end of life, thoughts on control*, and *living the last part of your life in a nursing home.* The older persons in this study did not fear death; rather, they viewed it as a natural and inevitable part of life, but did worry about the dying process, particularly whether they would experience pain, adequate pain relief, and whether the death would be long and protracted (Tjernberg & Bökberg, 2020). Most residents expressed feelings regarding living in the nursing home as being boring, feeling isolated, being lonely, and lacking stimulation.

Further, residents who were cognitively healthy believed that individuals who were cognitively impaired did not belong there, since they required more care and there would not be enough time to care for those with dementia and manage the care needs of the others. Thoughts of control were linked to older people's association with aging and different kinds of losses, mainly loss of function and independence. These feelings were a source of frustration for the respondents. Several residents expressed a wish to remain healthy until the end of their lives.

In another study of nursing home residents, Osterlind and colleagues (2017) identified three themes: waiting for death (death as a release), subordinating oneself to values and norms of the staff (feeling offended and trapped), and keeping courage up. The older people in this study characterized their lives as being alone in an unfamiliar place where they encountered loneliness without opportunities to discuss their thoughts of life and death, including preparations for their passing. The researchers emphasized the need for professionals to respect older adults as human beings in their transition, before, during, and after they move to a nursing home.

Caregivers were also encouraged to develop strategies to support the maintenance of older adults' identity and well-being at the end of life. In a similar study, Sjöberg and colleagues studied the meaning of existential loneliness in 23 people who were 76 to 101 years old and living in long-term care. The researchers identified similar themes among **frail older adults** as in previous studies: being trapped in a frail and deteriorating body, indifference and feelings of having lives without meaning or purpose, and no one with whom to share their lives. The researchers concluded that health professionals should develop strategies to facilitate older adults' sense of connectedness and address their specific needs in vulnerable situations.

SUMMARY

Nurses who wish to provide culturally competent care to older adults must begin by carefully reflecting on their own values, attitudes, and beliefs about aging and issues that confront older adults at the end of life. Whether caring for 65-year-olds or those who reach 101, the nurse must meet the older adult wherever they are in their efforts to negotiate integrity versus despair. In clinical situations in the community, and in extended care facilities, nurses have an opportunity to facilitate the physical, emotional, and psychologic transitions that occur as one ages and approaches the end of life. Healthcare literature attests to the challenges many older adults experience including the loss of control, functioning, and independence, as well as feelings of loneliness and isolation. In some settings, older adults are met with indifference and an inability to share their thoughts about their life or feelings about death and dying with others. Often this is due to nurses' unwillingness or inability to broach these sensitive and anxiety-producing topics with older adult patients.

After first exploring their own attitudes and beliefs about aging, nurses can then assess their clients' needs for support. Being able to provide opportunities for patients to reminisce about positive and negative aspects of their past lives, to listen with empathy and compassion, to address spirituality needs, and to engage patients in activities that enrich their remaining life is critical, especially during the five stages of grief. Nurses should seek training that equips them with skills needed to accomplish these goals. With the increasing life expectancy and the rise in the number of older adults, this is an imperative for culturally competent care provision in the 21st century.

IMPORTANT POINTS

- Older adults age 65 or older represented nearly 17% of the U.S. population in 2022.
- The Erikson theory of human development states that the crisis adults who are 65 and older face is integrity versus despair.
- There are many myths and stereotypes about the older adult (e.g., they are all the same, they are all frail).
- Older adults are not a monolithic group and are represented by every racial and ethnic group in America with an age range from 65 to 100 and older.
- Older adults are sometimes classified as young older adults (age 55–74) and old older adults (age 75 and older).
- In 2022 in the United States, there were 97,104 people who were over 100 years of age.
- In 2020, individuals who reached age 65 had an average life expectancy of an additional 18.5 years, with 19 additional years for women and 17 for men.
- In 2020, 24% of persons age 65 and older were members of racial or ethnic minority groups: 9% were African Americans, 5% were Asian Americans, 0.6% were American Indians/Alaskan Natives, 0.1% were Native Hawaiians/Pacific Islanders, and 0.8% of persons identified as being of two or more races.
- Older adults often experience ageism in the workplace and the media.
- In 2021, 10.6 million adults over 65 were actively working or seeking employment, whereas 16% of older adults older than age 65 lived below poverty.
- COVID-19 resulted in higher morbidity and mortality rates for older adults than other age groups.
- Frailty is a state of increased vulnerability across multiple health domains that leads to adverse health outcomes. It is not a normal sign of aging.
- Perceptions about aging and death and dying vary among older adults.
- In 2020, 51% of Americans whow ere age 65 lived in nine U.S. states: California, Florida, Texas, New York, Pennsylvania, Ohio, Illinois, North Carolina, and Michigan.
- Many older adults express concerns about having feelings of loneliness, experiencing loss of life's purpose and meaning, being treated with indifference, and being unable to share their thoughts and feelings with others.
- The healthcare literature encourages nurses to seek training to prepare themselves to assist older adults in their transitions through the final stages of life by holding difficult conversations about patients' attitudes and beliefs about life, death, and dying.

CASE SCENARIO

Sally is an 80-year-old, African American, legally blind, retired schoolteacher who is accompanied by her fraternal twin sister, Evie, with whom she has lived for the past 10 years, since the death of Evie's husband. Sally sustained partial loss of her vision in an injury while she was a child. Evie has been Sally's primary caregiver, but she is no longer able to care for her at home. After several recent hospitalizations for congestive heart failure (CHF), Sally's condition has stabilized, but she remains a frail 80-year-old who is now being admitted to an extended care facility.

During her intake interview, Sally is alert and oriented but speaks very little in response to the nurse's questions; instead, Evie answers and supplements Sally's answers. She explains that she and Sally are the daughters of a physician and come from an upper middle-class background. She is a member of an elite international sorority. Sally taught anatomy and physiology basics at a local college preparatory high school for nearly 35 years and was beloved by her students and colleagues. After retiring, Sally worked as a volunteer until 6 months ago, when she developed CHF. She has offered financial support for community causes. Sally was still teaching general educational development (GED) courses on a part-time at a local prison facility when she became ill. Evie says proudly that Sally is also a poet; and recently, she and Evie self-published her book of poetry and donated the proceeds to their church. "Sally is usually quite talkative and vivacious, but she's just a little sad about leaving her home," Evie says.

On the following day, Betty, one of Sally's close friends, came to visit her. Before entering the room, she heard a woman screaming and calling out incoherently. On entering the double-occupancy room, she finds Sally lying in bed with tears streaming down her face, as she watched her roommate screaming for no apparent reason. Betty hugs Sally and reminds her of happier times spent together. They talk for a while about all Sally's great accomplishments as a leader in her teaching profession, her church, and of her many valued contributions to the community where she lives. While many of Sally's older friends have passed away, she still has many younger acquaintances who admire her. "Yes," Sally says, "but look at me now. I have always tried to educate myself and help educate others, but now I am living with someone who does not even know I'm alive, all she does is scream all day and all night."

WHAT NURSES NEED TO KNOW ABOUT THEMSELVES AND THE PATIENT

Application to Staircase Self-Assessment Model: Self-Reflection Questions

1. Where am I on the Cultural Competency Staircase? What actions can I take to progress?
2. What do I understand about older adults in Sally's age group and the diversity that exists between members of this population?
3. What assumptions or stereotypes do I hold about members of Sally's age group?
4. What do I know about Sally as an individual? What perceptions does she have regarding the crisis she is experiencing according to Erikson, integrity versus despair?
5. How do my attitudes and values regarding health, quality of life, and death and dying differ from Sally's?
6. How willing am I to identify ways to support Sally through this transition and ensure that she receives culturally competent care?
7. What strategies might be useful in addressing Sally's psychologic and emotional needs?

Responses to Self-Reflection Questions 2, 3, 4, 5, and 7

Response: What do I understand about older adults in Sally's age group and the diversity that exists between members of this population?

At 80, Sally belongs to the generation born between 1928 and 1945. At her age, she could be considered an oldest-older adult based on the classification one uses. The Pew Research Center refers to members of this group as the Silent Generation. In 2023, members of this group range from age 78 to 95. Besides belonging to this cohort, Sally is considered a frail, older adult, due to her comorbidities, frequent hospitalizations, and fall risk due to her partial blindness. Ethnically, Sally is an African American woman (only 9% of women over 65 were African Americans in 2020) and is highly educated (she holds a master's degree in biology; African Americans held 9.5% of all master's degrees in the United States in 2019). Sally has become a resident at an extended care community and, like many, is experiencing depression, loneliness, and isolation.

Response: What assumptions or stereotypes do I hold about members of Sally's age group?

What preassumptions, if any, have I made about Sally based on her age and her race? How do I reconcile the differences between what I believed and what I have learned about her as an individual?

How can I build a supportive, caring, and therapeutic rapport with her?

Response: What do I know about Sally as an individual? What perceptions does she have regarding the crisis she is experiencing according to Erikson, integrity versus. despair?

As an individual, Sally is an active member of her church. She still has many interests and friends with whom she was communicating until this admission to the care facility. Sally is civic-minded and has been generous in sharing her time volunteering to help others. Sally is partially blind but can still get around with assistance. Based on her physical assessment, Sally is without any cognitive impairments, but is considered frail, due to her comorbidities, frequent hospitalizations, and fall risk due to her partial blindness. As Sally's sister indicated, she is usually a vivacious, talkative person who enjoys being with others. However, she has been depressed since being transferred to the care facility. She has expressed feelings of loneliness and isolation in her present situation.

Response: How do my attitudes and values regarding health, quality of life, and; death and dying differ from Sally's?

Sally has been a very active octogenarian until now. She has valued being active in her church and community. She is aware of her current limitations and is struggling with having to change to a more sedentary lifestyle. As a nurse, consider your values regarding quality-of-life issues as compared to Sally's attitudes and beliefs

Response: What strategies might be useful in addressing Sally's psychologic and emotional needs?

Sally's psychologic and emotional needs would be enhanced by first placing her with a different roommate as soon as space is available. The patient with whom she shares a room has dementia and is unable to communicate with her. Sally may be experiencing sleep deprivation due to her roommate's screaming throughout the night. This is unfair to Sally and was probably done based on their similar ages without consideration of Sally's cognitive ability. In addition, the nurse can conduct a spiritual assessment to determine if Sally would like to see a clergyman from her congregation or involve herself remotely with her church. Many churches today offer services online. Does the care facility have a chapel where Sally can visit? Nurses can also encourage Sally to participate in any recreational activities at the facility that capitalize on Sally's talents and skills and incorporate her desire to assist others.

NCLEX®-TYPE QUESTIONS

1. According to the U.S. Department of Health and Human Services (DHHS), in 2020 older adults who reached age 65 had an average life expectancy of:
   A. An additional 10 years
   B. An additional 18.6 years
   C. 20 additional years
   D. 25 additional years

2. Which statement is true regarding the diversity among older adults? *Select all that apply.*
   A. All individuals who reach age 65 have more commonalities than differences.
   B. Women have a longer life expectancy after age 65 than men.
   C. The level of one's ability to function cognitively varies among older adults.
   D. There are more men over 65 in the United States than women.

3. What percent of older adults live below the poverty line?
   A. 16%
   B. 9%
   C. 25%
   D. 30%

4. In 2020, what percent of persons age 65 and older are members of racial minority groups?
   A. 24%
   B. 30%
   C. 35%
   D. 40%

5. The state with the highest number of older adults is:
   A. Florida
   B. California
   C. Texas
   D. New York
   E. Pennsylvania

6. What crisis does the Erikson theory of human development say older adults must resolve?
   A. Identity versus role confusion
   B. Generativity versus stagnation
   C. Industry versus inferiority
   D. Ego integrity versus despair

7. According to healthcare literature, what are the most common concerns for older adults over age 65? *Select all that apply.*
   A. Loneliness and isolation
   B. Fear of death
   C. Fear of pain during the dying process
   D. Inability to share thoughts and feelings with others

8. What percent of older adults living in the community are considered frail?
   A. 15%
   B. 20%
   C. 30%
   D. 40%

9. In 2020, what percent of the over 65 population represented African Americans?
   A. 7%
   B. 9%
   C. 12%
   D. 15%

10. According to the literature, nurses can ensure culturally competent care to older adults through which of these nursing actions? *Select all that apply.*
    A. Demonstrating respect and acceptance of older adults as unique individuals
    B. Primarily focusing on older adults' shared cultural values
    C. Providing an assessment of older adults' psychologic, emotional, and physical needs
    D. Considering the nurse's own attitudes about aging, death, and dying
    E. Integrating cultural and spiritual considerations in care planning

ANSWERS TO NCLEX-TYPE QUESTIONS

1. B
2. B and C
3. A
4. A

5. B
6. D
7. A, C, and D
8. A

9. B
10. A, C, D, and E

AMERICAN ASSOCIATION OF COLLEGES OF NURSING COMPETENCIES ADDRESSED IN THIS CHAPTER

1. Apply knowledge of social and cultural factors that affect nursing and healthcare across multiple contexts.
2. Use relevant data sources and best evidence in providing culturally competent care.
3. Promote achievement of safe and quality outcomes of care for diverse populations.
4. Advocate for social justice, including commitment to the health of vulnerable populations.

 A robust set of instructor resources designed to supplement this text is located at http://connect.springerpub.com/content/book/978-0-8261-8302-6. Qualifying instructors may request access by emailing textbook@springerpub.com.

REFERENCES

Administration for Community Living. (2020). *2020 profile of Hispanic Americans age 65 and older.* https://acl.gov/sites/default/files/Profile%20of%20OA/HispanicProfileReport2021.pdf

Administration of Community Living. (2022). Profile of older Americans. https://acl.gov/aging-and-disability-in-america/data-and-research/profile-older-americans

Allison, R., 2nd, Assadzandi, S., & Adelman, M. (2021). Frailty: Evaluation and management. *American Family Physician, 103*(4), 219–226. https://www.aafp.org/pubs/afp/issues/2021/0215/p219.html

Bergeron, C. D., & Lacace, M. (2021). On the meaning of aging and ageism: Why culture matters. *University of Toronto Quarterly, 90*(2), 140–154. https://doi.org/10.3138/utq.90.2.06

Caplan, Z. (2023, May 25). *U.S. older population grew from 2010 to 2020 at fastest rate since 1880 to 1890.* U.S. Census Bureau. https://www.census.gov/library/stories/2023/05/2020-census-united-states-older-population-grew.html

Cherry, K. (2023). *Integrity vs despair in psychosocial development.* verywellmind. https://www.verywellmind.com/integrity-versus-despair-2795738

Clark, J. L., Phoenix, S., Bibrrey, A. C., McManus, T., Escal, K. A., & Arulanantham, R. (2018). Cultural competency in dementia care: An African American case study. *Clinical Gerontologist, 43*(3), 255–260. https://doi.org/10.1080/07317115.2017.1420725

Emiliussen, J., Engelsen, S., Christiansen, R., & Klausen, S. H. (2023). The good life in care homes—a qualitative investigation with residents, relatives, care workers and managers. *Ageing International, 48*, 16–40. https://doi.org/10.1007/s12126-021-09438-6

Fitzgerald, M. (2022). These are the nations with the most people over 100. *U.S. News & World Report.* https://www.usnews.com/news/best-countries/articles/2022-07-15/nations-with-the-most-people-over-100

Kurnat-Thoma, E. L., Murray, M. T., & Juneau, P. (2022). Frailty and determinants of health among older adults in the United States 2011–2016. *Journal of Aging and Health, 34*(2), 233–244. https://doi.org/10.1177/08982643211040706

Luo, M. S., Li, L. W., & Chui, E. W. T. (2020). Self-perceptions of aging and control of life in late adulthood: Between-person and within-person associations. *Journal of Aging and Health, 32*(9), 1275–1281. https://doi.org/10.1177/0898264320917303

Luo, M. S., Li, L. W. & Hu, R. X. (2021). Self perceptions of aging and domain specific health outcomes among midlife and later-life couples. *Journal of Aging and Health, 33*(1–2), 155–166. https://doi.org/10.1177/0898264320966263

Makita, M., Mas-Bleda, A., Stuart, E., & Thewal, M. (2021). Ageing, old age and older adults: A social media analysis of dominant topics and discourses. *Ageing & Society, 41*(2), 247–272. https://doi.org/10.1017/S0144686X19001016

Newsham, T. M. K., Schuster, A. M., Guest, M. A., Nikzad-Terhune, K., & Rowles, G. D. (2021). College students' perceptions of "old people" compared to "grandparents." *Educational Gerontology, 47*(2), 63–71. https://doi.org/10.1080/03601277.2020.1856918

Österlind, J., Ternestedt, B. M., Hansebo, G., & Hellström, I. (2017). Feeling lonely in an unfamiliar place: Older people's experiences of life close to death in a nursing home. *International Journal of Older People Nursing, 12*(1), e12129. https://doi.org/10.1111/opn.12129

Sjöberg, M., Beck, I., Rasmussen, B. H., & Edberg, A. K. (2018). Being disconnected from life: Meanings of existential loneliness as narrated by frail older people. *Aging & Mental Health, 22*(10), 1357–1364. https://doi.org/10.1080/13607863.2017.1348481

Stibich, M. (2022). *How to deal with death as you age.* https://www.verywellmind.com/how-to-deal-with-death-and-dying-as-you-age-2223446

Tjernberg, J., & Bökberg, C. (2020). Older persons' thoughts about death and dying and their experiences of care in end-of-life: A qualitative study. *BMC Nursing, 19*(1), 123. https://doi.org/10.1186/s12912-020-00514-x

Verghese, J., Ayers, E., Sathyan, S., Lipton, R. B., Milman, S., & Barzilai, N., & Wang, C. (2021). Trajectories of frailty in aging: Prospective cohort study. *PLoS ONE, 16*(7), e0253976. https://doi.org/10.1371/journal.pone.0253976

Williams, R. D., II, Shah, A., Doty, M. M., Fields, K., & FitzGerald, M. (2021, September 15). *The impact of COVID-19 on older adults: Findings from the 2021 International Health Policy Survey of Older Adults.* The Commonwealth Fund. https://www.commonwealthfund.org/publications/surveys/2021/sep/impact-covid-19-older-adults

IMPORTANT WEBSITES

AARP. Retrieved from https://www.aarp.org/

Healthy People 2030. Retrieved from https://health.gov/healthypeople

National Center for Health Research. Retrieved from https://www.center4research.org

National Council on Aging. Retrieved from https://www.ncoa.org

National Institutes of Health. Retrieved from https://www.nih.gov

8

Cultural Considerations When Caring for the Patient Who Is Terminally Ill

Gloria Kersey-Matusiak

Let us touch the dying, the poor, the lonely, and the unwanted according to the graces we have received, and let us not be ashamed or slow to do the humble work.

—MOTHER TERESA

LEARNING OBJECTIVES

After this chapter, the reader will be able to
1. Examine beliefs about death and dying and their influence on care provision to members of culturally diverse groups.
2. Discuss variations in attitudes regarding advance directives, life support, disclosure of diagnosis, and the designation of decision-makers during terminal illness.
3. Identify variations in beliefs, practices, and traditions during death and dying experiences between culturally diverse groups.
4. Assess the psychologic, cultural, spiritual, and/or religious factors influencing the death-and-dying experience of members of culturally diverse groups.
5. Examine selected cultural practices related to the care of the body and burial after death.
6. Describe the impact of factors impacting the death and dying experience of patients with communicable diseases like COVID-19.
7. Analyze the role of the nurse in assisting culturally diverse patients during death, dying, and grieving experiences.

KEY TERMS

Acculturation

Advance directive

AID

Culture

Espiritista

Hospice

Life support

MAID

Palliative care

Quality of life

Terminal illness

LIFE EXPECTANCY IN THE UNITED STATES

In 2021, the Centers for Disease Control and Prevention's (CDC) National Center for Health Statistics reported U.S. life expectancy at 76.4 for both sexes, broken down further with 73.5 for men and 79.3 for women (Murphy et al., 2021). In 2023, the United Nations (UN) charted U.S. life expectancy at 79.11 years, a 0.08% increase from 2022. Despite these slight increases, the United States continues to be ranked at the bottom half of developed countries in life expectancy, behind many that are much poorer than the United States (Ingraham, 2017; Rakshit et al., 2022); even so, the United States remains a top spender regarding healthcare costs. In addition, "[s]ince 2015, the United States has seen an historic decline in life expectancy driven by first the opioid epidemic and then the COVID-19 pandemic" (Klobucista, 2022, para. 1). The decline in life expectancy affected racial and ethnic groups differently. For example, while Black and Hispanic Americans were hit harder during the first year of the pandemic, White Americans saw a sharper drop in 2021. In 2020 to 2021, among American Indian and Alaska Native communities, life expectancy was shortened by 2 years. Their life expectancy now is the same as the total U.S. population in 1944 (Klobucista, 2022). The United States also ranks lower among the groups in the Organization for Economic Cooperation and Development (OECD) regarding the share of people fully vaccinated. That low ranking has been driven by reluctance and resistance, caused by misinformation and political polarization (Klobucista, 2022; Ubel, 2018). Consequently, increases in death due to COVID-19 accounted for more than half of the decline in the life expectancy (CDC, n.d.-a).

Another problem that contributes to the lower life expectancy is the high rate of homicide due to the public's easy access to guns. Moreover, tobacco use, obesity, and violence are all included among factors that help explain the United States' lower ranking on life expectancy. Despite these sad facts, the proportion of the U.S. population older than age 65 is increasing. In the United States, approximately 16.8% of the population, or 55.8 million people, is older than 65 years of age (Caplan, 2023). For example, the Associated Press (AP, 2023) in a recent report, reminded us of the longevity and resilience of a former U.S. president, Jimmy Carter who now resides in a nursing home in hospice at age 99.

CAUSES OF DEATH

In the discussion of the terminally ill in this chapter, the author will generally focus on the age group 65 and older, recognizing that many adults will become diagnosed with terminal illnesses long before age 65. In a CDC chart for 2018 listing the 10 leading causes of death for people ages 54 to 64, the top 10 causes of death are similar, but with malignant neoplasms occupying the number one position in the 54 to 64 age group, followed by heart disease (CDC, n.d.-b; see also CDC Chart of Causes of Death by Age in the Important Websites section).

In 2020, the CDC listed the 10 leading causes of death in the United States among all races of people aged 64 to 85 years old (CDC, 2023). In descending order, they were heart disease, malignant neoplasms, COVID-19 (which replaced chronic lung diseases), cerebrovascular disease, Alzheimer disease, chronic low respiratory disease, diabetes mellitus, unintentional injuries, nephritis, influenza, and pneumonia.

Among older adults, chronic diseases, especially cardiovascular diseases, and cancer are the leading causes of death (lung cancer leads among cancer deaths), with chronic respiratory diseases like emphysema and chronic bronchitis, Alzheimer disease, renal diseases, and infectious diseases included among them. About 10% of individuals die from sudden, unexpected events such as a myocardial infarction (MI) or an accident.

While there has been a gradual decline in overall coronary mortality, sudden death from cardiac arrest has stayed fixed or actually increased as a percent of the total mortality. However, more than 90% of persons who are ill die from an extended life-threatening or chronic illness that includes a "relatively short terminal phase" (CDC, 2021; Vitas Healthcare, 2020). In 2018, when considering deaths from all causes, 35.1% occurred in a hospital; 26.8% in long-term care facilities, including **hospice** and nursing homes; and 31.4% in the decedent's home (CDC, 2020). The literature attests to the fact that most patients prefer to die at home (Spelten et al., 2019).

Preparing for End of Life

The time during which a **terminal illness** is identified or when death is anticipated by the patient and/or the family is a challenging time of great indecision for many caregivers and family members. Even when the patient's wishes have been previously discussed, it is difficult to have these conversations when someone is seriously ill. However, it is important to discuss these matters before the patient is unable to make end-of-life (EOL) decisions. Vitas Healthcare (n.d.) suggested that everyone should have an **advance directive**. Advance directives include living wills and a medical power of attorney (National Institute on Aging, 2018). These measures afford individuals opportunities to discuss with others the medical treatments they want near the EOL. Vitas observed that while 90% of people say talking with loved ones about EOL care is important, only 27% had done so. Additionally, only 26.3% of Americans report having an advance directive; 80% say that if they had a serious illness they would want to talk to their doctor about EOL care, but only 7% have actually had an EOL conversation with their doctor and only 25% of doctors knew that their patients had advance directives on file (Vitas Healthcare, 2016).

In America, a tension often exists between the battle to sustain life through technology and the legal right of the patient to refuse treatment or let nature take its course. Medical research suggests a "patient-centered approach" that goes beyond having advance directives, which direct the patient's treatment during the EOL. Instead, more in-depth communication between the healthcare providers and patients, especially patients and families, is recommended. During such encounters, doctors relinquish domination over the encounter and focus on the patient's psychosocial needs to promote a deeper understanding of what the patient wishes. Ideally, family members should be included in this exchange; however, confronting the impending death of a loved one may be emotionally challenging for all concerned. To ensure that patients who are dying receive care that enhances, rather than detracts, from their **quality of life**, the healthcare provider's and the patient's views about the care that should be provided must be congruent. At the EOL, nurses are the largest and most likely group of professionals to play a critical role in ensuring that the wishes and goal of patients are met.

THE ROLE OF THE NURSE

One of the most challenging roles of the nurse is caring for patients who are terminally ill. As the cultural diversity of the U.S. patient population increases, nurses caring for terminally ill patients face the added challenge of providing terminal care that meets their patients' specific cultural needs. As a result, nurses will need to become knowledgeable about the important cultural aspects of care to address during these experiences. Moreover, members of culturally diverse groups will vary in their preferences for aspects of nursing care and place a different emphasis on religion and/or spirituality during the process of death and dying.

That is why caring for a patient at the EOL is one of the most fulfilling yet challenging roles a nurse can perform. It is fulfilling to know that as a nurse you are assisting someone in the final and most difficult stage of their life. It is challenging emotionally because it is the inevitable stage we all must one day pass through, so when caring for patients at the EOL, nurses are confronted with their own mortality.

Whether the patient is cared for at home, in a nursing home, hospital, or hospice unit, the nurse caring for someone who is dying must meet the patient's needs in four areas: physical comfort, mental and emotional needs, spiritual needs, and practical tasks (National Institute on Aging, 2022). There are many factors that contribute to the patient's discomfort throughout a terminal illness, including pain, breathing problems, digestive problems, temperature sensitivity, or fatigue (National Institute on Aging, 2022). The nurse must monitor the patient carefully to detect signs of discomfort, as sometimes patients who are experiencing chronic pain are used to it and/or are unwilling or too tired to discuss it with their caregivers. Pain is easily managed by administering ordered medication like opiates; usually MSO4 is given because it has an added benefit of controlling shortness of breath as well. Other strategies to ease the work of breathing include repositioning to better facilitate the patient's breathing, checking the pulse oximetry to determine a need for oxygen, using a humidifier, opening a window, or providing a fan.

The ability of the nurse to effectively address the mental and emotional needs of a terminally ill patient depends on the nurse's willingness to examine their own beliefs and attitudes about death and dying. The literature tells us that nurses and other healthcare professionals at all levels of experience have expressed uneasiness about discussing death and dying experiences with patients (Figueiredo & Assis, 2023) because they feel unprepared to do so. Yet, the literature also reminds us that many patients at the EOL wish to have those discussions with a willing listener. Patients' emotions may range from sadness to depression, fear and anxiety, and grief in anticipation of multiple losses including their own sense of a loss of identity. At times, episodes of confusion at EOL can lead to deeper feelings of isolation and despair. At these times, there is much that nurses can do to alleviate some of these feelings.

Researchers suggest providing physical contact by holding hands or offering a gentle massage if this is culturally gender appropriate. Using soft lighting or playing music at a low volume can help some patients relax (National Institute on Aging, 2022). In a study of perceptions of terminally ill cancer patients about the quality of life in a hospice-based and home-based palliative care setting, researchers found that the provision of palliative care in both settings was viewed positively by participants in the domain of social and emotional dimensions. The respondents in this study were especially pleased with the "good communication practices by staff members . . . which were a great source of comfort to them" (Patel et al., 2023, p. 61). The doctors and nurses were sensitive, supportive, and compassionate, very kind and respectful.

Kastbom and colleagues (2017) interviewed 66 adult patients with cancer in the palliative care phase who were either at home or in the hospital to determine what EOL patients consider a "good death." Respondents indicated that a "good death" meant preparing for death and dying comfortably, and dying quickly, with independence, with minimized suffering, and with social contacts intact. The researchers concluded that healthcare staff caring for palliative care patients should consider asking them to describe what they consider a "good death" to determine goals of care because the term means different things to different patients.

What the patient values and how those values are prioritized during this phase of life can be determined through an appropriate cultural assessment by the nurse. That assessment should then be utilized in establishing mutually agreed-upon goals among the patient, the nurse, and all members of the healthcare team to provide care that optimally meets the needs of patients and their families during this significant period in their lives. Nurses can facilitate such encounters by creating an open, safe, and supportive space in which the conversation can take place (Vitas Healthcare, 2020). Attentive listening to enable the patient's voice to be heard is a critical element of this process to reduce the psychologic and spiritual distress of persons who are terminally ill.

The American Nurses Association's (ANA's) revised position statement on the RN's role at the end of a patient's life reminds nurses that "interaction between the RN and the patient occurs within the context of the values and beliefs of the patient and the nurse" (Stokes, 2019). The nurse's own cultural values, attitudes, and beliefs about death and dying often set the tone for assisting patients during this significant period in their lives.

However, the ANA encourages nurses to be "mindful of the patient's cultural and spiritual beliefs and to advocate for them without personal bias." To ensure the delivery of culturally sensitive care to individuals and families, nurses need to have an awareness of their own attitudes and beliefs about terminal illness and the process of death and dying. Having this knowledge enables nurses to consider potential differences between their own and their patient's view of appropriate care at the EOL. Gurdogan et al. (2019) found that reducing nursing students' death anxiety helped to increase their positive attitudes toward caring for dying patients. By focusing on what the patient and their families value, nurses avoid imposing their own cultural attitudes and beliefs during death and dying experiences. In 2017, the ANA in collaboration with the Hospice and Palliative Nurses Association (HPNA) partnered to issue a call for action: Nurses lead and transform palliative care by ensuring palliative care can be provided in any setting where care is needed.

Nurses can begin the process of planning EOL care for culturally diverse groups by first expanding their perspective about what **culture** means. In a study that examined dying in hospitals, the researchers warned nurses against limiting the concept of culture to refer only to ethnicity. Rather, they urged nurses to consider culture in its broadest sense and to view the patient and the family holistically and in "their total context." This means including gender identity, age, race, immigration status, social position, sexual orientation, and so on (CDC, n.d.-c). For example, Medline Plus (2023) offers information about health-related issues specifically impacting persons who are LGBTQIA. Additionally, the researchers encouraged nurses to include an examination of the culture of the healthcare setting as well as that of biomedicine when trying to explore the patient's healthcare context. Having this expanded view affords nurses an opportunity to consider factors within the healthcare setting that may influence EOL decision-making. From this perspective, nurses and doctors examine the entire context in which patients make EOL healthcare choices and gain a better understanding of why these choices are made.

Assessing the Healthcare Environment

When exploring a particular healthcare institution's capacity for delivering culturally appropriate EOL care, nurses and other healthcare providers can ask themselves several important questions. For example: Does the institution have available resources and personnel to effectively respond to the needs of culturally diverse terminally ill patients? Are there language or attitudinal barriers that might need to be addressed before the hospital or a particular group of staff members can perform a cultural assessment or provide information to patients in their own language? Are the patients who utilize the hospital services coming from communities of affluence or poverty that may impact their access to care? For example, Isaacson and Lynch (2018) studied palliative care options for American Indians and Alaskan Natives and found that indigenous populations experience higher rates of death than the dominant U.S. culture. Regarding biomedicine, are the doctors who are prescribing medicine mindful of some patients' use of herbal medicine or other folk practices that potentially interact with prescribed medications? Are the doctors also aware of variations among some ethnic groups in their responses to Western medicine? Acknowledging barriers to communication between patients and providers is the first step in finding ways to resolve them.

Barriers to End-of-Life Communication

Older people vary in their medical status, cognitive ability, views, and preferences.

Besides language barriers between healthcare professionals and patients who speak languages other than English in their homes (see Chapter 3), other factors create barriers that may interfere with effective communication during interactions between healthcare professionals and patients about EOL issues. For example, older patients with a terminal illness may also experience cognitive problems, confusion, or disorientation that disrupts their decision-making ability (Khizar & Harwood, 2017). "People face multiple obstacles when experiencing a life-limiting condition" (Miller, 2023, p. 78). Often, they have not yet clarified their own values and priorities around the death and dying experience when learning of a terminal diagnosis. Therefore, "the patient needs to feel safe enough to be vulnerable when discussing end-of-life care" (Miller, 2023, p. 78). Nurses can set the tone by providing quiet, private spaces in which to hold these discussions and eliminate distracting noises from phones and other devices, and conversations.

Vitas Healthcare (2020) identified barriers to talking about death for healthcare providers, but these communication skills can also be learned, practiced, and utilized by nurses and other health professionals within their scope of practice. Barriers identified include concern for how the patient will react, concern about the healthcare professional's own reaction, concern that the healthcare provider can't do enough, and anxiety about leading such discussions. Regarding the health professional's concerns about how the patient will react, nurses recognize that although patients express an interest in transparency and truth-telling from their doctors and nurses, it is sometimes met with emotional or physical displays based on the idea of the patient's loss of control, changing self-image, and loss of life. Although these situations are uncomfortable, the nurse can prepare for this kind of exchange by first reflecting on their own concerns, attitudes, and beliefs about death and dying. The nurse should keep in mind that the purpose of such interactions are to ascertain the goals and wishes patients have for their care. Second, seeking information from the patient about what they have learned from the physician and understand about the diagnosis and prognosis is a good place to begin any discussion. Third, the nurse accepts the patient's perspectives and feelings about their circumstances without judgment or imposing the nurse's own attitudes and beliefs. Throughout the interaction between the healthcare professional and the patient, the nurse demonstrates empathy, kindness, and compassion, and intermittently seeks permission to continue the conversation by asking if the patient wishes to continue the dialogue or postpone it to a later date, especially if the patient seems excessively stressed by the encounter.

Cultural Variations at End of Life

Variations exist between and among culturally diverse groups in their attitudes about aspects of death and dying, including disclosure of the diagnosis and its prognosis; advance directives; use of **life support**; beliefs, practices, and traditions around grief; care of the body after death; and burial procedures. Within-group variations are based on patients' cultural and demographic characteristics, level of **acculturation**, and knowledge of EOL treatment options. For this reason, it is critical that nurses not make assumptions or predictions about the care needs of individuals based on their knowledge of a particular cultural group. Despite having some knowledge of cultural tendencies among members of a particular group, the nurse confers with patients and their families to determine their specific preferences. When caring for patients at the EOL, nurses have both the privilege and responsibility of ensuring that the final goals and wishes of the patient are met. To ensure culturally competent care, nurses are expected to listen attentively; initiate honest, open, and compassionate discussions with families; and assess patients' psychosocial as well as physical symptoms to determine anxiety, depression, sense of loss, grief, feelings of isolation, and/or spiritual distress. At end of life nurses must focus on the provision of the best care possible for their patients under the circumstances (American Association of Critical Care Nurses [AACN], 2021).

Cain and McClesky (2019) discussed the process by which a patient with a terminal illness may request MAID (medical assistance in dying) or **AID (assistance in dying)**, which has become legal in eight jurisdictions in the United States and all of Canada. However, in 40 U.S. states, MAID is considered illegal. Cain and McClesky found variations across three racial and ethnic groups: African American, Latinx, and White Californians. Participants in this study also differed in their ideas about what constitutes a "good death." Several elements were common to Western ideals of a "good death": relief, acceptance, mending of familial and other relationships, and not being a burden to others. From healthcare providers' perspectives, good deaths also avoid unnecessary treatment that cause suffering, are timely, and do not involve conflict with families. The authors acknowledge that the meaning of a "good death" is a cultural construction, and neither good nor bad. One dominant message in palliative care is acceptance of death, which the authors say "deindividualizes, and does not consider diversity" (p. 1176). The dominant definition of "good death" is not for everyone. For some, the concept of acceptance of death is contrary to the value placed on instead fighting for one's life.

Many groups consider AID/MAID controversial, since AID permits persons expected to live to 6 months or less to request a prescription for medication to hasten death. According to the authors, in a Gallup poll in 2017, 73% of Americans supported doctors assisting someone with a terminal illness to end their life painlessly. However, public opinion is based on the way the issue is framed. Medical actions that let nature take its course are more widely accepted than actively taking one's own life. Lower rates of acceptance are based on religious and cultural views.

Opponents argue that for people who are already vulnerable because of their age, lack of resources, or marginalized social status, AID might be viewed as an obligation, which may be felt when interacting with providers asked to determine the value of life-saving interventions and within families when older dependent adults require more care (Cain & McClesky, 2019). There are also the concerns that racial and ethnic minorities might not receive the same quality of EOL care and will instead be encouraged to use AID or not be given information about its availability.

Nursing generally has its own set of goals for patients who are terminally ill. Such goals are based on American culture and traditions as well as the ethical standards that guide nursing practice. One example is the primary goal of **palliative care**, which is to prevent and relieve suffering and to support the best quality of life for patients and their families regardless of their stage of disease or need for other therapy (World Health Organization [WHO], 2020). However, there are times when nursing goals may differ from those of the patient. For example, nurses in the United States strive to maintain patients' autonomy in healthcare decision-making. Yet, some cultural groups do not wish the patient to know of the seriousness of a diagnosis and/or its prognosis. For example, Rising (2017) explored the concept of truth-telling as it relates to telling patients about a poor prognosis in terminal illnesses. The researcher discussed truth-telling based on cultural values and beliefs of Asian and Latin American cultural traditions as compared to U.S. or Western values. In Asian cultures, withholding a poor prognosis is based on the cultural principles and the beliefs of beneficence and nonmalfeasance that are linked to the Confucian emphasis on family harmony over the beliefs of an individual. "Similarly in Latin American traditions there is an emphasis on the role of family in protecting elders and providing a "benevolent deception" to prevent emotional or psychologic harm and loss of hope (Rising, 2017, p. 49). In both belief systems, the action of withholding truth is justified as an ethical decision based on these principles. In the United States, emphasis on truth-telling is based on the need to maintain patients' autonomy and self-determination. However, in cases where nurses find themselves in conflict when families request that information be withheld from the patient, they may experience serious moral distress. Based on this study, the researcher Rising (2017) concluded that nurses should consider the equal validity of truth-telling and withholding a prognosis, based on principles of beneficence and nonmalfeasance versus autonomy, to mitigate potential moral distress. In this article, Rising (2017) also reminded nurses of the intercultural variability of Asian and Latin American populations and suggested that focusing on beliefs of the individuals regardless of patients' background is most important. When caring for patients from diverse backgrounds at EOL, nurses are encouraged to first determine whether the patient has the capacity and desire to speak for themself, or has designated a surrogate to do so. If so, the nurse supports the decision of the patient and/or the patient's designee and acts accordingly.

The challenges of caring for the terminally ill are experienced by nurses and other healthcare providers around the world. Most importantly, in this effort nurses should strive to assist patients in finding personal meaning in the dying and death experiences. To enable nurses to sustain their ability to carry on the day-to-day tasks required of them during this challenging time in patients' lives, strategies like those mentioned earlier must be incorporated in their daily lives. In addition, maintaining one's own spiritual and physical well-being is an important aspect of this process if the nurse is to be effective in delivering culturally relevant care.

In hospice and palliative care settings, the nurse appreciates the need for psychologic and spiritual care and looks on the process of dying as a normal aspect of life. Nurses in other healthcare settings may also find themselves having to deliver care for patients who are dying. For example, Oak and Sun-Kim (2020) discussed the ICU as an important place where hospice and palliative care is provided. At such times, nurses should seek the guidance and expertise of these hospice and palliative nurse colleagues. Nurses who have a clear understanding of their patients' beliefs and attitudes about the death experience are better able to make each nurse–patient encounter meaningful from the patient's cultural perspective. The nurse has several opportunities to listen actively to determine what the patient wishes during the dying experience. This nursing behavior is particularly useful when significant others are not available to act as resources for the staff.

CULTURAL FACTORS AND SPIRITUALITY

The ability of patients who are dying to negotiate this often lonely and frightening final stage of their life is influenced by the cultural and spiritual values they hold. Research supports the idea that cultural factors play a major role in determining patients' decisions about EOL care (Abbasi et al., 2022; Anderson & De Souza, 2021; Townsend & Kimball, 2017).

Abbasi and colleagues (2022), in a thematic analysis of available studies in the literature, explained several dimensions of spiritual care. The researchers found that spiritual care includes various and numerous dimensions and identified 10 main themes related to spiritual care: (1) spiritual and religious assessment; (2) developing a structure for providing spiritual care; (3) establishing effective and supportive communication with the patient; (4) training the patient and answering questions; (5) encouraging, maintaining, and developing social communication; (6) encouraging the patient to live happily; (7) helping the patient achieve peace and relaxation; (8) supporting spiritual rituals and activities; (9) supporting and training the patient's family; and (10) supporting the dying patient (see Chart 8.1). The authors of this study concluded that effective and supportive communication is an essential component of spiritual care. They emphasized maintaining and reinforcing the spiritual beliefs of patients.

As Erikson's work suggests, at the EOL, people experience a final crisis of psychosocial identity characterized as ego integrity versus despair as they transition from terminal diagnosis to death. Self-identity is challenged by bereavement. Rituals enable people to transition through life crises like these. Prayers are a form of ritual that are used throughout life and at EOL. Although prayers may differ in form, practice, and behaviors, most EOL prayers have a common theme of focusing on acceptance of death and providing hope for the family and friends left behind (Anderson & De Souza, 2021). As Anderson and De Souza (2021) explained, the form prayer rituals take varies across cultures and religions, yet each provides comfort to patients and families at EOL. Some examples are the surrounding of family and friends who must stay through the final moments of life among those practicing Judaism, family and friends reciting various prayers from the Quran for persons practicing Islam, the recital of various mantras in the presence of family and friends for Hindus during separation rites, or meditation and chanting various scripture for followers of the Buddhist tradition.

CHART 8.1 ■ DIMENSIONS OF SPIRITUAL CARE.

SPIRITUAL DIMENSIONS
1. Spiritual and religious assessment
2. Developing a structure for providing spiritual care
3. Establishing effective and supportive communication
4. Training the patient and answering questions
5. Encouraging, maintaining, and developing social communication
6. Encouraging the patient to live happily
7. Helping the patient achieve peace and relaxation
8. Supporting spiritual rituals and activities
9. Supporting and training the patient's family
10. Supporting the dying patient

Source: Abbasi, M., Eskandari, N., Heidari, A., Heidari, M., Yoosefee, S., Adeli, S.-H., & Kazemi, A. (2022). A thematic analysis of dimensions of spiritual care. *Iranian Journal of Nursing and Midwifery Research, 27*(5), 452–460. https://www.ncbi.nlm.nih.gov/pmc/articles/PMC9745858

Townsend and Kimball (2017) discussed faith as it relates to acceptance of hospice services in the African American community. In this study, the researchers explored reasons why African Americans choose aggressive, curative medical treatments over hospice after a terminal medical diagnosis. Through a qualitative study using focus groups with 34 members of two African American churches, researchers identified six major themes. The top two themes were (a) lack of knowledge about hospice and (b) spirituality. The remaining themes identified in the study were (c) cultural competence, (d) hospice is synonymous with death and elicits fear of death, (e) hospice prepares families for death, and (f) hospice provides comfort and support for patients and families. Based on these findings, the researchers concluded that partnerships between hospices and African American churches to provide hospice education would benefit the African American community and increase the use of hospice services.

Within the realm of cultural considerations, the nurse examines the patient's spiritual needs. The Oncology Nursing Society (ONS) takes the position that sensitive and appropriate spiritual care issues are assessed and integrated into the nursing care plan to promote adequate coping for patients, families, and significant others. Yet, while patients with life-threatening illnesses believe that psycho-spiritual support during a terminal illness is critical, it is often overlooked by many healthcare providers (Stephenson et al., 2022). As the patient experiences the dying process, the nurse may need to utilize the expertise of the patient's identified spiritual counselor or religious leader. Priests, ministers, rabbis, lay ministers, **espiritista**, and others are among the many religious leaders with whom a patient may wish to confer. These individuals can assist the nurse in providing support for patients and their families during grieving or other times of spiritual need. For patients who are religious, spiritual leaders can also assist them during sacred times.

Today, nurses can also utilize a screening tool like the State of Spirituality Scale (SOS) to assess patient's spiritual well-being in the moment. The scale allows patients who are receiving hospice care to illustrate their current spiritual state on several dimensions (Stephenson et al., 2022). Having this knowledge enables nurses to address the specific spirituality needs of patients at EOL.

Even patients who are religious will vary in their desire to incorporate prayer into their daily routine. Nurses can ask patients about their need for solitude, companionship, or for special religious items to assist them in prayer rituals. When a dying patient's anxiety is high or when grief is overwhelming, some patients welcome the opportunity for the nurse to sit quietly with them during prayer. In today's hectic healthcare environment, the nurse needs to be proactive and identify patients' care needs early and plan to incorporate strategies to address them into their daily schedule. Most hospitals have a generic place of worship to direct patients' families who wish to have private moments for meditation or prayer. Healthcare facilities usually have at least a lay minister to call on to meet the spiritual needs of patients. The ONS's position statement encourages nurses to provide interpreter services and culturally sensitive materials in the patient's own language. These services enable patients to make the optimum use of spiritual services that are available.

Because there are such wide variations in preferences around death and dying experiences, nurses must utilize a careful cultural assessment of their terminally ill patients and include their significant others in the process. Gathering information that is specific and relevant to the patient is the best way to ensure that the patient's desired outcomes are achieved.

IMPORTANT POINTS

- Caring for patients who are terminally ill requires nurses to first confront their own beliefs and attitudes concerning death and dying.
- Traditional and ethical goals of nursing may differ from those of the terminally ill patient.
- Anxiety, fear, and depression often accompany the death and dying experience.
- Differences exist between culturally diverse groups in their attitudes toward advance directives, life support, disclosure of diagnosis, and the designation of the decision-maker.
- A variety of health practices and rituals related to death and dying are found among culturally diverse groups.
- The nurse will need to assess the patient's psychologic, cultural, spiritual, and religious views when caring for terminally ill patients.
- When providing EOL care to members of diverse groups, the nurse should remember there is variability of beliefs and attitudes within groups and strive to identify individual values and beliefs.
- The nurse should utilize a variety of resources to assist in providing culturally competent care to patients who have terminal illnesses.
- A primary goal of palliative care is to prevent and relieve suffering and to support the best quality of life for patients and their families regardless of their stage of disease.

CASE SCENARIO

Ms. Vera Talsford, a 65-year-old widow, mother of two daughters, and grandmother of two young boys, arrived in the ED of a busy metropolitan trauma center complaining of a severe headache with increasing pain, dizziness, and nausea with movement. After the physical examination, the physician ordered a CT scan, which revealed a left occipital mass. Ms. Talsford was admitted with a brain tumor. During the next few days, MRI studies, a PET scan, and other tests revealed that Ms. Talsford had lung cancer with metastases to her brain. A friend of the family was with the patient when the doctor spoke with her. He asked Ms. T, as everyone called her, if it was okay to speak about her situation while the visitor was present. Ms. T said that was okay with her. The doctor spoke encouragingly and told Ms. T that everything would be done to remove the tumor from her brain. Over several days, Ms. T made a slow neurologic recovery from the surgery, but became more despondent after being told about the severity of her illness. She was starting to eat less each day and lost 20 pounds in a short period. Ms. T was well liked and had a room full of visitors each day. The nurses on the unit were confused about how to best care for Ms. T. They were not sure if she appreciated the significance of her diagnosis. One day Karen, one of the staff nurses, asked Ms. T if she would like to see a minister or other clergymen during her hospitalization. Ms. T stated, "Well, I'm not really the religious type." Karen was stunned by Ms. T's comments and replied, "Okay, I'll be back in a little while." She left the room perplexed about what to do next to assist Ms. T.

WHAT NURSES NEED TO KNOW ABOUT THEMSELVES

Application of the Staircase Self-Assessment Model: Self-Reflection Questions

1. Have you considered the significance of your own death?
2. Do you believe in life after death?
3. Where are you on the Cultural Competency Staircase when caring for patients who are terminally ill? How will you progress to the next level?
4. How comfortable are you caring for this patient and discussing issues related to the death and dying process with her and/or her family?
5. What cultural information about the patient will you need to obtain to provide culturally sensitive care during the EOL?
6. What kinds of psychologic, emotional, and spiritual support would you need if given a similar diagnosis?

Responses to Self-Reflection Questions

Response: Have you considered your own death? Life after death? Where are you on the Cultural Competency Staircase?

There are many exercises to help nurses explore their feelings and attitudes about death and dying that can be found on the web. Getting in touch with one's true feelings can open the mind toward understanding others' attitudes and beliefs. The authors recommend these exercises as a first step in assisting patients who are terminally ill during grieving stages of illness.

Response: How comfortable are you caring for this patient and discussing issues related to the death and dying process with her and/or her family?

As stated earlier, nurses begin by exploring their own attitudes about death and dying. One opportunity, which can be found at www.durbinhypnosis.com/deathdying.htm, is Paul Durbin's (2004) tribute to Dr. Elisabeth Kübler-Ross (*Death & Dying, Death & Grief: A Tribute to Dr. Kübler-Ross*). Other nursing actions include reviewing the content provided by nursing and medicine on principles guiding cross-cultural EOL care.

Several websites are recommended that provide relevant content on this subject, and can be found at the end of this chapter.

Response: What cultural information about the patient will you need to obtain to provide culturally sensitive care during the EOL?

Nurses caring for patients at the EOL will need to be aware of the patient's knowledge and understanding that the illness is terminal. This may or not be culturally appropriate based on the patient and family's cultural perspectives about sharing this information. Nurses should also explore what resources and coping mechanisms are available to the patient. It is particularly useful to determine the patient's religious attitudes and beliefs regarding what constitutes a happy or peaceful death; the patient's attitudes about life after death might also be discussed if the patient wishes.

Response: What kinds of psychologic, emotional, and spiritual support would you need if given a similar diagnosis?

This is very individual and will depend on the results of your cultural assessment. The degree to which people need supportive care depends on family support, and their psychologic, emotional, and spiritual preparation and personal readiness for death. When speaking with the patient and the family, the nurse can determine if the patient wishes to see a clergyperson or other spiritual leader or counselor. If desired, the nurse should afford the patient private time for prayer as needed on a routine basis.

NCLEX®-TYPE QUESTIONS

1. The nurse begins planning care for a patient newly diagnosed with pancreatic cancer. The patient has not yet been told of the diagnosis. The initial action by the nurse is to:
   A. Conduct a cultural assessment to determine the needs of the patient
   B. Reflect on personal beliefs and attitudes regarding terminal illness
   C. Offer the patient spiritual reading material
   D. Disregard the diagnosis and treat the patient like any other patient

2. The primary role of the nurse in caring for patients who have terminal illnesses is to ensure that:
   A. The patient has a happy death
   B. Pain is minimized and controlled
   C. The patient is protected from unnecessary stress
   D. The patient's goals and wishes related to death and dying are addressed

3. A terminally ill patient states that she believes the pain associated with her illnesses is God's way of purifying her of her sins before death; consequently, she is refusing pain medication. What statement by the nurse caring for a patient who is terminally ill suggests a need for further staff development?
   A. "That statement makes no sense; I believe we should add pain meds to her food."
   B. "The patient has a right to decide the care they receive as long as they are cognitively sound."
   C. "Let's continue to offer the medication just in case she changes her mind."
   D. "Perhaps we can offer some magazines or music therapy to divert her attention from her pain."

4. The staff development nurse conducts a workshop on caring for terminally ill patients. What statement by the nurse is accurate about culturally diverse groups and terminal illness?
   A. Members of the same cultural, racial, or ethnic groups generally share the same attitudes about death and dying.
   B. The nurse can assume there are variations among culturally diverse groups regarding death and dying beliefs and practices.
   C. Members of the same religious group share beliefs about postmortem procedures.
   D. To avoid confusion, it is best to care for all patients in the same way.

5. The hospice nurse comes to visit a terminally ill patient who has just been placed in her care. The nurse asks the patient whether he wishes to enter a hospice care facility or receive care at home. The nurse recalls that current research reveals most terminally ill patients prefer:
   A. Staying in the hospital where they feel safe
   B. Being discharged from nursing care, because they cannot expect a cure for their illness
   C. Going to a long-term care or rehabilitation facility
   D. Going home to die in the presence of their loved ones

6. The literature suggests that nurses caring for terminally ill patients will need to find ways to avoid burnout. Which of the following is an appropriate strategy? *Select all that apply.*
   A. Eat a healthy diet.
   B. Get adequate sleep.
   C. Limit conversations about death and dying with the patient.
   D. Exercise regularly.

7. In the United States, ideas about death and dying are most often a result of America's focus on the medical model of care and:
   A. One's personal view of death
   B. A desire to engage in the afterlife
   C. An effort to fight against death
   D. A concern for a peaceful death

8. Which statements are accurate about cultural variations in attitudes about issues at the end of life? *Select all that apply.*
   A. Variations exist between diverse groups about disclosure of diagnosis and advance directives.
   B. Witholding a poor prognosis is based on belief in beneficence among some Asian groups.
   C. Many African Americans are adverse to palliative or hospice care.
   D. Experiencing pain at end of life (EOL) is looked upon as a sign of a bad death by all patients.

9. During a cultural assessment, the nurse learns that a patient is a member of the Cherokee Nation. What *initial* action by the nurse is *most* appropriate?
   A. The nurse plans care for the patient based on personal knowledge about Cherokee Indians.
   B. The nurse performs a cultural assessment to learn about the individual care needs of the patient.
   C. The nurse plans to get an interpreter to speak with the patient.
   D. The nurse will review a cultural competency textbook to learn more about the Cherokee Nation.

10. A Muslim patient who is terminally ill refuses to eat during Ramadan. What statement by the nurse demonstrates a good understanding of providing culturally competent care to patients who are terminally ill?
    A. "You don't have to honor Ramadan at your stage of illness."
    B. "Fasting will only make you sicker. You must really try to eat something."
    C. "Your health is the most important consideration at this time."
    D. "I will bring you a tray after sundown."

ANSWERS TO NCLEX-TYPE QUESTIONS

1. B	5. D	9. B
2. D	6. A, B, and D	10. D
3. A	7. C	
4. B	8. A, B, and C	

AMERICAN ASSOCIATION OF COLLEGES OF NURSING COMPETENCIES ADDRESSED IN THIS CHAPTER

1. Apply knowledge of social and cultural factors that affect nursing and healthcare across multiple contexts.
2. Use relevant data sources and best evidence in providing culturally competent care.
3. Promote achievement of safe and quality outcomes of care for diverse populations.
4. Advocate for social justice, including commitment to the health of vulnerable populations and the elimination of health disparities.
5. Participate in culturally competent development.

A robust set of instructor resources designed to supplement this text is located at http://connect.springerpub.com/content/book/978-0-8261-8302-6. Qualifying instructors may request access by emailing textbook@springerpub.com.

REFERENCES

Abbasi, M., Eskandari, N., Heidari, A., Heidari, M., Yoosefee, S., Adeli, S.-H., & Kazemi, A. (2022). A thematic analysis of dimensions of spiritual care. *Iranian Journal of Nursing and Midwifery Research, 27*(5), 452–460. https://www.ncbi.nlm.nih.gov/pmc/articles/PMC9745858

American Association of Critical Care Nurses. (2021). *AACN position statement: Ethical triage and end-of-life-care.* https://www.aacn.org/policy-and-advocacy/aacn-position-statement-ethical-triage-and-end-of-life-care

American Nurses Association. (2017). *American Nurses Association and Hospice & Palliative Nurses Association call for palliative care in every setting.* https://www.nursingworld.org/news/news-releases/2017-news-releases/american-nurses-association-and-hospice--palliative-nurses-association-call-for-palliative-care-in-every-setting

Anderson, D., & De Souza, J. (2021). The importance and meaning of prayer rituals at the end of life. *British Journal of Nursing, 30*(1), 34–39. https://doi.org/10.12968/bjon.2021.30.1.34

Associated Press. (2023). Jimmy Carter, 98, is in "good spirits" three months after entering home hospice care, where ex-president enjoys ice cream and time with beloved wife Rosalynn, 95: Grandson says he could live 'til fall. *Daily Mail.com.* https://www.dailymail.co.uk/news/article-12116791/Jimmy-Carter-3-months-hospice-aware-tributes-enjoying-ice-cream.html

Cain, C., & McCleskey, S. (2019). Expanded definitions of the "good death"? Race, ethnicity, and medical aid in dying. *Sociology of Health and Illness, 41*(6), 1175–1191. https://doi.org/10.1111/1467-9566.12903

Caplan, Z. (2023, May 25). *U.S. older population grew from 2010 to 2020 at fastest rate since 1880 to 1890.* U.S. Census Bureau. https://www.census.gov/library/stories/2023/05/2020-census-united-states-older-population-grew.html

Centers for Disease Control and Prevention. (n.d.-a). *National Center for Health Statistics: Life expectancy.* https://www.cdc.gov/nchs/fastats/life-expectancy.htm

Center for Disease Control and Prevention. (n.d.-b). *National Center for Health Statistics. Leading causes of death.* https://www.cdc.gov/nchs/fastats/leading-causes-of-death.htm

Centers for Disease Control and Prevention. (n.d.-c). *Stigma and discrimination.* https://www.cdc.gov/msmhealth/stigma-and-discrimination.htm

Centers for Disease Control and Prevention. (2020). QuickStats: Percentage of deaths, by place of death - National Vital Statistics System, United States, 2000–2018. *Morbidity and Mortality Weekly Report, 69*(19), 611. https://doi.org/10.15585/mmwr.mm6919a4

Centers for Disease Control and Prevention. (2021). *Mortality in the United States, 2021.* NCHS Data Brief. https://www.cdc.gov/nchs/data/databriefs/db456.pdf

Centers for Disease Control and Prevention. (2023, December 5). Leading causes of death for 2020. *National Vital Statistics Report, 72*(13). https://www.cdc.gov/nchs/data/nvsr/nvsr72/nvsr72-13-tables.pdf

Figueiredo, C. S., & Assis, M. G. (2023). Death and dying in long-term care facilities: The perception of occupational therapists. *Journal of Death and Dying, 87*(1) 177–193. https://doi.org/10.1177/00302228211019206

Gurdogan, E. P., Kinici, E., & Aksoy, B. (2019). The relationship between death anxiety and toward the care of dying patients in nursing students. *Psychology, Health, and Medicine, 24*(7), 843–852. https://doi.org/10.1080/13548506.2019.1576914

Ingraham, C. (2017, December 27). Americans are dying younger than people in other rich nations. *The Washington Post.* https://www.washingtonpost.com/news/wonk/wp/2017/12/27/americans-are-dying-younger-than-people-in-other-rich-nations/?utm_term=.d54a8a553291

Isaacson, M. J., & Lynch, A. R. (2018). Culturally relevant palliative and end-of-life-care for U.S. indigenous populations: An integrative review. *Journal of Transcultural Nursing, 29*(2), 180–191. https://doi.org/10.1177/1043659617720980

Kastbom, L., Milberg, A., & Karlsson, M. (2017). A good death from the perspective of palliative cancer patients. *Support Care Cancer, 25*(3), 933–939. https://doi.org/10.1007/s00520-016-3483-9

Khizar, B., & Harwood, R. (2017). Making difficult decisions with older patients on medical wards. *Clinical Medicine, 17*(4), 353–356. https://doi.org/10.7861/clinmedicine.17-4-353

Klobucista, C. (2022, September 8). *U.S. life expectancy is in decline. Why aren't other countries suffering the same problem?* Council on Foreign Relations. https://www.cfr.org/in-brief/us-life-expectancy-decline-why-arent-other-countries-suffering-same-problem

Medline Plus. (2023). *LGBTQIA+ Health.* https://medlineplus.gov/lgbtqiahealth.html

Miller, J. (2023). Case management for patients nearing end of life. *Hospital Case Management, 31*(5), 78–79. https://www.reliasmedia.com/articles/case-management-for-patients-nearing-the-end-of-life

Murphy, S. L., Kochanek, K. D., Jiaquan, M. A., & Arias, E. (2021). *Mortality in the United States, 2020.* https://www.cdc.gov/nchs/products/databriefs/db427.htm

National Institute on Aging. (2018). *Advance care planning: Healthcare directives.* http://www.nia.nih.gov/health/advance-care-planning-healthcare-directives

National Institute on Aging. (2022). *Providing care and comfort at the end of life.* https://www.nia.nih.gov/health/providing-comfort-end-life

Oak, Y., & Sun-Kim, Y. (2020). Attitudes toward death, perceptions of hospice care, and hospice care needs among family members of patients in the intensive care unit. *Korean Journal of Palliative Care, 23*(4), 172–182. https://doi.org/10.14475/kjhpc.2020.23.4.172

Patel, D., Patel, P., Ramani, M., & Makadia, K. (2023). Exploring perceptions of terminally ill cancer patients about the quality of life in hospice based and home based palliative care: A mixed method study. *Indian Journal of Palliative Care, 29*(1), 57–63. https://doi.org/10.25259/IJPC_92_2021

Rakshit, S., McGough, M., Amin, K., & Cox, C. (2022). *How does U.S. life expectancy compare to other countries?* Health System Tracker. https://www.healthsystemtracker.org/chart-collection/u-s-life-expectancy-compare-countries

Rising, M. L. (2017). Truth telling as an element of culturally competent care. *Journal of Transcultural Nursing, 28*(1), 48–55. https://doi.org/10.1177/1043659615606203

Spelten, E., Timmis, J., Heald, S., & Duijts, S. F. A. (2019). Rural palliative care to support dying at home can be realized; experiences of family members and nurses with a new model of care. *Australian Journal of Rural Health, 27*(4), 336–343. https://doi.org/10.1111/ajr.12518

Stephenson, P., Sheehan, D., & Hansen, D. (2022). The State of Spirituality Scale as a screening tool for spiritual distress. *Clinical Journal* of *Oncology Nursing, 26*(6), 593–596. https://doi.org/10.1188/22.CJON.593-596

Stokes, L. (2019). ANA position statement: The nurse's role when a patient requests medical aid in dying. *The Online Journal of Issues in Nursing, 24*(3), https://doi.org/10.3912/OJIN.Vol24No03PoSCol02

Townsend, A., & Kimball, J. (2017). Can faith and hospice coexist: Is the African American church the key to increased hospice utilization for African Americans? *Journal of Transcultural Nursing, 28*(1), 32–39. https://doi.org/10.1177/1043659615600764

Ubel, P. (2018). Where you live in America determines when you die. *Forbes.* https://www.forbes.com/sites/peterubel/2018/01/24/where-you-live-determines-when-you-die-inequality-in-american-life-expectancy/#3230e34829c7

Vitas Healthcare. (n.d.). *Infographic: The importance of talking about end-of-life care.* https://www.vitas.com/hospice-and-palliative-care-basics/end-of-life-care-planning/having-a-conversation-about-the-end-of-life/importance-of-talking-about-end-of-life-care

Vitas Healthcare. (2016). *The state of hospice in America, 2016.* https://www.vitas.com/resources/hospice-care/infographic-state-of-hospice-in-america

Vitas Healthcare. (2020, April 2). *Suggesting hospice to your patients with advanced illness.* https://www.vitas.com/for-healthcare-professionals/making-the-rounds/2018/june/suggesting-hospice-to-your-seriously-ill-patients

World Health Organization. (2020). *Palliative care: Key facts.* https://www.who.int/news-room/fact-sheets/detail/palliative-care

IMPORTANT WEBSITES

American Academy of Family Physicians Position Paper on Cultural Proficiency. Retrieved from www.aafp.org/about/policies/all/cultural-diverse-populations.html

American Association of Colleges of Nursing: Peaceful Death: Recommended Competencies and Curricular Guidelines for End of Life Care. Retrieved from https://files.eric.ed.gov/fulltext/ED453706.pdf

Centers for Disease Control and Prevention: Leading Causes of Death 2020. Retrieved from https://www.cdc.gov/nchs/fastats/leading-causes-of-death.htm

U.S. Department of Health and Human Services, National Center for Health Statistics. https://www.cdc.gov/nchs/index.htm

9

Cultural Considerations When Working With LGBTQ+ Patients

Claire L. Dente

This is what Yahweh asks of you: only this, to act justly, to love tenderly and to walk humbly with your God.

—MICAH 6:8

LEARNING OBJECTIVES

After this chapter, the reader will be able to

1. Identify and understand who comprises the LGBTQ+, intersex, asexual, agender and ally population.
2. Articulate the importance of evolving language distinctions in understanding sexual orientation and gender identity and expression.
3. Gain knowledge of the healthcare concerns and institutional barriers facing the LGBTQ+ population.
4. Identify personal gaps in knowledge, skills, and comfort in working with members of the LGBTQ+ community.
5. Develop awareness of strategies to increase competence in working with the LGBTQ+ population.

KEY TERMS

Agender	Genderism
Ally	Genderqueer
Asexual	Heteronormativity
Binary	Heterosexism
Bisexual	Heterosexual/Straight
Cisgender	Homophobe
Cisnormativity	Homophobia
Cissexism	Homosexuality
Coming out	Intersex
Dead name/Deadnaming	Lesbian
Gay	LGBTQIA/LGBTQ+
Gender identity	Misgendering

Nonbinary	Terf
Pangender	Transgender
Pansexual	Transphobe
Queer	Transphobia
Sexual orientation	

OVERVIEW

When Dr. Gloria Kersey-Matusiak asked me to write this chapter for the first edition of this book several years ago, the chapter focused primarily on sexual orientation. In the second edition, I expanded this chapter to include emerging information related to gender identity and expression that had not previously been available. As I began editing this chapter for a third time, my exploration revealed much-needed advancement in scholarship addressing LGBTQ+ care, particularly inclusive of gender- and nonbinary-related research. Knowledge of the needs of LGBTQ+ individuals and best practices for providing inclusive care continue to unfold. Issues for LGBTQ+ people evolve within social, behavioral, medical, political, religious, scientific, linguistic, and advocacy contexts. External factors including acceptance, bias, prejudice, fear, and hatred can impact the health and mental health of LGBTQ+ individuals. Prevailing cultural beliefs, faith systems, and political perspectives undergird societal approaches to LGBTQ+ people which both limit and advance access to care.

Most of us give little thought to our own **sexual orientation** or **gender identity**. This is especially true if we identify as **heterosexual/straight** (those individuals who are attracted to members of the opposite sex), or **cisgender** (those individuals whose gender identity matches the sex/gender assigned to them at birth). Straight people do not have to come to terms with their attraction to members of the opposite sex or explain to friends and family that they are different from the majority. Cisgender people do not have to address the deep disconnect of the gender they feel themselves to be from the sex/gender assigned to them at birth. Straight people and cisgender people do not have to *come out* (disclose that one is lesbian, gay, bisexual, transgender, **queer**, questioning, intersex, **asexual,** or **LGBTQIA/LGBTQ**+) to self, family, friends, workplace colleagues, or a faith system again and again in each new context, uncertain of the response they will receive. As you consider LGBTQ+ individuals, what are your own beliefs and attitudes about working with individuals whose sexual orientation or gender identity or expression may differ from yours? If you identify as LGBTQ+, how might your views and experiences differ from other LGBTQ+ people? The following pages will encourage you to deepen your self-awareness of how you think and feel about LGBTQ+ people, while refining your skills in working with LGBTQ+ patients and colleagues.

This chapter presents an overview of some of the key issues facing LGBTQ+ patients. It includes a glossary of terms and cases where sexual orientation, gender identity, and gender expression are important elements in treatment considerations for patients and in professional nursing relationships. In accordance with the Staircase Self-Assessment Model, we will explore self-reflection questions as they relate to sexual orientation and gender identity and expression. Finally, we include references and resources that may assist you in expanding your knowledge and clinical skills when working with LGBTQ+ individuals.

THE IMPORTANCE OF LANGUAGE UNDER THE LGBTQ+ UMBRELLA

Evolving discourse has separated sexual orientation and gender identity into two different constructs. Most readers will know the following terms, but here is a quick overview. My *sexual orientation* is to whom I am attracted: emotionally, sexually, and romantically.

My *sexual identity* refers to how I define myself within that attraction. In general, we identify men who are attracted to women and women who are attracted to men as *heterosexual*. Men who are attracted to men usually identify as **gay** (though the term *gay* can be used more broadly), and women who are attracted to women as **lesbians**; men or women who are attracted to both men and/or women identify as **bisexual**. People who identify as **pansexual** can be attracted to a person of any sexual orientation or gender identity, while **pangender** has little to do with sexual orientation, and may describe an individual who identifies with multiple genders or something beyond traditional gender identities. It is important to consider how patients define themselves, rather than assuming we know.

My *gender identity* differs in that it refers to how I identify myself along a gender continuum: as masculine/male, feminine/female, **transgender, genderqueer, nonbinary, agender**, pangender, or another term. Language has evolved to accommodate our growing understanding of identities. Distinctions exist between sex and gender, and these distinctions are meaningful to LGBTQ+ people. The term *biological sex* was historically used to refer to the physical body with which an individual was born; this language has evolved in recent years. It is now common to discuss "sex assigned at birth" when referring to the way an individual was "labeled" at birth by the healthcare provider who delivered that baby. Sex assigned at birth differs from gender identity. Individuals who are born with an internal sense of their gender matching their sex assigned at birth (usually initially determined by external physical genitalia presentation) are referred to as *cisgender*. Individuals who feel an inconsistency between their internal sense of gender and the sex assigned to them at birth or matching their external body and genitalia may identify under the umbrella of transgender, genderqueer, nonbinary, agender, and/or pangender. **Intersex** individuals are those people who are born with a physical presentation that may be unclear, or they may have any one of numerous genetic and/or hormonal conditions that affect the clarity of their sex.

Sex and Gender Language Contexts

It is important to remember that these constructs have emerged within a society that has prioritized **binary** (male and female) understandings of sex and gender. Medicine, the social and behavioral sciences, LGBTQ+ advocates, and our culture have deepened exploration of the nuances of sex and gender. As noted, our binary culture has historically assigned a sex of male or female at birth and conflated that sex with gender, such that children grew up with *either* male or female gender/sex identification. Our society has used the terms *gender* and *sex* interchangeably, but this is not accurate. While sex generally refers to physical and physiologic components, gender refers more to socially constructed roles, expression, and behaviors (Canadian Institutes of Health Research, 2023). While assigning a gender of male or female at birth historically provided an opportunity for a child to live in a binarily gendered society with a binary gender identity, this process forced the individual to "fit" into societal sex and gender definitions that may never have fit for some intersex individuals, or later proved inaccurate as this child grew in awareness of their own gender identity. Individuals who experienced this sex and gender disconnect often delved deeper into themselves to understand their identity, with many ultimately self-identifying as transgender, gender diverse, genderqueer, gender nonbinary, pangender, or gender nonconforming. While society provided a gender label of male or female at birth, this label did not match their internal sense of identity. If you are cisgender, imagine for a moment what that experience might feel like. Consider the experiences a person faces and the ways they might cope in our very gendered society when the external world is telling you that you are one sex/gender, while inside you know and feel differently. Think about the stressors at play and their impact on one's physical and mental health.

These situations raise questions about how society might respond differently to the gender diversity that exists. What would it mean to remain open to a person's lived experience and development in the maturation process? Advocates have questioned if it is even necessary to label a person's identity at birth. Some individuals who identify as transgender or intersex would prefer that they had an opportunity to live without any specific gender assignment, rather than having to live with one that is incorrect. There are numerous accounts of individuals assigned to a gender identification that years later proved erroneous. As some children grew, they identified with another gender or experienced hormonal changes at puberty indicating the initial sex assignment was wrong. This has prompted advocacy for approaches that include nonbinary options to create space for those whose gender identity may be unclear at birth (according to the male/ female binary) and who gain clarity through maturation and development. A core question emerged that sits at the root of stances toward gender and transgender rights: Are sex and gender fixed or fluid?

Transgender advocates believe that sex and gender are not fixed, while others may tend to view sex and gender as clear from birth and fixed from that point forward. LGBTQ+ individuals will tune into the language that is used in healthcare settings to gauge a sense of your knowledge and support; hence, nurses will benefit from greater understanding and awareness of their own words. Language has evoked much vivid discussion that spills over into the legal and political realm. The term *sex assigned at birth* acknowledges that gender relates to an individual's internal sense of self and can be an entirely different construct from sex (see J. A. Clarke, 2022, for a helpful history and legal analysis of these constructs and their implications in resolving disputes in court). *Biological sex* suggests that sex is fixed and unchangeable; as J. A. Clarke (2022) has noted, this language is often used to counter transgender rights. Many others may use these terms interchangeably, with challenging implications for researchers (Colineaux et al., 2022). Some scholars challenge the idea of needing to categorize people at all, calling for a review of the labels in use and a "taxonomical renaissance" to upend categorization of identities (Amin, 2023, p. 92). Many healthcare organizations have adapted paperwork to include additional gender and sexual orientation options, and it is important to feel comfortable talking with patients about their identities and experiences.

As a society, we have historically been operating out of the idea that sex and gender are fixed at birth. Reconsidering this idea and the implications this has for our societal approach to transgender and nonbinary people is a significant shift, sometimes eliciting visceral reactions. We have observed responses to "the bathroom issue" for transgender people result in currents of opposition (Platt & Milam, 2018). This has included unfounded concerns of sexual assault, formal legislation requiring use of bathrooms aligned with sex assignment at birth, and, at times, outright hysteria. The increasing knowledge about nonbinary and gender-nonconforming identities has raised visibility, awareness, and advocacy. Sometimes this has polarized views along political, religious, and cultural spectra, with some scholars describing the ensuing upheaval against transgender and nonbinary people as a creation of "moral panic" (Pepin-Neff & Cohen, 2021, p. 646). As scholars, advocates, and gender-nonconforming people have brought light to these issues, others are exploring how our social processes and environments may need to accommodate the diversity of individuals. The tension between the focus on the individual or the environment has contributed to much of the passionate discourse today related to gender, transgender, and nonbinary rights, and the overall treatment of LGBTQ+ people.

Some advocates have sought legal support for a gender-neutral alternative to the binary classification of male or female on documents such as driver's licenses and birth certificates in numerous states (Migdon, 2022). Internationally, the United States of America and other countries, including Canada, Australia, India, Malta, Nepal, and New Zealand, have also permitted a gender-neutral passport designation (Hernandez, 2022). As informed professionals, we must stay current on this issue to keep our practices, policies, forms, and procedures relevant and sensitive to the needs of LGBTQ+ patients. How can nurses support a family or child growing up with gender diversity? How can nurses create informed and welcoming spaces for individuals and families to receive healthcare without judgment? With continuously evolving knowledge and language amidst passionate discourse, it is important for nurses to access current scholarship on sex, gender, and sexual orientation, and ways to implement this knowledge with patients, providers, healthcare systems, and broader society.

DIAGNOSTIC AND STATISTICAL MANUAL OF MENTAL DISORDERS, FIFTH EDITION, TEXT REVISION

The LGBTQ+ community encompasses a broad range of diversity across sexual orientation, gender identity, and gender expression. The American Psychiatric Association has also evolved its language in addressing sexual orientation and gender identity and expression.

In 2013, the fifth edition of the *Diagnostic and Statistical Manual of Mental Disorders (DSM-5)* removed Gender Identity Disorder (GID) from its pages (American Psychiatric Association, 2013). Gender Dysphoria was added in place of GID. As a category in the *DSM-5*, and later in its text revision, the *DSM-5-TR*, Gender Dysphoria reflects that a gender identity that is not male or female is not a disorder; rather, emphasis shifted to the discomfort between sex assigned at birth and one's sense of one's own gender identity. Gender Dysphoria removed pathology from a nonbinary gender identity and focused on alleviating the tension and conflict an individual might face (Turban, 2022) as nonbinary in our binary society. This move was akin to removing **homosexuality** from the *DSM* in 1973; thus, a gay, lesbian, or bisexual sexual orientation is also not a mental illness (Drescher, 2015). Some transgender people find having a diagnosis of Gender Dysphoria helpful for obtaining medical care and insurance coverage or for challenging discrimination, while others consider it problematic to require a diagnosis to seek hormones, surgery, or other interventions and support.

Most recently, the American Psychiatric Association (2022) updated the *DSM-5-TR* to incorporate language changes to reflect differentiation between sex and gender and to loosen the concept of gender as fixed. These revisions aimed to use more culturally sensitive language that is less stigmatizing, such as using "experienced gender" in place of "desired gender," and replacing "cross-sex medical procedure" with "gender affirming medical procedure" (American Psychiatric Association, 2023, p. 1). This language change suggests the need for a significant shift of responsibility to our environments in creating supportive contexts for the well-being of transgender and nonbinary people, rather than assigning dysfunction to the individual who is "different."

Evolving Identity Language

In the past, the term *queer* was a slur aimed at LGBTQ+ people. Many LGBTQ+ people have reclaimed and freely use the word *queer,* and it is now seen and heard with positive connotations. While many LGBTQ+ (particularly younger) people embrace this word as liberating and its positive use has grown, others still may feel that it reaffirms a negative depiction of LGBTQ+ individuals. Older generations may recall greater trauma associated with this term; thus, nurses should gauge the use of the term *queer,* as it could be conceived differently depending on the generation using it. Similarly, the term *homosexuality* bears a loaded history. As a diagnosis in the original *DSM,* having this term removed from the *DSM* was a relief to many gay, lesbian, and bisexual people. Many LGBTQ+ people dislike this term, although it continues to surface in clinical contexts and in the language of those who do not support LGBTQ+ people.

Our understanding of sex and gender, and its meaning to LGBTQ+ people, continually evolves. Transgender people differ from each other and there is a great amount of intra-group diversity. Nurses must approach each person as a unique individual in their identity. Not all who identify as transgender or nonbinary undergo hormonal or surgical interventions. Others do seek surgery and transition on multiple levels. As noted, some people identify as gender nonconforming or agender, where they do not identify as or adhere to "typical" gender expression as defined by culture. How do we even define "typical"?

This is both an exciting and scary time for people who may have had to conceal their true selves and now can live with an integrated sense of self. LGBTQ+ people make decisions each day whether to come out about who they love or how they identify. It is important to respect that LGBTQ+ patients may or may not come out to you as their nurse or to other healthcare providers until they feel they are safe, that you as the provider can be trusted, and that they feel accepted by you. For individuals transitioning or **coming out**, identity is significant; how we refer to people can affirm or negate that identity. LGBTQ+ people can feel particularly vulnerable in the early stages of transitioning or coming out.

Pronouns and New Names

Language is a powerful tool. For transgender, gender diverse, nonconforming, and nonbinary people, pronouns are *extremely important*. It can sometimes be confusing for cisgender people to understand the significance of a pronoun or using a person's new name. Even caring, sensitive individuals may ask, "What is the big deal?" Yet, for a transgender/nonbinary person, it is very much a "big deal." It may have taken years to reach their level of self-understanding, acceptance, and a decision to be open or to transition. Using the wrong pronoun or gender connotes **misgendering**; it can feel invalidating to a person. Similarly, if a person has changed their name to a new name or asked you to use a new name, yet you persist in calling them by their previous name, this is referred to as misnaming by using their **dead name**, or **deadnaming**.

Nurses can create safer spaces for patients to receive care by adding gender-inclusive language on forms and by learning more about culturally sensitive language. Nurses can ask patients the name they wish to be called and the pronouns they use, as some medical records contain legal names only. The patient may not have legally changed their name for multiple reasons, ranging from personal decision to cost. They may not intend to change it ever, or they may still be in that process. If a healthcare agency already asks patients to identify their pronouns and name, nurses should make every effort to adhere to the patient's responses. This may seem cumbersome and obvious, and perhaps even awkward. Nurses for whom it feels unfamiliar to ask about pronouns should practice asking trusted colleagues these questions to achieve greater comfort. While cisgender patients may not care or understand why a nurse would ask these questions, a transgender patient will appreciate that they are included and relevant. Displaying supportive symbols, and *not* displaying symbols associated with anti-LGBTQ+ sentiments, are also important for creating safer healthcare spaces that reflect acceptance and support (Clary et al., 2022).

Some individuals identify and embrace their identity as male *and* female or as a combination of genders; some identify as two-spirit or third gender. Using the pronouns "they/their/them" may seem more accurate. Sometimes, it can be challenging for cisgender providers to understand the use of traditionally plural pronouns when there is one individual standing before them, but it is important to respect the patient's identity. It can also be a challenge for those of us who have been deeply entrenched in binary language for many years. Everyone can make mistakes. When we are well-meaning but forget or "get it wrong," most recommend a simple acknowledgement and apology that you used the wrong name or pronoun, that you recognize how important this is to the person, and that you will work to do better.

Some cisgender people have argued that using "they/them" pronouns is grammatically incorrect, but even *Merriam-Webster* supports the use of "they" (Merriam-Webster, n.d.). Advocates have proposed using "they/them" with patients when unsure, and simply asking the person what pronouns they use. Language evolves with new generations and new knowledge, and just when you think you are confident in the terminology, you can be assured it will change again! Complacency is not an option. Attend to emerging language for LGBTQ+ patients, especially our youth. They will call you out if you do not! Remember also that each person is different in their identity; this language can and *will* change with time.

STRENGTHS, CHALLENGES, AND WELL-BEING

Isms, "Normativity," and Phobias

You can read my name at the beginning of this chapter; yet, standing alone, my name does not tell you much about me. You do not know my skin color, ethnicity, age, or ability status; you do not know my sexual orientation, gender identity, or gender expression. For most of us, unless we are tuned in to consider that people may have diverse identities we cannot see, we often presume they are the majority: straight and cisgender. **Heterosexism** presumes someone is straight; similarly, when these assumptions are based on gender identity, the process describes **cissexism**. We could argue that the number of LGBTQ+ individuals is significantly smaller than the general population. While statistically true, we want to avoid making this error with patient identities. Just like universal precautions can keep everyone healthier, universal practices, such as avoiding presumptions until you ask, can respect all, especially LGBTQ+ patients.

Heteronormativity and **cisnormativity** extend the concepts of heterosexism and cissexism. They involve presumptions of "straight and cisgender." Intentionally or not, this then ranks these identities as "better than" LGBTQ+ identities. **Genderism** describes the preference for having only two binary genders of male and female recognized, with these two considered superior to gender variance. Thus, under a culture of heteronormativity and cisnormativity, a heterosexual sexual orientation and cisgender identity are often both presumed and preferred over LGBTQ+ identities. Heteronormativity and cisnormativity can result in **homophobia**, the discomfort, dislike, and even hatred an individual or community has toward nonheterosexual people, while **transphobia** describes this same fear and hatred directed to transgender people. People who are hostile to transgender individuals are sometimes referred to as **"transphobes"** or **"terfs"** in the vernacular, while those hostile to LGB people may be referred to as **"homophobes."** Unsupportive social environments created by these concepts at work consciously or unconsciously contribute both to internal and external suffering, poorer health outcomes and well-being, and even violence for LGBTQ+ people. When growing up and living in unsupportive climates, LGBTQ+ people can develop *internalized homophobia* or *internalized transphobia*. This refers to the concept of recognizing one's own diverse sexual orientation, gender identity, or gender expression and then directing the societal hatred and loathing inward to oneself. This link between affect and behavior can have implications for the quality of life of LGBTQ+ people. How do you view gender diversity? Jones and Becker (2023) found that the more positively individuals evaluated transgender people, the more likely they were to support transpositive policies, and that this support increased among those who were more politically aware. More supportive policies create safer environments for transgender people. Thus, it is important to understand gender-diverse people and the experiences they may face in broader society that impact their well-being and access to healthcare.

Health and Well-Being

In a society where stigma and bias continue to negate LGBTQ+ people, suicide, mental health challenges, and violence rates are higher for LGBTQ+ individuals than for their straight and cisgender counterparts. This includes stigma and hate crimes directed at LGBTQ+ people (Colliver & Silvestri, 2022; Flores et al., 2022), challenges accessing gender-affirming healthcare during the COVID-19 Pandemic (Kia et al., 2022), increased social anxiety and mental health challenges (Ghassabian et al., 2022; Mahon et al., 2022), sexual assault and teen dating violence (Coulter & Gartner, 2023; López et al., 2023), and a complexity of suicidality circumstances, intersections, and protective factors (Drescher et al., 2021; Patten et al., 2022; Rivas-Koehl et al., 2020). LGBTQ+ patients of color may face unique challenges at this intersection of racial violence and suicide with sexual orientation and/or gender-nonconforming identities.

Stigma, discrimination, and oppression have negative consequences on the health and well-being of LGBTQ+ people (Clark, 2014; Rodríguez-Díaz et al., 2016). It is important to note contributions of the theory of intersectionality (Crenshaw, 1991) and minority stress theory (Meyer, 2003). The impact of compounded stressors can have negative impacts for LGBTQ+ people and people of color across their lifetime (Collet et al., 2022; Parra et al., 2022; Ramirez & Paz Galupo, 2019). The theory of *intersectionality* facilitates the understanding of how oppression can occur within coexisting marginalized identities such as race, ethnicity, and age (Kum, 2017). People experiencing stigma, discrimination, and oppression in society who then face this also when seeking healthcare may experience extensions of this psychologic distress and trauma. Thus, approaching LGBTQ+ patients and families with sensitivity requires awareness of these intersecting identities and proactive strategies for effective practice. It is especially important to recognize the distinct experience one LGBTQ+ patient may have from another LGBTQ+ patient. A lesbian who is an older adult, a Black woman of color who identifies as female, has a different life experience than an older White or Latinx gay man. Each lived through the Civil Rights Movement of the 1960s, the feminist movement of the 1970s, and marriage equality in the 21st century, but each experienced these differently because of their unique identity constellation. The concepts of intersectionality and minority stress recognize that these individuals live with stressors and health effects that differ for individuals with identities that may have privileged or marginalized their experiences in other ways. Each patient seeks healthcare within the context of their identities and experiences.

Other factors also influence LGBTQ+ well-being. In some cases, cultural identity affects parental acceptance of their LGBTQ+ children (Teran et al., 2022). Family support is tremendously important; it has been identified as one of the most significant factors for reducing depression and suicidality in sexuality and gender minority youth in the United States (Rivas-Koehl et al., 2020). Lower income and socioeconomic challenges can influence safer sex health practices (Harrison et al., 2022), food insecurity (Russomanno & Jabson Tree, 2020), and other social factors including poverty and unhoused status.

Coping With Substances

Stressors and stigma can invite unhealthy coping methods. Historically, many LGBTQ+ people met at bars and clubs, or used substances to deal with rejection, depression, unhoused status, and coping in general. While there is greater acceptability of LGBTQ+ identities, stigma, discrimination, and hostility remain. For some LGBTQ+ people, these and other factors contribute to using substances in unhealthy ways. As with many communities, powerfully addictive substances including opioids have reached the LGBTQ+ population. Researchers have explored risks, motivation, and decision-making in LGBTQ+ youth substance use to identify preventative measures (Mata et al., 2022; Schuler & Evans-Polce, 2022). Others have specifically examined mental health, e-cigarette use, and methamphetamine use in sexual minorities with housing instability (Azagba et al., 2022; Blackwell & López Castillo, 2020; A. Leonard et al., 2022). Treatment and recovery programs have been developed that specifically embrace LGBTQ+ individuals to assist them with the complexities of substance use, particularly where this may relate to their LGBTQ+ identity. Nurses can familiarize themselves with local and regional LGBTQ+ recovery and treatment resources to provide referrals for their patients who may need these services. It is also important to advocate for increased funding to support treatment centers that are sufficient in number to meet the needs of the community. Long waiting lists, insurance challenges, and a shortage of treatment programs with staff trained to understand the specific needs of the LGBTQ+ population can impede access to care.

Nurses should also consider youth access to medications on the internet and through the black market. While not substance use in the traditional conception of using alcohol and other drugs to obtain a "high," obtaining hormones, puberty blockers, PrEP (preexposure prophylaxis), and other medications through the internet or the black market can be dangerous on many levels. Youth who are unable to access supportive healthcare environments to obtain accurate information on gender identity and transitioning may utilize this strategy. Lack of support from parents, healthcare providers, and school; limited insurance coverage; and cold, hard fear can all contribute to how a young person chooses to access information. While the internet has been a resource for providing connection and access to information for LGBTQ+ youth, it also poses challenges and dangers. Information gleaned on the internet is not necessarily accurate and certainly is not specific to an individual's own health status. It is not uncommon for youth to obtain hormones from unclear sources and without the guidance of a medical professional. These youth may be taking powerful medications without an informed understanding of proper dosage, side effects, and their impact. The medications may have been altered or mixed with other substances. Other youth may be at risk of adverse drug reactions, particularly when they lack awareness of drug interactions with other medication they take, alcohol or other substance use, and other medical conditions they may experience. Accessing these substances may cost the individual not only in money, but perhaps in *quid pro quo* goods for services arrangements and even human trafficking scenarios. Youth engaged in black market access face the inherent dangers of procuring illicit substances, legal risks, and possible exposure to exploitation, physical harm, or violence. This practice further makes the case to provide accessible information in supportive healthcare settings that encourage young people to ask questions and receive accurate responses.

Youth, Schools, and Education

School settings have traditionally presented difficult environments for LGBTQ+ youth. In *The 2021 National School Climate Survey*, Gay, Lesbian, Straight Educator's Network (GLSEN; 2021) reported the continued presence of anti-LGBTQ+ bullying, harassment, assault, and discrimination in schools. Furthermore, GLSEN (2021) identified that only about 10% of LGBTQ+ students reported school staff intervention against negative homophobic remarks, and less than 10% of LGBTQ+ students reported staff intervention against negative comments about gender expression (GLSEN, 2021). In contrast, those students who observed staff or other students intervening against homophobic remarks, and those surrounded by positive LGBTQ+ representation in school, were more likely to model this positive behavior and intervene in other situations (Ioverno et al., 2022). Thus, school staff, including school nurses, must speak out against anti-LGBTQ+ rhetoric, as intervening improves climate. LGBTQ+ students and school health professionals have also reported challenges in unmet health needs including access to bathrooms and safe spaces, identifying specific needs for information on gender transitioning, violence, sexual harassment, and racism (Sava et al., 2021).

Other questions have arisen regarding transgender students on sports teams at all levels. In the United States and internationally, groups like the NCAA and International Olympic Committee (IOC) have issued guidelines that generally aim for fairness and support of transgender athletes (IOC, 2021; NCAA, 2021). The World Athletics Council, which oversees track and field events, has limited participation of transgender women who transitioned after experiencing male puberty (Kim, 2023). High stakes competitions will continue to generate dialogue as science unfolds; yet, consider youth who play baseball, football, soccer, or basketball on the playground, in youth leagues, and in K–12 grades with their friends. In some districts, these students are excluded from organized sports and recreation. How might nurses advocate for transgender and nonbinary children who want to participate in sports activities? Discrimination and bias can interfere with play in youth leagues, where sports provide multiple benefits to a child's physical health, social skills, acceptance, and overall well-being.

Despite these challenges, there are positive steps being taken in schools. Leonard (2022) elicited five areas of focus from transgender students that they reported to have had a positive impact on their school experience. These included the importance of accurate language, support from individual teachers, "whole-school approaches" (trainings, clubs), community connections (outside transpositive connections), and personal strengths including humor and self-advocacy (Leonard, 2022). Nurses can reinforce these areas in schools and in other contexts where they work. McGowan and colleagues (2022) found similar themes of desire for acceptance and validation in secondary school transgender students. Gender and Sexuality Alliances (GSAs) provide opportunities for supportive groups in school settings where nurses can bring their knowledge and skill set to provide information and validation while reducing isolation (Boyd et al., 2022). Numerous protective and risk factors specific to rural youth can impact well-being and mental health (Elliott et al., 2022). In isolated and rural regions, nurses in the community can develop virtual networks to build support for youth that reduce isolation and establish connections (Martinez et al., 2022).

Legislation, Policy, and Advocacy

In some jurisdictions, school boards and legislators have begun to discriminate openly against LGBTQ+ youth through bans on books and educational materials that contain LGBTQ+ content. In many areas, this is part of a larger political wave to dampen diverse representation and silence voices reflecting the experiences of Black, Asian, Latinx, and LGBTQ+ students. Faculty, staff, and students can be banned from posting LGBTQ+ positive symbols such as rainbow flags and other images that designate supportive environments and "safer spaces" for LGBTQ+ students. Helping professionals, including nurses, and the public should not take this lightly. Students who see positive images of people like themselves tend to lead happier and healthier lives. These political trends, as well as emerging school policies and legislation, aim to render LGBTQ+ students, faculty, and staff invisible. When you are invisible, you no longer matter. For those youth who may still be questioning and exploring their identity, invisibility and hostility place a stigma on LGBTQ+ identities. It is not safe. For those who are out and identified or even *perceived* to be LGBTQ+ through societally imposed definitions of gender expression, it is also not safe. Harassment, bullying, and violence increase when certain groups are not acknowledged and intentionally excluded, erasing them from the learning community or rendering them as disordered. These practices reinforce heterosexism and cissexism, where sexual orientation is presumed as straight, gender identity is presumed as male/female only, and gender expression must fit "traditional" societal norms. These approaches present LGBTQ+ identities as unhealthy and inferior and are occurring in both schools and the broader society.

In many states, legislative bills are being introduced under the guise of preserving parental rights. In 2022, Florida passed the "Parental Rights in Education" bill (referred to as the "Don't Say Gay" bill by opponents) which prohibited public schools from discussing sexual orientation or gender identity in grades K–3. Proponents of the bill stated that it supported parental determination of when and how to discuss these topics with their children (Diaz, 2022). In 2023, the Florida House passed HB 1069 which expanded the law to include grades K–8 and created laws around the use of pronouns, stating that "It shall be the policy of every public K–12 educational institution…that a person's sex is an immutable biological trait and that it is false to ascribe to a person a pronoun that does not correspond to such person's sex" (Parental Rights in Education, 2023, Subsection 9 of Section 1, 1000.21, p. 4). Notably, this legislation conflates sex and gender and views these as unchangeable components of biology. The legislation also gives parents the right to sue school districts who violate the law.

LGBTQ+ supportive caregivers and professionals have been targeted by this recent wave of discrimination and attacks. What are the consequences for nurses, teachers, social workers, psychologists, counselors, and others who post an LGBTQ+ positive sticker in their office, keep LGBTQ+ books on their shelves, or provide gender-affirming care? Will they be disciplined, fired, or even lose their license? Most professional standards and codes of ethics mandate nondiscrimination and equal access to care; professionals may now face ethical and legal dilemmas with severe consequences. This places professionals between the "rock and a hard place" of adhering to their professional standards versus adhering to the policies of their employers and laws of local, county, or state jurisdictions who may be swayed by political or religious perspectives instead of informed by the medical, social, and behavioral sciences. What will you do in this type of situation? These are complex situations requiring advocacy through the collaborative efforts of multiple professional associations. In an era of inflation, banking crises, mortgages, and student loans, most professionals cannot afford to be fired or quit their job without severe consequences to themselves and their own families, nor does this solve the problem of anti-LGBTQ+ bias and discrimination.

Parents and caregivers also face tremendous challenges when jurisdictions promote anti-LGBTQ+ policies and legislation. States across the United States are banning gender-affirming care, and, in some cases, criminalizing parents, caregivers, and medical professionals. In 2022, the Texas Supreme Court ruled that child welfare agencies could investigate families for child abuse where parents were providing gender-affirming care to their trans children, such as administering hormones and puberty blockers (Chappell, 2022, May 13). In some cases, parents and caregivers have made difficult decisions to leave the supports of family, career, community, and neighborhood to move to other states where they and their LGBTQ+ child can live in a safer environment with access to gender-affirming care.

Multiple states are passing these and other anti-LGBTQ+ legislation. The American Civil Liberties Union (ACLU) identified areas where lawmakers are targeting LGBTQ+ people (ACLU, 2023). As noted on the ACLU website, these included documentation challenges, such as making it harder to change the gender on one's birth certificate, driver's license, and other legal identification (ACLU, 2023). Civil rights challenges include using freedom of religion arguments to support discrimination against LGBTQ+ people by refusing goods and services. Challenges to free speech and expression involve book bans and bans on drag performances while challenges to healthcare include the previous discussions along with eligibility for coverage of gender-affirming care, medications, surgeries, and so on. Public accommodation challenges are those that limit bathroom and locker room usage, while attacks on schools and education include the content noted earlier. It is also significant to be aware that some lawmakers propose forced "outing" by teachers and other school professionals, a damaging practice where the adult shares an LGBTQ+ student's sexual orientation or gender identity without their permission (ACLU, 2023). Incidents such as these create stress in the lives of LGBTQ+ people. As is now widely known, stress responses results in higher levels of the hormone cortisol, and those with chronically higher levels of cortisol can experience long-term deleterious effects to their health and well-being.

Adulthood, Parenting, and Families

LGBTQ+ people may experience typical developmental milestones with an additional layer of questions, needs, or concerns unique to their identities. Meeting life partners and maintaining relationships, choosing to have families, and parenting may be impacted by how "out" each person in the relationship is, support from their family of origin, and the process of becoming a parent. LGBTQ+ people become parents through previous relationships, giving birth, infant adoption, co-parenting, and foster care to adoption. Some have chosen parenthood as single or coupled. Reproductive health for LGBTQ+ individuals may involve fertility treatments and artificial insemination. The World Professional Association for Transgender Health (WPATH) published international *Standards of Care (SOC) for the Health of Transsexual, Transgender, and Gender Nonconforming People* to guide care for transgender and gender-nonconforming individuals (Coleman et al., 2022; wpath. org/publications/soc).

In the not-so-distant past, LGBTQ+ people were not legally permitted to adopt children or to participate in second parent adoption, and engaging with reproductive health and fertility clinics was awkward and uncomfortable. While these situations have largely progressed with greater inclusivity and sensitivity to LGBTQ+ people, bias and discomfort can persist, as when a transgender male chooses to birth a child. How does the medical facility approach this patient? While many transgender people can seek gender-affirming healthcare in areas where there are multiple healthcare systems, sometimes rural individuals are faced with limited healthcare options that may not be as welcoming or supportive. LGBTQ+ people who are raising children while supporting their own parents and older relatives also comprise the "sandwich generation." Others must question whether a certain school district will welcome their children, or if a neighborhood will be safe for their family. Where to live, work, study, and travel are often vetted through a lens of safety which becomes more complex with financial challenges.

An important distinction for LGBTQ+ patients is the experience they bring of never quite knowing how another person will respond to their sexual orientation, gender identity, or gender expression. We know that nursing has identified care for LGBTQ+ people as an important cultural competency consideration, that LGBTQ+ people may hesitate to come out to providers, and that folks have felt marginalized, invisible, stigmatized, and unhappy with care in the past (see my chapter in the second edition of this text). Transgender people often avoid EDs despite a need for care. The National Center for Transgender Equality is currently processing data gathered from its more recent survey conducted in late 2022, and the Center expects to release an updated report of their findings in 2023. The Center identified several health concerns for transgender people in the previous *Report of the 2015 U.S. Transgender Survey* (James et al., 2016). These included general healthcare issues as well as concerns related specifically to the transitioning process and ongoing care. Transgender patients face many barriers and challenges to care, including lack of health insurance, unmet care needs, and less routine care (Lambda Legal, 2023). Transgender youth also faced challenges, including accessing trained pediatric providers, inconsistent protocols, inaccurate use of names and pronouns, lack of care coordination, challenges accessing pubertal blockers and cross-sex hormones, and insurance coverage (Gridley et al., 2016). Questions about sexual orientation and gender identity, the use of medications like preexposure prophylaxis (PrEP), decisions about how to become a parent and pregnancy, parenting skills, routine health screenings for breast or prostate cancer, and other issues arise for LGBTQ+ people.

Aging and Older Adults

The older LGBTQ+ population may have experienced life far differently than current LGBTQ+ youth. Growing up in eras where LGBTQ+ identities may have been illegal, immoral, or considered a mental illness, many were closeted about their identities. It would be easy to label an older LGBTQ+ person's concern for privacy as secretive or "paranoid" behavior, but the costs for many older adults were real: losing one's job or housing, safety concerns, violence, arrest, bullying, assault, and sometimes death. Common scenarios included dishonorable discharge from the military, inability to visit a sick or dying partner, losing one's children, and rejection by one's family, coworkers, and faith system. In caring for older LGBTQ+ adults, it is important to recognize the resilience it took to navigate and survive these difficult situations.

Although society has grown more accepting of LGBTQ+ people, older adults may have internalized homophobia/transphobia, or still have family and peers who are uncomfortable with their identities. Others may be incredibly open and out. Because many LGBTQ+ older adults experienced rejection, shunning, and cut-off from their families of origin, many built social networks that became their family of choice. These networks are important. Past experiences of discrimination and bias can also influence older LGBTQ+ adults in the decisions they make about their needs. Some LGBTQ+ people may avoid senior centers where they could receive free or low-cost healthcare, exercise classes, recreation, and lunch. For others, the past may inform decisions about future care; this proactive approach is a strength in selecting care. While approximately 78% of older LGBTQ+ adults anticipated discrimination in long-term care, many of these same individuals expressed a preference to receive care from LGBTQ+ providers or care specifically directed to LGBTQ+ people (Dickson et al., 2022). Are you prepared to work with them?

LGBTQ+ older adults expressed hesitation and concerns related to coming out, discrimination, caregiver training, and other support when pursuing palliative care (Roberts et al., 2022; Rosa et al., 2022). Lack of LGBTQ+ cultural competency in healthcare systems, and a hesitancy to pursue support because of past experiences, impacted the decisions of LGBTQ+ dementia caregivers to seek supports (Di Lorito et al., 2022). Dementia and other neurocognitive disorders also may present unique challenges for LGBTQ+ older adults in assessments normed on binary populations (Scharaga et al., 2021).

Other Populations

Nurses may encounter other LGBTQ+ people with unique circumstances that impact their experiences or their ability to seek healthcare. Individuals on the autism spectrum also seek gender-affirming care. They may bring a constellation of needs that arise with neurodivergent social interaction and communication styles, mental health concerns, and a desire for gender-affirming healthcare (Genovese et al., 2022; Strang et al., 2022). Other attention has focused on transgender refugees, noting that these vulnerable and marginalized identities may leave an individual at this intersection rejected both by other refugees and other transgender people who may be competing for resources and validation (Camminga, 2022). LGBTQ+ forced migrants face tremendous challenges and stressors in moving to a new country, while also demonstrating resilience and strengths that nurses can support to enhance their health and well-being (Gottvall et al., 2023). Kurdyla (2022) noted the challenges of cisnormativity in detention centers where transgender immigrants may be held. This cisnormativity may be used to discriminate against transgender people, calling forth advocacy from nurses and healthcare providers working within these systems. During the COVID-19 pandemic, pandemic responses negatively impacted transgender prisoners' mental health through increased solitary confinement and decreased access to gender-affirming care (Suhomlinova et al., 2023). LGBTQ+ populations enter our schools, hospitals, medical offices, prisons, detention facilities, and other locations where nurses provide healthcare services. It is important to assess each context to consider proactively how LGBTQ+ patients can receive appropriate care.

LGBTQ+ INTERSECTIONS WITH FAITH, RELIGION, AND AFFIRMING CARE

Multiple influences form our beliefs and thinking: our family system, education, neighborhood, friends, culture, historical era, political influences, and, for some of us, faith, religion, and/or spirituality. These factors influence our approach to sexual orientation, gender identity, and gender expression. Many of us were raised in spaces that have not been affirming and welcoming of LGBTQ+ populations, while others of us had more positive exposure to LGBTQ+ diversity. This chapter is written from an affirming perspective that supports competent, sensitive care to LGBTQ+ populations as ethical and just practice. Nurses should know that while some faith systems do not support LGBTQ+ identities, others offer inclusive, welcoming, and nurturing space to their LGBTQ+ members. Nonetheless, institutional religion in many denominations has been unsupportive of LGBTQ+ people, and at times has served to promote outright oppression and intolerance (Human Rights Campaign, 2023a). For this reason, many LGBTQ+ individuals are cautious when approaching formal religious institutions. Challenges can arise when hospitals and healthcare systems are affiliated with faith traditions that have historically offered limited or no support and even presented barriers to LGBTQ+ patients.

Sexual Orientation and Gender Identity Change Efforts

Some religious traditions that view LGBTQ+ sexual orientation and gender identity as an illness or as sinful support interventions that claim to "cure" an individual's sexual orientation or gender identity such that the individual can then presumably live as a heterosexual and cisgender person (American Psychological Association, n.d.). These efforts have been known as reparative or conversion therapies, and transformational or ex-gay ministries within some faith communities. In viewing sexual orientation or gender identity as something to be "fixed," these stances view LGBTQ+ identities as disordered. Considering LGBTQ+ identities as disordered is in direct contrast to the practices and ethics of the medical, social, and behavioral sciences and health professions. Most professional associations have issued public policy statements opposing sexual orientation change efforts, reparative and conversion therapies, and transformational or ex-gay ministries (Human Rights Campaign, 2023b). Professional organizations first began issuing objections in 1999 (Just the Facts, 1999/2006; National Association of Social Workers & National Committee on Lesbian, Gay, Bisexual and Transgender Issues, 2015), and the American Nurses Association also opposes these efforts (Stokes, 2018). As of this writing, 20 states and the District of Columbia have banned the use of conversion therapy with minors, while six states partially ban it with minors (Movement Advancement Project, 2023). Twenty-one states have no state law or policy banning conversion therapy (Movement Advancement Project, 2023). It is important to note that while approximately half of the states in the United States responded to education and advocacy with complete or partial bans on conversion therapy, Alabama, Georgia, and Florida are currently in federal judicial circuit with a preliminary injunction that prevents the enforcement of a ban on conversion therapy, despite the lack of evidence for the effectiveness of conversion therapies (Movement Advancement Project, 2023). While bans against the use of conversion therapies with youth have increased, these therapies generally remain an option for adults.

LGBTQ+ advocates have raised concerns about a recent trend claiming a phenomenon labeled "rapid-onset gender dysphoria" (ROGD). No such formal diagnosis exists in the *DSM-5-TR* or *International Classification of Diseases* (*ICD*), and ROGD is not supported by the medical or behavioral health professions (Bauer et al., 2022). Nurses should be cautious, as this hypothesis has not been vetted through rigorous scientific inquiry. The concept initiated from one online study of parents that was challenged for its limitations and participant selection bias. In brief, ROGD involves an idea that some youth suddenly experienced gender dysphoria as teens through peer social influences and contagion, and that it particularly affected teens with mental health concerns and family conflicts. The study suggested that youth might later regret gender-affirming care they received as teens. This approach implied transgender identity as disordered and as "a phase," thus invalidating experiences of transgender youth. The use of clinical language to define this hypothesis without scientific data to support it may involve a reactive approach to greater visibility of transgender youth and their need for gender-affirming care (Ashley, 2020).

Other challenges occur when LGBTQ+ people encounter faith-based institutions with unsupportive tenets of LGBTQ+ identities. Recent legislation and United States Supreme Court rulings have strongly supported religious freedom over antidiscrimination laws. The Supreme Court ruled in favor of Catholic Social Services, who sued the city of Philadelphia, Pennsylvania, when it lost its contract to provide foster care because it would not consider married LGBTQ+ couples in screening for foster parents (Totenberg, 2021, June 17).

Other LGBTQ+ opponents have utilized this amendment to argue that they should not have to provide their services (e.g., wedding cakes, photography services, etc.) to LGBTQ+ people when their religion opposed LGBTQ+ identities. Although LGBTQ+ people often choose to avoid these interactions, in some cases it is not possible. Some areas may have one major health center that happens to be part of a faith-based tradition, which will limit access to LGBTQ+-affirming care. Transgender people may not be able to access hormones, surgery, or other treatments at faith-based institutions. Perhaps a specialist is located within that healthcare system for any health need such as cardiology or ophthalmology, but the LGBTQ+ person hesitates to seek care there based on a fear of discrimination or of receiving inferior care.

It is common to summon pastoral care services when patients are very ill, dying, or coping with a challenging family health situation. Hospice care and specialized hospital care areas (ICU, NICU, ED) often integrate pastoral care. Healthcare facilities should include LGBTQ+-affirming pastoral care providers on their teams who understand LGBTQ+ experiences and are familiar with their needs. Despite past history, many LGBTQ+ people are deeply spiritual and will want to speak with someone, so it is important to know that while some LGBTQ+ people are definitely not interested, others most certainly would like to have pastoral care for religious or spiritual needs. Like many people, some LGBTQ+ people belong to faith traditions and have deep spiritual connections, while others do not. Some participate actively in faith communities and reap the social and spiritual benefits of these affiliations, while other LGBTQ+ patients may not participate in traditional religious institutions at all because of the oppression and alienation they have experienced. In any case, although many mainstream denominations are taking steps toward the inclusion of LGBTQ+ people into full participation, many congregations remain divided over their openness to accept the full participation of LGBTQ+ people. Thus, nurses need to accept that each patient brings their own experience of the interplay of liberation and oppression from organized religion.

Likewise, each nurse brings their own experience and view of LGBTQ+ people as formed by each one's own unique religious tradition and the experience of living in a culture built on certain dominant religious traditions. Some nurses may find it difficult to reconcile their own personal and religious beliefs that view LGBTQ+ sexual orientation and gender identity as sinful with providing culturally sensitive care to LGBTQ+ patients. It is important for nurses to be aware of their own beliefs. How might these beliefs subtly affect patient care with LGBTQ+ patients? A first step is to validate any discomfort you may have and to recognize that working with LGBTQ+ patients will require extra attentiveness to the potential impact your discomfort could have on patients and their families. The patient's well-being—physical, psychosocial, and spiritual—should not be at risk. Additional training, professional workshops, and reading nursing journals can inform and educate nurses about any misconceptions. What is most essential is that nurses provide competent, sensitive care to all patients, including those who are LGBTQ+.

IMPORTANT POINTS

1. The LGBTQ+ population consists of different individuals. They range in socioeconomic status, education, ability, race, ethnicity, age, religion, gender, political beliefs, and veteran status.
2. Gender identity (how a person identifies as male, female, transgender, etc.) differs from gender role or expression (how one chooses to present oneself in dress, style, mannerisms, etc.). An individual's gender identity and gender expression may or may not match one's sex assigned at birth (one's anatomical configuration). Sexual orientation (to whom one is attracted) and sexual behavior (with whom one chooses to be sexual) may or may not match how one views the self in terms of sexuality and attraction (sexual identity).

(continued)

IMPORTANT POINTS

(continued)

3. Historically, individuals who have identified as LGBTQ+ have experienced oppression and discrimination from health and mental health providers, and from religious institutions. This experience has resulted in reluctance to seek healthcare, wariness of service providers, and lack of disclosure (coming out) to one's healthcare providers. For this reason, many LGBTQ+ individuals consciously seek providers who appear knowledgeable and educated on their needs and concerns. They are also sensitive to those providers who dismiss their concerns or where they feel invisible.

4. Cultural identities such as race, ethnicity, age, and religion may affect an individual's decision to disclose to a healthcare provider. Healthcare concerns change at different developmental points across the life span for LGBTQ+ individuals. The social and political climate toward LGBTQ+ people may negatively or positively affect their access to care, available resources, and stressors to well-being.

5. Heterosexism, cissexism, homophobia, and transphobia may affect service delivery of care to LGBTQ+ individuals. Nurses need to understand these concepts and reduce discrimination or prejudice against all patients, including those identified as LGBTQ+.

6. Health and mental health organizations do not view sexual orientation as a "choice." They reject conversion, reparative, transformational ,and ex-gay therapies as forms of treatment to "change" one's sexual orientation to heterosexuality or one's gender identity to cisgender. These organizations view sexual orientation and gender diversity as a variation of "normal," in the same way one might view left-handedness in a right-hand-dominated world.

7. Knowledge of the interaction between gender, gender identity, gender expression, sex assigned at birth, sexual orientation, sexual identity, and sexual behavior continues to unfold. Thus, culturally sensitive practice with LGBTQ+ individuals is an ongoing process informed by research in health, mental health, advocacy, and the social science professions.

CASE SCENARIO

Case Analysis

Nurses should be aware of the health risks, trends in healthcare service delivery, and needs that may be higher for LGBTQ+ individuals. Barriers to healthcare (e.g., provider bias and psychotherapeutic issues), chemical dependency, and its relationship to internalized homophobia, as well as lesbian health concerns related to breast cancer, gynecologic problems, HIV and women, physical and sexual abuse, and mental health, require attention. Transgender individuals have specific healthcare needs at different developmental periods of their life related to transitioning, puberty, hormone use, and possibly surgeries. An understanding of the concerns of high-risk sexual behaviors, substance abuse, HIV infection, intimate partner violence, and coping with many levels of stressors is also essential. Taking universal precautions has helped to avoid targeting specific patients based on LGBTQ+ identity. It is important for nurses to understand risk and protective factors for health conditions more prevalent among LGBTQ+ people. While these are important, this case material focuses primarily on the cultural sensitivity required of nurses in a professional healthcare setting when working with or delivering healthcare to individuals who are LGBTQ+.

The following cases reflect a composite of issues that affect LGBTQ+ individuals who seek healthcare services. Consider the following scenarios:

Scenario 1: Samuel/Samantha (Sam)

Sam is 10 years old and in fifth grade. Sam was born with a penis, and Sam's sex assigned at birth was male. Ever since Sam was a small child, Sam liked wearing "girl clothes" and wanted long hair. Sam self-identified as a girl and insisted that people refer to her as "Samantha" or "Sam"; Sam referred to herself using the pronouns "she" and "her." Sam's parents initially viewed Sam's behavior as "a phase." In school, Sam wanted to play with the girls, and use the girls' bathroom and locker room. Sam wanted to participate on the girls' sports teams. Sam became upset when the health teacher and school nurse did not allow her to attend the presentation about menstruation with the other girls in class. Sam's parents have been struggling with this issue as Sam asserts her gender identity. Sam has been a patient since birth at the pediatric practice where you work.

Scenario 2: Pablo

Pablo is strong academically in school and excels in sports. At 16 years old, he loves soccer and is the high scorer on his high school team. Pablo always knew there was something different about himself. He liked boys growing up, and when adolescence hit, he never found himself attracted to girls in the way the other boys did. In high school, Pablo became more aware of his attraction to males, but said nothing and tried to hide his feelings. His Roman Catholic Latinx family believed that being straight is the only acceptable sexual orientation, and both his ethnic and religious cultures condemned same-sex behavior. Pablo began to struggle with depression as he realized his family would never accept him. He knew there was a counselor at school, but he dared not ask for help or discuss this with her, fearing his parents would learn of his identity. Recently, Pablo had an encounter that involved kissing a teammate on the soccer team, which brought his feelings to light. He felt shame and guilt that overwhelmed him, and worried what might happen if anyone ever found out. Pablo attempted to take his own life. He was admitted to an inpatient facility for treatment. He was ashamed of the disgrace he believed he had brought to his family in being hospitalized for a suicide attempt, and in what they still did not know about him. He does not know if he can or should trust anyone, including the nurses and counselors at the hospital or at school.

WHAT NURSES NEED TO KNOW ABOUT THEMSELVES

Application of the Staircase Self-Assessment Model: Self-Reflection Questions

1. Where am I on the Cultural Competency Staircase? What do I need to do to progress to the next level?
2. How many interactions have I had with people who identify as LGBTQ+? Would I have known at the time that my patient was LGBTQ+? How might these experiences have prepared me for interactions with patients like Sam and Pablo?
3. What assumptions, stereotypes, or generalizations shape my beliefs about the individuals in these case scenarios or other members of the LGBTQ+ community? Do I hold any bias against them?
4. How much have I communicated with patients like Sam and Pablo? How much do I understand the need for recognition and affirmation of identity (Sam), or for an appreciation of shame (Pablo)? Do I minimize these concerns and the experiences of these patients?

5. How do I present myself to patients who are LGBTQ+? Do I seem comfortable and accepting, or nervous and unsure?
6. What steps can I take to improve my ability to be genuine, sincere, and interested in the concerns of my LGBTQ+ patients?
7. Do heterosexism, cissexism, homophobia, and transphobia really exist? In what ways do I participate in heterosexism/cissexism, and what does it mean for me personally to be homo/transphobic?
8. Do I make insensitive statements to or about LGBTQ+ people, or laugh at jokes others tell that involve these individuals?
9. What is the most sensitive way to elicit information about health practices that allows the LGBTQ+ patient to answer questions honestly and enables the nurse to complete an effective assessment? Do I believe I currently have the skills needed to do this?
10. Do I have knowledge of the LGBTQ+ patient's experiences and attitudes toward healthcare? What do I know about LGBTQ+ culture as it varies by generation and subgroups, and the health risks and behaviors of LGBTQ+ patients?

Responses to Self-Reflection Questions

Response: Where am I on the Cultural Competency Staircase? What do I need to do to progress to the next level?

Review the Staircase Self-Assessment Model presented in Chapter 1. Identify where you are in this model regarding sexual orientation and gender identity and expression. What specific steps can you take to progress to the next step?

Response: How many interactions have I had with people who identify as LGBTQ+? Would I have known at the time that my patient was LGBTQ+? How might these experiences have prepared me for interactions with patients like Sam and Pablo?

How many LGBTQ+ people do you know? Take a moment to recall any LGBTQ+ patients for whom you have cared in your training or work experiences. How did you know that you were working with an individual who was LGBTQ+? Although there are some stereotypical behaviors that people assign to LGBTQ+ people based on media representations, most LGBTQ+ people look like everyone else. It is most probable that you have worked with many more LGBTQ+ people than you know about, but perhaps you were unaware of their sexual orientation or gender identity because they did not come out to you. Have you automatically presumed that everyone you know, care for, and work with is heterosexual/cisgender? How can you be more aware and sensitive in your encounters with LGBTQ+ people.

Response: What assumptions, stereotypes, or generalizations shape my beliefs about the individuals in these case scenarios or other members of the LGBTQ+ community? Do I hold any bias against them?

Each person is a product of the society in which we exist. Our communities, family, religious traditions, political and personal experiences, and societal values inform our belief systems. Take a moment now to make a list of everything that comes to mind when you think of LGBTQ+. What enters your consciousness as you jot down your ideas? Did you think of clinical terms and stereotypes, or pride and slogans like "love makes a family"? You may have focused on positive or negative images, or perhaps both, such as social oppression, political issues, marriage equality, bathroom laws, or hate-crimes legislation. How many derogatory terms came into your mind? Do you believe that Sam was acting out behaviorally, "going through a phase," or psychologically ill? Do you have strong religious beliefs that shape your understanding of LGBTQ+ people? How do you feel about Pablo and his family, whose Latinx and Roman Catholic background will affect their perceptions of his gay sexual orientation?

It is important to consider your own starting point in your understanding of sexual orientation and gender identity. Identify your own beliefs—do you think that people "choose" their sexual orientation and gender identity? The science in these two areas is exploding with new knowledge. How do you inform your understanding of gender and sexual orientation to keep up with all that is unfolding? Let us presume in Scenario 2 that Pablo was admitted to a hospital in a religiously sponsored healthcare system, or attended a religiously affiliated school with doctrines that do not endorse LGBTQ+ identities. Most likely, Pablo would have heard negative messages in school, and some may even have come from teachers or the school nurse. Statements indicating that sexual orientation is a choice suggest a belief that it is not "natural" to be gay and view the issue of same-sex attraction as a moral issue, where an individual chooses "bad" behaviors. Identifying your own beliefs will help you to be aware of the perspective you take. Your beliefs can influence your attitudes and treatment of your patients. It is important to base your beliefs on accurate knowledge of the facts about sexual orientation and gender identity. Professional health and mental health associations offer a wealth of information and can serve as resources for reliable research on understanding sexual orientation and gender identity.

Response: How much have I communicated with patients like Sam and Pablo? How much do I understand the need for recognition and affirmation of identity (Sam), or for an appreciation of shame (Pablo)? Do I minimize these concerns and the experiences of these patients?

When we are uncomfortable with something or someone, we may tend to avoid that topic or person. Avoidance can affect communication styles. It is important to use good communication skills to engage patients and their families, including both verbal and nonverbal communication strategies.

Nurses working with clients like Sam and Sam's family will send a message in the moment the issue of transgender identity becomes apparent; thus, it is important to think about this type of scenario before the first time it occurs. How comfortable am I in talking with patients and families about sexual orientation and gender identity? Do I limit, dismiss, minimize, change topics, or say too much or not enough? What do I say to parents who express feelings that their child, like Sam, may be transgender?

Consider if Pablo was in college and his friend, Maria, a lesbian, went to the health center for bronchitis and sees a nurse practitioner (NP) there. Reading Maria's medications on her laptop, the NP asks her if she uses birth control when she does not see it listed. Maria replies no, and the nurse asks why not. Maria states she does not need it, but the NP persists. Maria does not want to come out to a "stranger," but the NP pushes more until Maria finally shares that she is a lesbian. Maria berates herself on the ride home that she did not stand her ground and instead came out to a stranger who immediately typed this information into her medical record. Mostly, nurses treat patients with the utmost respect; they would not intend to convey messages of diminished value or disrespect to patients. Yet, LGBTQ+ patients might have prior negative experiences that heighten their sensitivity to subtle nuance, innuendo, and other meanings, so it is important for nurses to convey respect and genuine concern in communications. A simple yes/no question for heterosexual, cisgender women might have layers of meaning for LGBTQ+ patients.

Response: How do I present myself to patients who are LGBTQ+? Do I seem comfortable and accepting, or nervous and unsure?

It cannot be stated enough how important it is to present oneself as professional. Although this most importantly includes knowledge of one's nursing tasks and duties, it also involves speaking with confidence and respect. Patients will perceive the confidence and dignity professionals convey about them. What they do not know does not threaten or intimidate confident professionals; rather, they are curious to understand so that they can provide a higher level of service. Patients who identify as LGBTQ+ often have experienced negative and rejecting messages about their identity at some point in their past. Many will be particularly adept at picking up signals a nurse may send that being LGBTQ+ is not okay, awkward, or uncomfortable. LGBTQ+ patients sometimes find themselves in the role of reassuring the provider when they do not know how to approach the patient, which is not acceptable. Nurses must assume responsibility for competent practice. Thus, it is important that nurses present a positive, informed, and confident demeanor to LGBTQ+ patients.

It is important to remember that there is great variation among healthcare contexts. Some nurses work in large urban settings with extensive resources and services covering all aspects of healthcare; others may be the only nurse in a rural school setting. Some settings are fast paced, leaving little time with patients. Consider that a transgender man will still need Pap smears. He will probably have to present at a gynecologist's office, sit in the waiting room with mainly heterosexual women, and enter an office that has probably not seen too many other transgender men that day. How comfortable are you in working with this patient? More importantly, how comfortable can nurses make that experience for that patient?

Response: What steps can I take to improve my ability to be genuine, sincere, and interested in the concerns of my LGBTQ+ patients?

This question taps into your fundamental awareness of your feelings about LGBTQ+ people and your core desires about your role as a nursing professional. Most nurses feel drawn to the nursing profession because of a concern for and desire to help others. How much do I care about the needs of people who experience social marginalization and legal discrimination? What attitudes might I need to change to be more accepting of LGBTQ+ patients on my unit? A genuine desire to learn more about the specific needs and healthcare issues facing the LGBTQ+ population will help nurses to provide more competent, sensitive care. Education is power. Attending workshops and trainings about specific needs of LGBTQ+ patients, such as conferences for transgender health and webinars that cover LGBTQ+ health and well-being, can build knowledge, and knowledge builds competence. Meeting LGBTQ+ people in genuine exchanges can also expand sincere interactions.

Response: Do heterosexism, cissexism, homophobia, and transphobia really exist? In what ways do I participate in heterosexism/cissexism, and what does it mean for me personally to be homo/transphobic?

Perhaps the concepts of hetero/cissexism are new for you. Do you believe they exist, or do you scoff at the idea? Think back to the last patient you met. Many healthcare workers do not even consider that a patient might be LGBTQ+. If the patient was wearing a traditional wedding ring, how did you know the person was not in an LGBTQ+ relationship? Consider how you speak to your patients and the presumptions you might be making about them. As noted earlier, Maria was frustrated by her experience with an NP who presumed she needed birth control (heterosexism). While nurses should always ask required questions, they also must be listening to the patient's replies. Patients need to feel accepted and comfortable so that they can entrust you with their care. The way in which nurses ask questions can make a difference in how friendly or hostile the patient perceives the environment. If a nurse mistakenly presumes a patient's identity, this sends a message to the patient that their identity or presence is not the norm. If a nurse believes that heterosexual/cisgender people are somehow better, preferred or "more normal" than LGBTQ+ people, they may alienate LGBTQ+ patients and discourage them from seeking healthcare information or reporting new symptoms.

In considering your awareness about your presumptions and biases around sexual orientation and gender identity, it is important to assess your own comfort level with LGBTQ+ people. Do you know someone personally who is LGBTQ+, such as a family member or close friend? Such individuals are more likely to be accepting of that person, to feel comfortable around them, and are less likely to feel threatened by their identity as LGBTQ+. If you suspect that someone might be LGBTQ+ but that person has not come out to you, why might they have avoided coming out to you? Certainly, it is challenging for LGBTQ+ people to know to whom they can come out, but in focusing on your own self-awareness, note if you are giving off subtle messages that you are "not okay" with such information. Your own discomfort may be sending messages loud and clear that you are uncomfortable with or disgusted by the idea of LGBTQ+ identities. It is possible that Pablo's school nurse also embraced the faith system of his school. Was she giving off nonverbal messages that being gay was unacceptable? Her own knowledge, belief system, and lack of comfort about individuals who are gay could heighten her fears, disgust, and avoidance of gay students. She may not desire to learn more or to challenge her current knowledge of what it means to be LGBTQ+.

Response: Do I make insensitive statements to or about LGBTQ+ people, or laugh at jokes others tell that involve these individuals?

Sometimes insensitive statements or jokes result from surprise, insecurity, lack of knowledge, or not knowing how to handle a situation in the moment. Did the nurse tell Sam's parents not to worry because it was probably "just a phase"? Did Sam's parents and healthcare providers continue to refer to Sam as "he" despite Sam's insistence that her gender identity was "a girl"? We can only wonder how the different staff at the pediatrics office responded to Sam, from the receptionist and the nurse to any others the family encountered. Most of the team probably focused solely on providing the best care possible for their patient in need. Yet, it is possible that someone uncomfortable with Sam's identity may have snickered or made a sarcastic comment or some other insensitive statement. Such comments may have evoked a level of discomfort in some of the other nurses in the office who felt that it was not their role to pass judgment, but instead to provide medical care to Sam. It would not be surprising for an individual like this to refer to transgender people in a derogatory manner. These insensitive statements reflect biases and beliefs that LGBTQ+ people are somehow flawed or that Sam was "just going through a phase."

Although many professionals are not likely to be as overt, even the most sensitive people can still unintentionally create dissonance between themselves and LGBTQ+ patients. The more interactions with LGBTQ+ patients nurses have, the more aware they can be to increasing sensitivity to the unique needs of this population. The desire to understand the oppression and discrimination faced by LGBTQ+ people can help nurses to see that insensitive comments and jokes can be harmful to their well-being.

Response: What is the most sensitive way to elicit information about health practices that allows the LGBTQ+ patient to answer questions honestly and enables the nurse to complete an effective assessment? Do I believe I currently have the skills needed to do this?

Imagine that you are the nurse reviewing Maria's medical record in the doctor's office or Sam's health visits. What is the most sensitive way to obtain needed information? Some nurses feel uncomfortable requesting personal information from any patient, but especially in areas related to sexuality, sexual orientation, and gender identity. Rehearsing your interviewing skills with a clinical supervisor or a trusted colleague will help you to reduce your discomfort. Strategies for effective interventions can help to reduce healthcare disparities for LGBTQ+ people. Practice asking questions that make you feel uncomfortable until you can ask them smoothly and without judgment or hesitation.

There are specific strategies that a nurse can use to identify a patient's support system without putting those questions in a hetero/cisnormative context. For example, the nurse can ask if the individual is in a significant relationship and with whom. Some LGBTQ+ patients have been married in traditional heterosexual relationships in the past, even though they may now be in a gay, lesbian, bisexual, or pansexual relationship. It is clinically appropriate in certain contexts to know a woman's sexual history, as certain activities may put the woman at risk for different forms of cancer or other diseases. Asking a woman if she is straight or gay may not elicit this information; rather, the nurse can inquire about the patient's prior behaviors. Effective communication requires skillful interviewing, knowledge about the healthcare needs relevant to this population, and experience through relationships with individuals; these help nurses increase their comfort level in providing care to individuals who do not fit "traditional" family constellations and relationships.

Response: Do I have knowledge of the LGBTQ+ patient's experiences and attitudes toward healthcare? What do I know about LGBTQ+ culture as it varies by generation and subgroups, and the health risks and behaviors of LGBTQ+ patients?

It is important for nurses to know some of the history of gays and lesbians and the healthcare system. It was not until 1973 that the American Psychiatric Association transitioned from its view of homosexuality as a mental disorder in the *DSM* and began to classify "homosexuality" as an orientation or expression. Prior to this, gay and lesbian patients were subject to numerous interventions, ranging from institutionalization to electroconvulsive shock therapy. Intersex individuals often grew up having had a doctor determine their sex/gender, and transgender people were often treated as if their status was purely a mental health disorder. Given this historical background and negative social attitudes, it is not difficult to understand why many LGBTQ+ individuals might approach the healthcare system with caution and hesitation, particularly older generations who lived through many of these experiences.

The case of Sam demonstrates the ambivalence and concern of LGBTQ+ patients and families in how to complete admission forms and paperwork that ask for gender. Depending on their own comfort and acceptance, the parents themselves might answer contrary to what Sam would say, or perhaps they are just confused on how to answer that they are not sure. Many forms now include an "unsure" or "other" box on paperwork, which can be helpful. If Sam needed an inpatient procedure, how do Sam's parents respond to the many questions they are asked? Perhaps they hesitate to share information because they fear a response or how Sam might be treated. If Sam was older, perhaps 16, and admitted to the floor, what is the hospital's policy about her room? Are there single accommodations for transgender patients, or is Sam placed in a room with another male or female patient? Sam must assess the safety of "coming out," and yet may not have much control over this. Sam may wonder of each nurse and aide who toilets her or helps her to bathe: Is this person safe? Will I experience discrimination? Do they view me as a curiosity? It starts again each time there is a shift change. The patient expends a lot of energy assessing each healthcare worker's attitude and acceptance, while other patients spend their energy on healing. For LGBTQ+ people, there is a cost to telling the truth and a cost to be holding back. If the patient is in a committed relationship, they may be worried about how their spouse or partner might be treated.

Generationally, it is important for nurses to recognize that older LGBTQ+ people may have different ways of identifying as LGBTQ+ than do younger people. Years of anti-LGBTQ+ policies such as "don't ask, don't tell" in the military and a lack of marriage equality for most of their lives may affect their comfort levels with disclosure. Younger LGBTQ+ people may speak more freely but still experience rejection. In Sam's case, her parents may hesitate to share their questions and concerns about her gender identity with their healthcare providers.

A FINAL WORD TO GAY, LESBIAN, BISEXUAL, TRANSGENDER, NONBINARY AND GENDER NONCONFORMING NURSES

Although readers may have approached the chapter as geared to heterosexual, cisgender readers, it is quite likely that LGBTQ+ nurses are reading this chapter as well. While mainly supported by the nursing profession, LGBTQ+ nurses can also face challenges. It is hopeful and reassuring that many caring LGBTQ+ nurses also work in various roles in the healthcare system and are sensitive to the issues faced by LGBTQ+ patients.

For LGBTQ+ nurses, one's identity can raise challenges in working with patients more than with coworkers. Will the patient not want me to provide care if my sexual orientation or gender identity is known? Stereotypes of LGBTQ+ people as highly sexualized, focused only on sex, and wanting to "hit" on everyone and anyone still abound, despite the absurdity of such beliefs. How will the patient react to me as a nurse if the patient learns of my sexual orientation or gender identity? Will the patient not want me to assist with toileting, bathing, and other activities of daily living, or with medical treatments?

With growing anti-LGBTQ+ sentiment related to recent political extremism and anti-LGBTQ+ rhetoric, workplace discrimination may also be a concern for the LGBTQ+ nurse. Will my coworkers treat me differently if they know that I am LGBTQ+? Will administration withhold promotions or compensations? If I make an error, will it be attributed to characteristics of my sexual orientation or gender identity? If I receive extra challenging work assignments, how will I know whether this is just my turn to receive a challenging assignment or whether someone has some hidden feelings against my sexual orientation or gender identity? These uncertainties challenge LGBTQ+ people in any workplace. As a microcosm of a larger society, the healthcare world reflects many of the same concerns found in other workplaces.

On a positive note, LGBTQ+ nurses can offer the healthcare workplace a wealth of knowledge and skills. As LGBTQ+ people themselves, these nurses are aware of issues of concern to LGBTQ+ patients. LGBTQ+ nurses can be a visible sign of safety to LGBTQ+ patients who may view such staff as sensitive **allies**, helpers, and advocates to the unique circumstances of their care. In some cases, LGBTQ+ nurses can serve as cultural translators to other healthcare providers unfamiliar with the challenges and fears faced by patients. They can provide education to staff, patients, and families of patients, and serve on committees to improve sensitivity to issues of concern for LGBTQ+ patients and staff.

SUMMARY

The case scenarios of Sam and Pablo highlight some of the key issues relevant to working with an LGBTQ+ individual. Hetero/cissexism and homo/transphobia can creep into the practice of even the most well-intentioned healthcare providers. It is important to promote a healthcare environment that accepts all people, regardless of sexual orientation or gender identity. The Staircase Self-Assessment Model can provide a structure for assessing the key areas of cultural competency as they pertain to sexual orientation and gender identity. Staff education can provide a valuable avenue for raising nurses' awareness, knowledge, and skill level in encounters with LGBTQ+ individuals. LGBTQ+ people exist across every age, ability status, religion, race, ethnicity, and political and socioeconomic status. Thus, nurses can expect to care for LGBTQ+ patients at some time in their career.

School nurses can work to promote safety in the schools, reduce harassment of LGBTQ+ students and the resulting physical and emotional injuries that occur because of it, and help young people just coming out or transitioning to feel supported and safe. Home-care nurses can be sure that patients are receiving sensitive care in their homes, and inpatient hospital unit nurses can help to raise awareness of LGBTQ+ patients' needs, both clinical and psychosocial.

NCLEX®-TYPE QUESTIONS

1. A culturally competent nurse leads a staff development workshop for nurses on the care of patients who are LGBTQ+. What statement by the nurse conveys the most accurate information about the acronym LGBTQ+?
   A. It is a term that describes an organization in support of gay people.
   B. It is an umbrella term for individuals who are antigay.
   C. It is an umbrella term that reflects both gender identity and sexual orientation identities.
   D. It is a term that refers only to males who are gay.

2. A nurse is assigned to care for a newly admitted patient who sustained multiple injuries in a car crash and requires complete care. The patient self-identifies as a lesbian and is accompanied by her partner of 10 years. What action by the nurse suggests a need for further staff development in the care of patients who are LGBTQ+?
   A. The nurse asks the patient's partner if she has any questions and allows her to assist the nurses by feeding the patient.
   B. The nurse reminds the patient's partner that visiting hours are not until 2 p.m., but only close members of the family will be permitted in to see the patient at that time.
   C. The nurse includes the patient's partner in the discussion during the interview when collecting information about the patient's medical history.
   D. The nurse documents the patient's partner's contact information on the chart.

3. A nurse is working on a pediatric unit where a 15-year-old male patient has confided to the nurse that he is uncomfortable sharing with his parents that he believes he is probably gay. On reflecting on this situation, the nurse considers that the young man has expressed a concern about what aspect of himself? *Select all that apply.*
   A. Gender identity
   B. Sexual orientation
   C. Attraction to members of the same sex
   D. View of himself as a female

4. What statement is true about the impact of attitudinal barriers on individuals who are LGBTQ+?
   A. The impact of stereotyping and discrimination is evident throughout the life span of persons who are LGBTQ+.
   B. Only teenagers and young adults who are LGBTQ+ and sexually active are affected by discrimination.
   C. The impact of discrimination against LGBTQ+ is most notable in midlife.
   D. Senior citizens who are LGBTQ+ are no longer impacted by discrimination toward persons who are LGBTQ+.

5. When giving the change of shift report to the other nurses on her unit, a young female nurse explains that a middle-aged male patient on the unit "appears to be gay." She further states that as a result she is uncomfortable caring for the patient until she is certain about his HIV status. The culturally competent nurse receiving the report appreciates that the nurse's comments probably reflect the younger nurse's:
   A. Ageism
   B. Heterosexism
   C. Homophobia
   D. Transphobia

6. A nurse states to one of her colleagues that she believes that any patient who self-identifies as being a member of the LGBTQ+ population is experiencing some type of psychologic problem. What statement by the nurse colleague offers the most appropriate response?
   A. "Psychologic problems are found among members of every cultural group."
   B. "Some gay and lesbian patients have psychologic problems, some do not."
   C. "Everyone has attitudes based on their own beliefs; however, the American Psychiatric Association removed homosexuality from the *Diagnostic and Statistical Manual of Mental Disorders* in the early 1970s."
   D. "This is probably true, but nurses should not judge anyone."

7. The nurse who expresses the belief that being gay is a choice made by individuals who are deviating from the normal or appropriate sexual behavior pattern is exemplifying what characteristic?
   A. Heterosexism
   B. Ethnocentrism
   C. Homophobia
   D. Centrism

8. The first action by nurses who are seeking to provide culturally sensitive care to patients who are LGBTQ+ is to:
   A. Gain an understanding of their own beliefs and attitudes about members of this group
   B. Seek information about the health risks in this population
   C. Attempt to learn about what it means to be LGBTQ+
   D. Involve themselves in advocacy groups to assist members of the group

9. What statement best describes the role of the culturally competent nurse in providing care to patients who are LGBTQ+? Culturally competent nurses:
   A. Abandon their own values and beliefs and adopt those of the patients for whom they are caring
   B. Recognize their personal discomfort level and refer patients to other resources when they are personally unable to assist them
   C. Seek training, professional workshops, and journals to explore information about topics related to patients who are LGBTQ+
   D. Advocate for patients and coworkers as the first step on the staircase of cultural competency

10. The ED nurse interviews a 32-year-old patient who has come to the ED alone complaining of severe headache. Her blood pressure is 160/110 and she is being admitted until her hypertension is stabilized. During the interview, the nurse asks if the patient is married or single. The patient hesitates and then responds, "I'm married." What statement by the nurse reflects an effort to be culturally sensitive in this situation?
   A. "What is your husband's name and cell phone number?"
   B. "Is there a significant person or family member you would like me to contact?"
   C. "Who is your next of kin? Are there children I might get in touch with?"
   D. "Are you sure? You seem hesitant."

ANSWERS TO NCLEX-TYPE QUESTIONS

1. C
2. B
3. B and C
4. A
5. C
6. C
7. A
8. A
9. C
10. B

AMERICAN ASSOCIATION OF COLLEGES OF NURSING COMPETENCIES ADDRESSED IN THIS CHAPTER

1. Apply knowledge of social and cultural factors that affect nursing and healthcare across multiple contexts.
2. Use relevant data sources and best evidence in providing culturally competent care.

3. Promote achievement of safe and quality outcomes of care for diverse populations.
4. Advocate for social justice, including commitment to the health of vulnerable populations and the elimination of healthcare disparities.
5. Participate in continuous cultural competence development.

A robust set of instructor resources designed to supplement this text is located at http://connect.springerpub.com/content/book/978-0-8261-8302-6. Qualifying instructors may request access by emailing textbook@springerpub.com.

REFERENCES

American Civil Liberties Union. (2023). *How state lawmakers are targeting LGBTQ rights*. Author. https://www.aclu.org/legislative-attacks-on-lgbtq-rights?state=PA

American Psychiatric Association. (2013). *Diagnostic and statistical manual of mental disorders* (5th ed.). https://doi.org/10.1176/appi.books.9780890425596

American Psychiatric Association. (2022). *Diagnostic and statistical manual of mental disorders* (5th ed., text rev.). https://doi.org/10.1176/appi.books.9780890425787

American Psychiatric Association. (2023). DSM-5-TR *fact sheets: Updated disorders: Gender dysphoria*. https://www.psychiatry.org/psychiatrists/practice/dsm/educational-resources/dsm-5-tr-fact-sheets

American Psychological Association. (n.d.). *Banning sexual orientation and gender identity change efforts*. Retrieved December 28, 2023, from https://www.apa.org/topics/lgbtq/sexual-orientation-change

Amin, K. (2023). Taxonomically queer?: Sexology and new queer, trans, and asexual identities. *GLQ: A Journal of Lesbian & Gay Studies, 29*(1), 91–107. https://doi.org/10.1215/10642684-10144435

Ashley, F. (2020). A critical commentary on "rapid-onset gender dysphoria." *Sociological Review, 68*(4), 779–799. https://doi.org/10.1177/0038026120934693

Azagba, S., Ebling, T., Adekeye, O. T., & Shan, L. (2022). Mental health condition indicators and e-cigarette use among sexual minority youth. *Journal of Affective Disorders, 319*, 1–7. https://doi.org/10.1016/j.jad.2022.09.032

Bauer, G. R., Lawson, M. L., & Metzger, D. L. (2022). Do clinical data from transgender adolescents support the phenomenon of "rapid onset gender dysphoria"? *The Journal of Pediatrics, 243*, 224–227. https://doi.org/10.1016/j.jpeds.2021.11.020

Blackwell, C. W., & López Castillo, H. (2020). Use of electronic nicotine delivery systems (ENDS) in lesbian, gay, bisexual, transgender and queer persons: Implications for public health nursing. *Public Health Nursing, 37*(4), 569–580. https://doi.org/10.1111/phn.12746

Boyd, M., Cygan, H. R., Marshall, B., Little, D., & Bejster, M. (2022). Supporting and establishing gender and sexuality alliances in Chicago public schools. *The Journal of School Nursing*, 10598405221142306. https://doi.org/10.1177/10598405221142306

Camminga, B. (2022). Competing marginalities and precarious politics: A South African case study of NGO representation of transgender refugees. *Gender, Place & Culture: A Journal of Feminist Geography*, 1–18. https://doi.org/10.1080/0966369x.2022.2137473

Canadian Institutes of Health Research. (2023, March). *What is gender? What is sex?* https://cihr-irsc.gc.ca/e/48642.html

Chappell, B. (2022, May 13). *Texas Supreme Court OKs state child abuse inquiries into the families of trans kids. NPR special series: Efforts to restrict rights for LGBTQ youth*. NPR. https://www.npr.org/2022/05/13/1098779201/texas-supreme-court-transgender-gender-affirming-child-abuse

Clark, F. (2014). Discrimination against LGBT people triggers health concerns. *Lancet, 383*(9916), 500–502. https://doi.org/10.1016/s0140-6736(14)60169-0

Clarke, J. A. (2022). Sex assigned at birth. *Columbia Law Review, 122*(7), 1821–1898. https://www.jstor.org/stable/27178460

Clary, K., Goffnett, J., King, M., Hubbard, T., & Kitchen, R. (2022). "It's the environment, not me": Experiences shared by transgender and gender diverse adults living in Texas. *Journal of Community Psychology, 51*(3), 1–18. https://doi.org/10.1002/jcop.22948

Coleman, E., Radix, A. E., Bouman, W. P., Brown, G. R., de Vries, A. L. C., Deutsch, M. B., Ettner, R., Fraser, L., Goodman, M., Green, J., Hancock, A. B., Johnson, T. W., Karasic, D. H., Knudson, G. A., Leibowitz, S. F., Meyer-Bahlburg, H. F. L., Monstrey, S. J., Motmans, J., Nahata, L., ... Arcelus, J. (2022). Standards of care for the health of transgender and gender diverse people, Version 8. *International Journal of Transgender Health, 23*(S1), S1–S260. https://doi.org/10.1080/26895269.2022.2100644

Colineaux, H., Soulier, A., Lepage, B., & Kelly-Irving, M. (2022). Considering sex and gender in epidemiology: A challenge beyond terminology. From conceptional analysis to methodological strategies. *Biology of Sex Differences, 13*(1), 1–10. https://doi.org/10.1186/s13293-022-00430-6

Collet, D. S., Kiyar, M., Martens, K., Vangeneugden, J., Mueller, S., & T'Sjoen, G. (2022). Minimal change in minority stress after a 6 month follow up in a transgender population. *Journal of Sexual Medicine, 19*(11), S65. https://doi.org/10.1016/j.jsxm.2022.08.072

Colliver, B., & Silvestri, M. (2022). The role of (in)visibility in hate crime targeting transgender people. *Criminology & Criminal Justice, 22*(2), 235–253. https://doi.org/10.1177/1748895820930747

Coulter, R. W. S., & Gartner, R. E. (2023). LGBTQ+ youth-generated intervention concepts for reducing teen dating violence inequities. *Health Promotion Practice, 24*(2), 252–257. https://doi.org/10.1177/15248399221137276

Crenshaw, K. (1991). Mapping the margins: Intersectionality, identity politics, and violence against women of color. *Stanford Law Review, 43*(6), 1241–1299. https://doi.org/10.2307/1229039

Di Lorito, C., Bosco, A., Peel, E., Hinchliff, S., Dening, T., Calasanti, T., de Vries, B., Cutler, N., Fredriksen-Goldsen, K. I., & Harwood, R. H. (2022). Are dementia services and support organisations meeting the needs of lesbian, gay, bisexual and transgender (LGBT) caregivers of LGBT people living with dementia? A scoping review of the literature. *Aging & Mental Health, 26*(10), 1912–1921, https://doi.org/10.1080/13607863.2021.2008870

Diaz, J. (2022, March 28). *Florida's governor signs controversial law opponents dubbed 'Don't Say Gay.' NPR special series: Efforts to restrict rights for LGBTQ youth.* https://www.npr.org/2022/03/28/1089221657/dont-say-gay-florida-desantis

Dickson, L., Bunting, S., Nanna, A., Taylor, M., Spencer, M., & Hein, L. (2022). Older lesbian, gay, bisexual, transgender, and queer adults' experiences with discrimination and impacts on expectations for long-term care: Results of a survey in the Southern United States. *Journal of Applied Gerontology, 41*(3), 650–660. https://doi.org/10.1177/07334648211048189

Drescher, C. F., Griffin, J. A., Casanova, T., Kassing, F., Wood, E., Brands, S., & Stepleman, L. M. (2021). Associations of physical and sexual violence victimisation, homelessness, and perceptions of safety with suicidality in a community sample of transgender individuals. *Psychology & Sexuality, 12*(1–2), 52–63. https://doi.org/10.1080/19419899.2019.1690032

Drescher, J. (2015). Out of DSM: Depathologizing homosexuality. *Behavioral Sciences, 5*, 565–575. https://doi.org/10.3390/bs5040565

Elliott, K. J., Stacciarini, J.-M. R., Jimenez, I. A., Rangel, A. P., & Fanfan, D. (2022). A review of psychosocial protective and risk factors for the mental well-being of rural LGBTQ+ adolescents. *Youth & Society, 54*(2), 312–341. https://doi.org/10.1177/0044118X211035944

Flores, A. R., Stotzer, R. L., Meyer, I. H., & Langton, L. L. (2022). Hate crimes against LGBT people: National crime victimization survey, 2017–2019. *PLoS ONE, 17*(12), 1–15. https://doi.org/10.1371/journal.pone.0279363

Gay, Lesbian, Straight Educators' Network. (2021). *The 2021 national school climate survey: The experiences of LGBTQ+ youth in our nation's schools.* Author. https://www.glsen.org/research/2021-national-school-climate-survey

Genovese, A. C., Singh, S. C., Casubhoy, I., & Hellings, J. A. (2022). Gender diverse autistic young adults: A mental health perspective. *Archives of Sexual Behavior, 52*, 1339–1343. https://doi.org/10.1007/s10508-022-02443-z

Ghassabian, A., Suleri, A., Blok, E., Franch, B., Hillegers, M. H. J., & White, T. (2022). Adolescent gender diversity: Sociodemographic correlates and mental health outcomes in the general population. *Journal of Child Psychology & Psychiatry, 63*(11), 1415–1422. https://doi.org/10.1111/jcpp.13588

Gottvall, M., Brunell, C., Eldebo, A., Johansson Metso, F., Jirwe, M., & Carlsson, T. (2023). Post-migration psychosocial experiences and challenges amongst LGBTQ+ forced migrants: A meta-synthesis of qualitative reports. *Journal of Advanced Nursing, 79*(1), 358–371. https://doi.org/10.1111/jan.15480

Gridley, S. J., Crouch, J. M., Evans, Y., Eng, W., McCarty, C., Ahrens, K., & Breland, D. J. (2016). Youth and caregiver perspectives on barriers to gender-affirming health care for transgender youth. *Journal of Adolescent Health, 59*(3), 254–261. https://doi.org/10.1016/j.jadohealth.2016.03.017

Harrison, S. E., Paton, M., Muessig, K. E., Vecchio, A. C., Hanson, L. A., & Hightow-Weidman, L. B. (2022). "Do I want PrEP or do I want a roof?": Social determinants of health and HIV prevention in the southern United States. *AIDS Care, 34*(11), 1435–1442. https://doi.org/10.1080/09540121.2022.2029816

Hernandez, J. (2022, April 11). U.S. citizens can now choose the gender "X" on their passport applications. *National Public Radio (NPR).* https://www.npr.org/2022/04/11/1092000203/gender-x-us-passport-applications

Human Rights Campaign. (2023a). *Faith positions.* https://www.hrc.org/resources/faith-positions

Human Rights Campaign. (2023b). *Policy and position statements on conversion therapy.* https://www.hrc.org/resources/policy-and-position-statements-on-conversion-therapy

International Olympic Committee. (2021, November). *IOC framework on fairness, inclusion and non-discrimination on the basis of gender identity and sex variations.* https://stillmed.olympics.com/media/Documents/Beyond-the-Games/Human-Rights/IOC-Framework-Fairness-Inclusion-Non-discrimination-2021.pdf

Ioverno, S., Nappa, M. R., Russell, S. T., & Baiocco, R. (2022). Student intervention against homophobic name-calling: The role of peers, teachers, and inclusive curricula. *Journal of Interpersonal Violence, 37*(21–22), NP19549–NP19575. https://doi.org/10.1177/08862605211042817

James, S. E., Herman, J. L., Rankin, S., Keisling, M., Mottet, L., & Anafi, M. (2016). *The report of the 2015 U.S. transgender survey.* National Center for Transgender Equality. https://transequality.org/sites/default/files/docs/usts/USTS-Full-Report-Dec17.pdf

Jones, P. E., & Becker, A. B. (2023). Affect toward transgender people, political awareness, and support for transgender rights. *American Politics Research, 51*(1), 76–80. https://doi.org/10.1177/1532673X221090488

Just the Facts Coalition. (1999; revised 2006). *Just the facts about sexual orientation & youth*. American Psychological Association. https://www.apa.org/pi/lgbt/resources/just-the-facts

Kia, H., Rutherford, L., Jackson, R., Grigorovich, A., Ricote, C. L., Scheim, A. I. & Bauer, G. (2022). Impacts of COVID-19 on trans and non-binary people in Canada: A qualitative analysis of responses to a national survey. *BMC Public Health, 22*, 1284 [Open Access]. https://doi.org/10.1186/s12889-022-13684-x

Kim, J. (2023, March 24). *Transgender track and field athletes can't compete in women's international events*. NPR: Sports.https://www.npr.org/2023/03/24/1165795462/transgender-track-and-field-athletes-cant-compete-in-womens-international-events

Kum, S. (2017). Gay, gray, black, and blue: An examination of some of the challenges faced by older LGBTQ people of color. *Journal of Gay & Lesbian Mental Health, 21*(3), 228–239. https://doi.org/10.1080/19359705.2 017.1320742

Kurdyla, V. (2022). Advocating for transgender immigrants in detention centers: Cisnormativity as a tool for racialized social control. *American Behavioral Scientist, 66*(13), 1777–1796. https://doi .org/10.1177/00027642221083531

Lambda Legal. (2023). *Fact sheets*. https://www.lambdalegal.org/publications/fact-sheets

Leonard, A., Broussard, J., Jain, J., Kumar, S., Santos, G., & Dawson, R. C. (2022). Prevalence and correlates of methamphetamine use in transitional age youth experiencing homelessness or housing instability in San Francisco, CA. *Journal of Nursing Scholarship, 55*(3), 711–720. https://doi.org/10.1111/jnu.12856

Leonard, M. (2022). 'It was probably one of the best moments of being trans, honestly!': Exploring the positive school experiences of transgender children and young people. *Educational and Child Psychology, 39*(1), 44–59. https://explore.bps.org.uk/content/bpsecp

López, G., Yeater, E. A., Veldhuis, C. B., Venner, K. L., Verney, S. P., & Hughes, T. L. (2023). Sexual assault, psychological distress, and protective factors in a community sample of Black, Latinx, and White lesbian and bisexual women. *Journal of Interpersonal Violence, 38*(1–2), NP1239–NP1260. https://doi .org/10.1177/08862605221090570

Mahon, C. P., Lombard-Vance, R., Kiernan, G., Pachankis, J. E., & Gallagher, P. (2022). Social anxiety among sexual minority individuals: A systematic review. *Psychology & Sexuality, 13*(4), 818–862. https://doi.org/10.1080/ 19419899.2021.1936140

Martinez, D., Jansen, N., Royer, G., & Kennedy, H. (2022). Creating a virtual network to support LGBTQIA+ youth in rural settings: Development of Colorado's queer youth network. *Health Promotion Practice, 24*(4), 606–608. https://doi.org/10.1177/15248399221142629

Mata, D., Korpak, A. K., Macaulay, T., Dodge, B., Mustanski, B., & Feinstein, B. A. (2022). Substance use experiences among bisexual, pansexual, and queer (Bi+) male youth: A qualitative study of motivations, consequences, and decision making. *Archives of Sexual Behavior, 52*(3), 1169–1181. https://doi.org/10.1007/ s10508-022-02447-9

McGowan, A., Wright, S., & Sargeant, C. (2022). Living your truth: Views and experiences of transgender young people in secondary education. *Educational & Child Psychology, 39*(1), 27–43. https://doi.org/10.53841/ bpsecp.2022.39.1.27

Merriam-Webster. (n.d.). They. In *Merriam-Webster.com dictionary*. Retrieved April 12, 2023, from https://www. merriam-webster.com/dictionary/they

Meyer, I. H. (2003). Prejudice, social stress, and mental health in lesbian, gay, and bisexual populations: Conceptual issues and research evidence. *Psychological Bulletin, 129*(5), 674–697. https://doi.org/10.1037/0033-2909.129.5.674

Migdon, B. (2022, May 31). Here are the states where you can (and cannot) change your gender designation on official documents. *The Hill (Changing America)*. https://thehill.com/changing-america/respect/diversity-inclusion/3507206-here-are-the-states-where-you-can-and-cannot-change-your-gender-designation-on-official-documents

Movement Advancement Project. (2023). *Conversion "therapy" laws*. http://www.lgbtmap.org/equality-maps/ conversion_therapy

National Association of Social Workers & National Committee on Lesbian, Gay, Bisexual and Transgender Issues. (2015). Position statement: *Sexual orientation change efforts (SOCE) and conversion therapy with lesbians, gay men, bisexuals, and transgender persons*. Author. https://www.socialworkers.org/LinkClick. aspx?fileticket=yH3UsGQQmYI%3D

NCAA. (2021). *Transgender student-athlete participation policy, p. 156*. https://www.ncaa.org/sports/2022/1/27/ transgender-participation-policy.aspx

Parental Rights in Education. (2023, March). *Florida HB 1069, subsection 9 of section 1, 1000.21, p. 4*. https://www .flsenate.gov/Session/Bill/2023/1069/BillText/c2/PDF

Parra, L. A., Spahr, C. M., Goldbach, J. T., Bray, B. C., Kipke, M. D., & Slavich, G. M. (2022). Greater lifetime stressor exposure is associated with poorer mental health among sexual minority people of color. *Journal of Clinical Psychology, 79*(4), 1130–1155. https://doi.org/10.1002/jclp.23463

Patten, M., Carmichael, H., Moore, A., & Velopulos, C. (2022). Circumstances of suicide among lesbian, gay, bisexual and transgender individuals. *Journal of Surgical Research, 270*, 522–529. https://doi.org/10.1016/j.jss.2021.08.029

Pepin-Neff, C., & Cohen, A. (2021). President Trump's transgender moral panic. *Policy Studies, 42*(5–6), 646–661. https://doi.org/10.1080/01442872.2021.1952971

Platt, L. F., & Milam, S. R. B. (2018). Public discomfort with gender appearance-inconsistent bathroom use: The oppressive bind of bathroom laws for transgender individuals. *Gender Issues, 35*(3), 181–201. https://doi .org/10.1007/s12147-017-9197-6

Ramirez, J. L., & Paz Galupo, M. (2019). Multiple minority stress: The role of proximal and distal stress on mental health outcomes among lesbian, gay, and bisexual people of color. *Journal of Gay & Lesbian Mental Health, 23*(2), 145–167. https://doi.org/10.1080/19359705.2019.1568946

Rivas-Koehl, M., Valido, A., Espelage, D. L., Robinson, L. E., Hong, J. S., Kuehl, T., Mintz, S., & Wyman, P. A. (2020). Understanding protective factors for suicidality and depression among U.S. sexual and gender minority adolescents: Implications for school psychologists. *School Psychology Review, 51*(3), 290–303. https://doi.org /10.1080/2372966X.2021.1881411

Roberts, N. J., Harvey, L. A., Poulos, R. G., Ní Shé, É., Dillon Savage, I., Rafferty, G., & Ivers, R. (2022). Lesbian, gay, bisexual, transgender and gender diverse and queer (LGBTQ) community members' perspectives on palliative care in New South Wales (NSW), Australia. *Health & Social Care in the Community, 30*(6), e5926–e5945. https://doi.org/10.1111/hsc.14024

Rodríguez-Díaz, C. E., Jovet-Toledo, G. G., Vélez-Vega, C. M., Ortiz-Sánchez, E. J., Santiago-Rodríguez, E. I., Vargas-Molina, R. L., Rodríguez Madera, S. L., & Mulinelli-Rodríguez, J. J. (2016). Discrimination and health among lesbian, gay, bisexual and trans people in Puerto Rico. *Puerto Rico Health Sciences Journal, 35*(3), 154–159. https://prhsj.rcm.upr.edu/index.php/prhsj/article/view/1337/1021

Rosa, W. E., Roberts, K. E., Braybrook, D., Harding, R., Godwin, K., Mahoney, C., Mathew, S., Atkinson, T. M., Banerjee, S. C., Haviland, K., Hughes, T. L., Walters, C. B., & Parker, P. A. (2022). Palliative and end-of-life care needs, experiences, and preferences of LGBTQ+ individuals with serious illness: A systematic mixed-methods review. *Palliative Medicine, 37*(4), 460–474. https://doi.org/10.1177/02692163221124426

Russomanno, J., & Jabson Tree, J. M. (2020). Food insecurity and food pantry use among transgender and gender non-conforming people in the Southeast United States. *BMC Public Health, 20*(1), 1–11. https://doi .org/10.1186/s12889-020-08684-8

Sava, L. M., Earnshaw, V. A., Menino, D. D., Perrotti, J., & Reisner, S. L. (2021). LGBTQ student health: A mixed-methods study of unmet needs in Massachusetts schools. *Journal of School Health, 91*(11), 894–905. https:// onlinelibrary.wiley.com/doi/10.1111/josh.13082

Scharaga, E. A., Chang, A., & Kulas, J. F. (2021). What happens when we forget our own narrative: Transgender dementia case study. *The Clinical Neuropsychologist, 35*(8), 1485–1497. https://doi.org/10.1080/13854046.2020.1766575

Schuler, M. S., & Evans-Polce, R. J. (2022). Perceived substance use risks among never users: Sexual identity differences in a sample of U.S. young adults. *American Journal of Preventive Medicine, 63*(6), 987–996. https:// doi.org/10.1016/j.amepre.2022.07.003

Stokes, L. (2018, November 19). Position statement: Nursing advocacy for LGBTQ+ populations. *The Online Journal of Issues in Nursing, 24*(1). https://doi.org/10.3912/OJIN.Vol24No01PoSCol02

Strang, J. F., Chen, D., Nelson, E., Leibowitz, S. F., Nahata, L., Anthony, L. G., Song, A., Grannis, C., Graham, E., Henise, S., Vilain, E., Sadikova, E., Freeman, A., Pugliese, C., Khawaja, A., Maisashvili, T., Mancilla, M., & Kenworthy, L. (2022). Transgender youth executive functioning: Relationships with anxiety symptoms, Autism Spectrum Disorder, and gender-affirming medical treatment status. *Child Psychiatry & Human Development, 53*(6), 1252–1265. https://doi.org/10.1007/s10578-021-01195-6

Suhomlinova, O., O'Reilly, M., Ayres, T. C., Wertans, E., Tonkin, M. J., & O'Shea, S. C. (2023). "Gripping onto the last threads of sanity": Transgender and non-binary prisoners' mental health challenges during the Covid-19 pandemic. *International Journal of Mental Health, 52*(3), 218–238. https://doi.org/10.1080/00207411.2022.2068319

Teran, M., Abreu, R. L., Tseung, E. S., & Castellanos, J. (2022). Latinx fathers of transgender and gender diverse people: Journey toward acceptance and role of culture. *Family Relations: An Interdisciplinary Journal of Applied Family Studies, 74*(4), 1908–1925. https://doi.org/10.1111/fare.12799

Totenberg, N. (2021, June 17). *Supreme Court rules Catholic group doesn't have to consider LGBTQ foster parents.* NPR: All Things Considered. https://www.npr.org/2021/06/17/996670391/supreme-court-rules-for-a-catholic-group-in-a-case-involving-gay-rights-foster-c

Turban, J. (2022, August). *What is gender dysphoria?* American Psychiatric Association. https://www.psychiatry .org/patients-families/gender-dysphoria/what-is-gender-dysphoria#section_3

IMPORTANT WEBSITES

American Academy of Pediatrics (AAP). Retrieved from www.aap.org

American Nurses Association (ANA). Retrieved from www.nursingworld.org

American Psychological Association (APA). Retrieved from www.apa.org

Centers for Disease Control & Prevention (CDC): Lesbian, Gay, Bisexual & Transgender Health. Retrieved from www.cdc.gov/lgbthealth/index.htm

Gay, Lesbian, Straight Educators' Network (GLSEN). Retrieved from www.glsen.org

GLMA: Health Professionals Advancing LGBT Equality (Previously Known as the Gay & Lesbian Medical Association). Retrieved from www.glma.org

Human Rights Campaign (HRC). Retrieved from www.hrc.org

Lambda Legal. Retrieved from www.lambdalegal.org

National Association of School Nurses. Retrieved from www.nasn.org/advocacy/professional-practice-documents/position-statements/ps-lgbtq

National Association of Social Workers (NASW). Retrieved from www.socialworkers.org

National Center for Transgender Equality (NCTE). Retrieved from www.transequality.org

Parents, Families, and Friends of Lesbians and Gays (PFLAG). Retrieved from www.pflag.org

Philadelphia Trans-Health Conference (PTHC). Retrieved from www.mazzonicenter.org/gender-affirming-care/philadelphia-trans-wellness-conference

World Professional Association for Transgender Health (WPATH). Retrieved from www.wpath.org

10

Cultural Considerations When Caring for the New Immigrant or Refugee

Gloria Kersey-Matusiak

The interests we share as human beings are far more powerful than the forces that drive us apart.

—BARACK OBAMA

LEARNING OBJECTIVES

After this chapter, the reader will be able to

1. Define the concepts and terms that are used to differentiate types of immigrants and nonimmigrants who reside permanently or temporarily in the United States.
2. State the geographical origins of most immigrants and migrant workers that currently come to America.
3. Discuss the cultural diversity that exists between and among immigrant populations and the implications for nurses.
4. Explain the role of the nurse when caring for members of immigrant populations.
5. Identify resources to assist the nurse and other healthcare providers when providing care for new immigrants.
6. Describe issues including myths and realities surrounding the debate for and against immigration in the United States and its impact on nursing.

KEY TERMS

Acculturation

Aliens

Asylee

Asylum

Customs and Border Protection (CBP)

Deferred Action for Childhood Arrivals (DACA)
    program

Department of Homeland Security (DHS)

Department of Justice (DOJ)

Deportation

Detainee

Green card

Immigration

Immigration and Customs Enforcement (ICE)

Immigration and Nationality Act (INA)

Lawful permanent resident (LPR)

Migrant

Naturalization

Nonimmigrant

Office of Refugee Resettlement (ORR)

Permanent resident status	Temporary protective status (TPS)
Permanent visa	Temporary visa
Pull factors	Undocumented unauthorized immigrant
Push factors	United States Citizenship and Immigration
Refugee	Services (USCIS)

MIGRATION VERSUS IMMIGRATION

The word **migration** usually refers to individuals who move from one country or region to another, but it can also refer to movement within one's borders from one location to another (internally displaced persons [IDPs]). The term **immigration** means movement across one's national borders to come into a new country and settle there. In 2021, there were 331.9 million people living in the United States (USA Facts, n.d.). Of that number, 14.2% or 46.2 million were immigrants (Camorota & Zeigler, 2021). Sometimes individuals need to move from a second neighboring country into a third country before they can settle there, because their initial place of refuge poses risks that are similar to those they encounter in their homeland.

Nurses who understand the why and how of immigration and its impact on the lives of millions of human beings that experience it each year are better prepared to be of meaningful service to the migrants they encounter in various healthcare settings. The migration experience is often fraught with psychologic as well as physical trauma. Having knowledge of what hardships individuals have endured enables nurses, social workers, and other healthcare professionals to understand the need for trauma-informed care and the importance of delivering care that is culturally sensitive to the emotional, psychologic, and physical needs of all patients.

WHY PEOPLE MIGRATE

The reasons individuals and families leave their homes for foreign lands are described as *push* and *pull* **factors.** Push factors are those that force individuals or families out of their countries of origin, which occur for a variety of reasons. Sometimes individuals are displaced due to changes in their environment, like hurricanes, earthquakes, or tornadoes, that destroy their homes, neighborhoods, and schools, forcing them to migrate. Other migrants are compelled to leave their homelands in search of religious, political, or social freedoms, or to escape violence (e.g., gang violence in Central America), or to flee persecution because of their membership in a particular social group. Even less fortunate are those suddenly faced with the perils of civil war or an unanticipated attack by another country on their native land, like the Russian war in the Ukraine of the early 2020s. Each of these situations places a migrant in an untenable position, especially when the individual or family is responsible for the lives of children as well as their own. Members of these groups have no other option but to seek a temporary or permanent place of refuge. According to the Universal Declaration of Human Rights, when people flee their place of nationality for any of the reasons mentioned previously, they are entitled to seek **asylum** in another country. Pull factors are those that draw immigrants and nonimmigrants to another country such as the promise of employment; better wages; freedoms not found in their homeland; and perceptions of acceptance as a member of a racial, religious, political, or social group that may likely be persecuted in their own country of nationality. In other words, many individuals leave their native lands in search of peace and justice elsewhere.

The Role of the United States in Global Immigration

The United States, through its signed agreement with the 1951 Refugee Convention and its federal immigration laws, regulations, and provisions, specifically the U.S. **Immigration and Nationality Act** (INA; 1952), United States Citizenship and Immigration Services (2019), has committed to abide by the principles of the Convention. The major principle holds that signees "recognize and protect people who flee their countries of nationalities because of persecution or conflict" (Asylum Access, 2021, para. 1). The 1951 Refugee Convention defined the term *refugee* and established core principles of nondiscrimination, nonpenalization, and nonrefoulement. Nonrefoulement means that no country can expel or return a refugee to a territory where their life or freedoms would be threatened. This agreement was initially intended for post-World War II refugees from Europe; however, the 1967 Protocol expanded the scope of the protections to apply them globally to those fleeing their countries due to credible fears of persecution or death. Since that time, 145 states have since approved the Convention's rules and indicated that they intend to comply. The United States resettlement program is the largest in the world, serving "at-risk women and children at risk, female-headed households, elderly, and survivors of violence and torture, and those with acute medical needs" (Song & Teichholtz, 2020, p. 2). In 2021, the United States resettled 12,500 refugees (UNHCR, 2022). However, not all immigrants enter the country as asylum seekers or refugees.

The following discussion describes the various types of immigrants that enter the United States.

Mexican Immigrant as Migrant Farm Worker

According to the World Health Organization (WHO; 2019), labor migrants constitute the largest group of migrants globally. This section focuses on the millions of individuals who choose to migrate to America on a seasonal and/or temporary basis for the purpose of providing a better life for their families through employment that is unattainable in their own country. One such group is the migrant farm worker. Since the 1940s, Americans have benefitted from the hard work and resilience of seasonal farm workers, especially those that come to the United States from Mexico. In the early days because of a temporary agreement between Mexico and the United States, migrants came from Mexico as part of the *Bracero* program that allowed them to travel back and forth to provide support for farmers in the southwest (National Center for Farmworker Health [NCFH], 2018; Paat et al., 2022). Although that program ended in 1964, today many farm workers continue to commute between Mexico and the United States. According to the U.S. Department of Agriculture (USDA), in 2021 the United States hosted 3 million farm workers, many of whom were family farm workers who also labored in the general agricultural force "growing, sowing, weeding, fertilizing, harvesting, handling, processing, and packaging crops" (Paat et al., 2022, p. 73). It is important to note that there is diversity among the groups we often refer to as migrant farm workers, as though they consist of a single group of workers. Males represent 73% and females 27% of all farm workers, with an average age of 44 years; 20% of farm laborers are under age 25. Another recent study (Paat et al., 2022) reported that 90% of workers were male and the average age was 62.9, with an age range of 28 to 84. In this study, about 42.5% reported having fewer than 3 years of elementary education. About 77% of these workers were employed full time and the participants reported daily salaries that ranged from 12 USD to 55 USD. More than half of these workers reported having been sick or injured while at work.

Hispanics, especially Mexicans, make up a large percent of the farm work force (57%); however, 44% of farm workers were born in the United States. The mix of Hispanic workers varies with the states where they work. For example, in California 92% of all farm workers are Hispanic. We recognize that, among farm workers, there are numerous individuals, nearly half of whom are undocumented workers who have lived and worked in the United States for many years. Across the nation, 69.5% of farm workers are White (67% were farm managers, inspectors, and supervisors), 3.9% were Black or African American, 1.2% were Asian, 1.2% were American Indian and Alaskan Natives, and 1.3% were an unknown race (USDA, Economic Research Service, 2022). Recall that individuals who are Hispanic may identify as members of any racial group.

Recruitment of Farm Workers

To obtain large numbers of low-cost farm workers to assist them during agricultural seasons, farm labor contractors will petition the U.S. government to obtain agricultural workers from certain countries through the H-2A visa program. These workers represent about 10% of agricultural labor in the country and have some legal protections based on immigration law. For example, H-2 permit holders must provide housing and transportation for workers but are not required to give them health insurance or medical leave. Farm contractors who are permit holders are required to adhere to the H-2 rules or be heavily fined for not doing so. However, there are less stringent fines for hiring unauthorized workers; therefore, many agricultural employers may choose this option rather than pay the housing and other costs dictated by the H-2 regulations. The farm workers are paid on an hourly or "piece rate" basis; consequently, many will continue to work while ill. Six states accounted for 55% of these workers, with each having at least 10,000 H-2A workers: California (9%), Florida (14%), North Carolina (8%), Louisiana (4%), Georgia (10%), and Washington (10%). The average duration of job offers is 168 days or 24 weeks (Martin & Rutledge, 2021).

A 2023 report indicates that 41% of farm laborers are **undocumented unauthorized immigrants** (Rosenbloom, 2023). An undocumented worker is someone who has entered the country through an unauthorized pathway and has avoided being inspected by **Customs and Border Protection (CBP)** at a port of entry. The reasons why some individuals choose this approach are many, but one of the main reasons is the complicated immigration system that requires many steps and months to years before an immigrant or nonimmigrant can legally enter the country. The H-2 process is a lengthy process and employers are encouraged to petition at least 60 to 120 days before the employee is needed. For the individual or family whose need for an income is urgent, the temptation to take the fastest route to employment may seem overwhelming.

General complaints among some workers include poor physical work conditions like crowded and unsanitary worksites, "sometimes there is no water . . ., bathrooms are removed... no food, and they (employers) do not treat us with dignity and respect." In a study of 100 H-2 workers during the SARS-CoV-2 (COVID-19) pandemic, one study found that among the hundred workers that had traveled from Vera Cruz, Mexico, to north central Florida, none of the workers wore masks and many contracted COVID-19. These researchers concluded that H-2 "face the same environmental [hazards] as all farmworkers but may be even more vulnerable because they have less control over their living and working environments" (Lauzardo et al., 2021, p. 571). Despite the fact that conditions are improving in some states for migrant farm workers, housing generally remains substandard and 78% of respondents report they live in crowded conditions.

Health of the Migrant Farm Worker

The U.S. Bureau of Labor Statistics stated, "agriculture is frequently ranked as one of the most dangerous industries in the nation" (NCFH, 2018). Injuries most often reported include exposure to the elements, symptoms of pesticide exposure in parents and children, farm equipment injuries, and heat stress.

Some of the factors that impede agricultural workers' access to healthcare and social services include poverty, frequent mobility, low literacy, language and cultural barriers, limited transportation, and the lack of time-efficient healthcare delivery methods and a medical referral system. Community-based health centers serve populations with limited access to healthcare and receive federal funding to provide health services to agricultural workers, among others. In 2015 the Health and Resources Services Administration of the U.S. Department of Health and Human Services reported providing services to 910,172 agricultural workers and their families (NCFH, 2018). The most common diagnosis reported for migrant workers and their families were as follows: overweight/obesity, hypertension, diabetes mellitus (DM), otitis media and Eustachian tube disorders, depression, and other mood disorders.

Despite all that migrant farm workers do to ensure that nutritious food arrives on American tables, and the ongoing demand for their labor, these workers, especially those from Mexico, face enormous socioeconomic and health challenges. These challenges make them more vulnerable to illness, injury, and poverty throughout their lives. As one writer notes, they are engaged in the "dirty, dangerous, and demanding (sometimes degrading or demeaning" jobs (Moyce & Schenker, 2018 as cited in Paat et al., 2022, p. 2) that few Americans would choose to do. One writer noted that when Americans were chosen to do these jobs, they lasted only 1 week (Roos & Rouhandeh, 2021). In addition, most of the time these workers are "hidden from the public," so many Americans do not regularly think about immigrants' important contribution to our society, nor consider the hardships they endure to do the work (Fleuriet, 2013; Saldanha, 2021).

Myths and Realities

At the same time, numerous myths prevail that suggest immigrants are lazy, looking for handouts, and are stealing jobs from citizens or that they represent a criminal element that poses a threat to society. The reality is that because of the high demands of the job, farm labor contractors seek individuals from among migrants who are the hardest work-ers with the strongest work ethics and who have the coping skills to be successful, despite working long hours in the hot sun for low wages. The work requirements and demands of a farm worker include time constraints;, having to understand new technology; danger-ous working conditions; occupational stress; fatigue; physical injuries; poor, overcrowded, and unsanitary living conditions; and exposure to pesticides. Additionally, some migrants' housing camps are frequently located in remote areas, which makes healthcare access dif-ficult for the workers and perpetuates their "invisibility" from the public. Often, there is also a language barrier that makes communicating health problems with care providers difficult even when they can interact with them. Ironically, food insecurity is also a prob-lem among farm workers in California. Between 40% and 70% of these farm workers and their families face food insecurity due to the low wages they receive that make it difficult for them to "buy the food they pick" (America: The Jesuit Review, 2017).

Moreover, discrimination and marginalization of Mexican farm workers is another com-mon theme in the literature. For example, as one researcher noted, "historically, migrant farm workers have experienced stigma and various forms of discrimination [due to] low educational attainment and limited English proficiency . . . skin color, immigration status, and national origin" (Paat et al., 2022, p. 2). Immigration reform is needed that responds humanely to the socioeconomic and health needs of U.S. farm workers to whom Americans are truly indebted for the contributions they make to our economy and nutritional well-being. As nurses and health professionals, keeping oneself informed about the impact of migration on migrant farm workers' health will enable nurses to view the plight of the migrant farm worker as a critical public health concern. Having that awareness, nurses can begin to identify specific healthcare and social needs of migrant workers and determine ways to advocate for them so that they ultimately receive the dignity, respect, and justice that they so deserve.

Asylum Seekers

Refugees and asylum seekers are individuals who are unable or unwilling to return to their country of origin or nationality because of a well-founded fear of persecution. They are eligible for protections based on race, religion, nationality, membership in a particular social group, or political opinion. In the United States, the major difference between a refu-gee and an asylum seeker is refugees are usually *outside* of the United States, while asylum seekers apply from *within* the United States. "Contrary to some perceptions that refugees rush to wealthy countries, 85% of refugees globally are hosted in developing countries" (WHO, 2019, #2,). Each year the president, in collaboration with Congress, determines the annual number of **refugees** permitted to enter the United States within a fiscal year. The

United States grants permission to a limited number of refugees seeking asylum to enter the country and apply for citizenship. Some of these individuals are given **green cards** that indicate their status as permanent residents who are free to live and work in the United States. **United States Citizenship and Immigration Services (USCIS)** processes between six and eight million applications and petitions each year. In 2017, USCIS granted asylum to 26,568 individuals. A total of 53,691 were admitted to the U.S. as refugees during 2017 (USCIS, 2019). Until 2018, the U.S. led the world in refugee resettlement and only fell behind with changes in policies during the Trump administration. In 2020, fewer than 12,000 refugees were resettled in the U.S., a decline from 70,000–80,000 annually a few years earlier (Monin et al., 2021).

The current Biden administration has made a commitment to increase the resettlement limit to 125,000 in FY 2022.

The risks taken by those seeking asylum in the United States is a sad testament to the conditions they must have experienced in the countries from which they are fleeing. As one writer reports, "the number of deaths in the Rio Grande is rising at an alarming rate" (Kanno-Youngs, 2019, para. 13).

Asylum seekers, once they reach the U.S. border, must prove that their fears and threats of persecution are credible to either an asylum officer or immigration judge. **Deportation**, which is removal from the United States, and/or detention (being held in custody by the CBP) until a decision is made are real possibilities that add to the arduous journey of a person seeking asylum. In addition, children without parents or a guardian are especially vulnerable and at risk for abduction, trafficking, and/or sexual exploitation. For these reasons, depression and anxiety are commonly reported, linked to lengthy asylum-seeking processes, poor socioeconomic conditions, and social isolation, with children being at greatest risks (WHO, 2019). In 2019, a total of 30,000 refugees were resettled in the United States. Most came from the Democratic Republic of the Congo, Burma (Myanmar), Ukraine, Eritrea, and Afghanistan. Smaller groups of refugees entered the United States from Syria, Iraq, Sudan, El Salvador, Columbia, and other countries (DHS, 2019). More than a quarter of these refugees settled in Texas, Washington, New York, and California in 2018. According to the UN Refugee Agency (n.d.), all 50 states have welcomed refugees into their communities.

THE IMMIGRATION STATUS OF MIGRANTS

It is beyond the scope of this text to discuss all the foreign-born groups now living in the United States as of this writing. However, this chapter focuses on selected groups as collectives coming from the same continent and sharing some commonalities. The term *foreign born* includes all documented and undocumented persons who were born outside of the United States. It is important to note that most immigrants are in the country legally (Budiman, 2020). As of mid-2020, the U.S. immigrant population was the highest in the world at 50.6 million, with new arrivals coming from more than 200 countries and territories (World Population Review, n.d.-a). However, the process of immigrating to America has become increasingly more difficult. Many immigrants come seeking to be reunited with their loved ones who are already living in the United States. In 2018, 11.2 million immigrants living in the United States were from Mexico, representing 25% of all U.S immigrants, followed by China at 6%, India at 6%, the Philippines at 4%, and El Salvador at 3%. Immigrants from Asia combined accounted for 28% of all immigrants (Budiman, 2020). The Pew Research Center (Budiman, 2020) predicts that Asians will replace Hispanics as the largest foreign-born group in America by 2055.

The U.S. **Department of Homeland Security (DHS;** 2017) reported that in fiscal year 2017, 1.13 million **aliens** obtained lawful **permanent resident status**, with each quarter showing a decrease in new arrivals: from 151,000 in the first quarter to 143,000 in the fourth quarter. By 2020, the United States granted 707,362 people legal permanent resident status, which was a significant drop from previous years. **Lawful permanent residents (LPR)** are green card recipients who have been granted lawful permanent resident status in the United States (DHS, 2016). A large percentage of this group is eligible for **naturalization**. An immigrant may apply for naturalization or citizenship after a 5-year residency in the United States. In fiscal year 2019, about 800,000 immigrants applied for naturalization (Budiman, 2020). Many LPRs are immigrants who have gained that status as immediate relatives of U.S. citizens who have come to the United States to be reunited with their family members.

However, not everyone who comes to America has the intention of making it a permanent home. For this reason, the USCIS issues both **permanent** and **temporary visas** to individuals coming from five regions around the world: Asia, Africa, Europe, Latin America, and Oceania, a group of Pacific islands. Currently, the largest groups of immigrants come to the United States from Latin America and Asia. In 2010, Mexico was the leading country, with 3.3 million emigrants or 26% of the LPRs who come to America. Table 10.1 illustrates the top 10 countries from which the United States receives immigrants: Mexico, the Philippines, the People's Republic of China, India, El Salvador, Vietnam, Cuba, the Dominican Republic, South Korea, and Guatemala. It is also noteworthy that some states lead the country in receiving immigrants, thereby becoming geographically more multicultural than others. California, Florida, Texas, New York, and New Jersey are the leading states for immigration, as illustrated in Table 10.2.

Other Types of Immigration Status

Nonimmigrants who enter the country with the intention of returning to their native lands are considered *foreign nationals* and are granted temporary entry into the United States for business or pleasure, study, temporary employment, or to act as a foreign governmental or organizational representative. In 2020, the DHS granted about 86 million nonimmigrant admissions to the United States. These admissions were down 51% from the average over the last 10 years. These lower numbers in 2020 reflect the policy and behavioral changes due to the pandemic. Nonimmigrant admissions included temporary visitors for business

TABLE 10.1 ■ PLACE OF BIRTH FOR THE FOREIGN-BORN POPULATION IN THE UNITED STATES

TOP 10 COUNTRIES	2020	2017	2010	2000	1990
Mexico	1,480,901	170,952	11,711,103	9,177,487	4,298,014
China	713,527	74,194	2,166,526	1,518,652	921,070
India	631,689	60,525	1,780,322	1,022,552	450,406
Philippines	496,361	49,134	1,777,588	1,369,070	912,674
Vietnam	333,900	38,191	1,240,542	988,174	543,262
El Salvador	214,390	25,107	1,214,049	817,336	465,433
Cuba	468,604	65,097	1,104,679	872,716	736,971
South Korea	197,791		1,100,422	864,125	568,397
Dominican Republic	481,183	58,560	879,187	687,677	347,858
Guatemala		13,236	830,824	480,665	225,739
Jamaica	196,552				
All of Latin America		79,164	21,224,087	16,086,974	8,407,837
All Immigrants		1,128,194	39,955,854	31,107,889	19,767,316

Source: World Population Review. (n.d.). *U.S. immigration by country 2024.* https://worldpopulationreview.com/country-rankings/us-immigration-by-country

TABLE 10.2 ■ NEW LAWFUL PERMANENT RESIDENTS BY STATE IN 2022

STATE	NUMBER
California	182,921
Florida	113,653
New York	111,309
Texas	109,720
New Jersey	54,958
Illinois	34,551
Massachusetts	32,885
Washington	31,835
Virginia	28,902
Pennsylvania	28,381

Source: Baugh, R. (2023). *U.S. lawful permanent residents: 2022.* https://www.dhs.gov/sites/default/files/2023-11/2023_0818_plcy_lawful_permanent_residents_fy2022_0.pdf

and pleasure (89%), temporary workers and their families (6.9%), and students and their families (2.5%; Meeks, 2021). Mexico, Canada, the United Kingdom, Japan, and South Korea represented the top five sending countries.

Detainees

"The USDHS is authorized to detain non-U.S. citizens who are alleged to have violated immigration laws to await legal proceedings or removal from the country, if their case has already been decided. Congress has mandated a daily minimum number of detention beds which has risen from 34,000 in 2010 to 52,000 in 2019 just before the pandemic. For example, "during an influx of migrants in June 2019, the Customs and Border Protection (CBP) held more than 15,000 detainees in crowded holding cells" intended to adequately house 4,000 (National Immigration Forum, 2021). **Detainees** may include those who have (a) entered the country without proper documentation, (b) received a final removal order, or (c) have been convicted of certain crimes. Although immigration crimes are civil ones, detainees are often incarcerated in local jails and prison facilities for extended periods of time. The average detention may be as long as 18 months. Several advocacy groups report that individuals in these facilities often receive inadequate physical and mental healthcare. Several deaths have been reported because of inadequate or inappropriate healthcare while immigrants were awaiting disposition. The United States has the largest system of immigration detention in the world with over 131 sites in states throughout the United States. Unaccompanied children who are apprehended must be taken into custody of the **Office of Refugee Resettlement (ORR)** within 72 hours, where there are several programs that include shelters, group homes, foster care, and therapeutic facilities.

Unauthorized Immigrants

The unauthorized-immigrant population, also referred to as undocumented or illegal immigrants, includes all foreign-born noncitizens who are not legal residents. Most of the unauthorized have entered the country without inspection or were admitted temporarily and remained past the date they were required to depart. This category also applies to those who had **temporary protective status (TPS),** were part of the **Deferred Action for Childhood Arrivals (DACA) program**, or who are awaiting removal proceedings in immigration court (DHS, 2021). The DHS estimated that in 2018, 11.4 million unauthorized persons were living in the United States, and of that total, about 15% entered in January 2010. Slightly fewer than 50% of unauthorized immigrants were from Mexico, compared to 55% in 2015, and 40% lived in Texas or California (Baker, 2021).

Generally, the numbers of unauthorized immigrants has declined due to increased immigration enforcement at the U.S border, reduced immigration from Mexico, and many Mexicans leaving the United States. Today, after the largest immigrant group coming from Mexico, the next largest groups are groups of people coming from the Northern Triangle, including El Salvador (700,000), Guatemala (640,000), Honduras (400,000), India (430,000), and the Philippines (360,000). Other regions from which America receives immigrants are Asia, North America, South America, and Europe.

THE IMMIGRANT EXPERIENCE

In the transition from their places of birth to their arrival to the United States, many immigrants endure the hardships of losing loved ones through illness and death or being permanently separated. Often, they must leave their culture and traditions behind and live in a society that devalues their cultural norms, traditions, religion, and language. For many immigrants, not speaking English poses the greatest challenge to their survival after their arrival to the United States. Although language ability varies among immigrant groups, in, 2018, half (53%) of immigrants were proficient English speakers, either speaking English very well (37%) or only speaking English at home (17%). The longer immigrants have lived in the United States, the greater the likelihood they are English proficient. Table 10.3 illustrates the English proficiency by country.

TABLE 10.3 ■ ENGLISH PROFICIENCY AMONG IMMIGRANTS TO THE UNITED STATES

ENGLISH PROFICIENCY	COUNTRY OR REGION
Mexico	34%
Central America	35%
East and Southeast Asia	50%
South America	56%
Canada	96%
Oceania	82%
Europe	75%
Sub-Saharan Africa	74%

Source: Budiman, A. (2020, August 20). *Key findings about U.S. immigrants.* Pew Research Center. https://www.pewresearch.org/short-reads/2020/08/20/key-findings-about-u-s-immigrants.

Some immigrants spoke English well or very well. On the other hand, 30.3% of all immigrants did not speak English at all or not very well. In any case, most new immigrants face numerous other problems. As the Center for Immigration Studies (CIS) reported, after an immigrant's arrival to the United States, those with children were more likely to experience living at or near poverty (47.6% vs. 31.1% of natives), living in crowded housing conditions (12.7% vs. 1.9% of natives), having no health insurance (34.1% vs. 13.8% of natives), and requiring Medicaid (50.2% vs. 28.5% of natives) or other welfare subsidies. These figures are mainly attributed to the low rates of high school completion among many immigrants, with 28% of the population having less than high school completion versus only 7.2% of natives. However, immigrants were just as likely as U.S.-born citizens to have a bachelor's degree or more (32% and 33%, respectively). Immigrant children now represent one in four public school students or approximately 18 million children (Children's Defense Fund, 2021). Since so many immigrant schoolchildren live in poverty and lack health insurance, 25.5% compared to 5.1% of native-born children, this poses a challenge for the nations' schools (CDF, 2021).

The Status of the Deferred Action for Childhood Arrivals (Dreamers)

The U.S. government has vacillated in its commitment to immigration reform.

In June 2012, with an executive order, President Obama created the DACA program. DACA was intended to protect the children of immigrants who were brought to the United States illegally when they were children, providing a renewable work authorization and a temporary program to defer deportation for eligible individuals. The goal of DACA was to allow "eligible individuals who did not pose a threat to national security or public safety" an opportunity to work (Barack Obama as cited in Robertson, 2018, para. 4) without fear of deportation, albeit temporarily. However, this program did not change the immigration status of those who qualified for it. To qualify for DACA, an individual had to be at least age 15, but younger than 31 years when applying; be younger than 16 years when entering the United States; be living continuously in the United States since June 2012; be in school or have completed high school or have been honorably discharged from the military; not convicted of a felony, a significant misdemeanor, or three or more misdemeanors; complete a seven-page application; and pay a fee of $495. Through this program, about 40,000 individuals became LPRs. However, nearly 72,000 applicants were denied. The largest numbers of recipients live in California (28%), Texas (16%), New York (5%), and Florida (4%; Robertson, 2018).

At this writing, several partisan and bipartisan bills regarding DACA have been proposed in Congress. Yet, no bill by either major party has been passed. According to the USCIS (2021), as it stands, individuals may continue to apply for DACA if eligible, but the fate of current DACA recipients remains undecided. As of this writing, dreamers still have no legal path to citizenship while living in the only country many of them have ever really known.

American Citizens' Attitudes Toward Immigration

Americans today are divided in their perspectives about immigration, mainly along political and ideologic lines (National Immigration Forum, 2019). Unfortunately, since the terrorist attacks of September 11, 2001, and the rise in terrorism, people throughout the world are experiencing a heightened sense of fear and anxiety. This fear has resulted in a significant reduction in the numbers of refugees and other immigrants that America and other nations are generally willing to accept. As a means of blocking unlawful entry into the United States, President Trump proposed the construction of a border wall at the southern border between the United States and Mexico. That proposal was supported by some, but criticized by others because of its anticipated costs and the implications for our relationship with Mexico, a U.S. ally. Other immigration controversies focused in part on whether persons who are undocumented should be granted a path to citizenship or be deported for breaking the law. According to Pew Research (McQueen, 2021), 60% of Americans oppose giving citizenship to illegal aliens. However, many believe that offering amnesty to those who are already living here would remove undocumented immigrants from the shadows, afford them legal employment, provide fairer wages, strengthen the economy, and enrich the nation's cultural diversity.

In addition, Americans hold diverse opinions about the immigration process, as well as its laws and policies, and these attitudes are also often divided along partisan lines. However, Americans have become somewhat more positive about immigrants and immigration. For example, in 2018 70% of Americans polled said the idea of being welcoming of people from different cultures was very important. In 2019, several polls conducted by various groups indicated that the majority of Americans (53%) said they thought immigrants made America better. There is also diversity of opinions between younger voters and Baby Boomers, Gen Xers, and Millennials, with younger voters being more positive. Americans are also divided on the issues of immigration reform, increasing or decreasing the numbers of immigrants allowed to enter the United States, providing a pathway to citizenship for those who are unauthorized (including DACA recipients), and on whether to allow the unauthorized to stay within the country or deport them.

Through the Eyes of the Immigrant

As stated earlier, the current immigration process is arduous, costly, and lengthy. For those who have taken the legal route to entering the United States at a port of entry, the wait may be as long as a decade to reunite with loved ones already living here. The same delays are encountered after applying for work-related visas. Because of the COVID-19 pandemic of 2020, there is a huge backlog of applicants waiting to receive long-awaited responses from Immigration Services. For others who are desperately attempting to flee untenable situations by seeking asylum at the border, there is the potential for them to be detained or immediately flown back to their country. In other unauthorized situations, there are also long waits as multitudes journey to the Mexican border, only to be apprehended by the CBP or by **Immigration and Customs Enforcement (ICE)** if they make it inside the country. These people are then returned to their country of origin or held indefinitely in crowded unhealthy settings. In any case, for the unauthorized immigrant who enters the country, the cost is high. Many desperate Mexicans and people coming from Central America travel across difficult desert terrain, placing themselves at risk of hazards for which they are physically and mentally unprepared. Many die in search of a "better life." For those who succeed in entering the country without inspection (undocumented), when they arrive they are likely to face unemployment, or receive low paying jobs, and are unqualified for social and medical benefits to which they would be entitled as legal immigrants. Some U.S. cities are designated "sanctuary cities" because their municipal laws tend to protect immigrants from deportation. Still, unauthorized entry into the United States also means living an underground existence in fear of discovery and deportation. Yet, for some immigrants, the dream of living in America is worth the risks when compared with the obstacles faced in their country of origin.

Today, there are increasing numbers of immigrants coming to the United States from around the world. The experience of living in America is different for each immigrant group and the quality of that experience is influenced in part by the group members' support systems and their ability to acculturate or assimilate into the American culture. Immigrants' success in the United States may also be affected by the attitudes held toward them by other members of the communities in which they live and work. Specifically, the attainment of health information, healthcare access, and healthcare treatment are by-products of an immigrants' successful navigation of unfamiliar territory, often with a language barrier complicating the process. Although the debates around the pros and cons of immigration continue, there is still the need for nurses to appreciate the diversity that exists among the various groups that immigrate to America and to realize that a vast number of immigrants enter the country legally.

Nurses can help address the challenges posed by immigration that impact the health and well-being of both citizens and immigrants who already live in the United States. The health and well-being of new immigrants is an important consideration for all healthcare providers in the prevention of disease and the maintenance of health in the general community. Another serious consideration is that of providing adequate and culturally appropriate healthcare for the large numbers of culturally diverse people who arrive and who already live in the United States.

HEALTH AMONG IMMIGRANTS: THE ROLE OF THE NURSE

In 2019, according to WHO, "migrants and refugees are likely to be healthy in general" (#3). However, they are at risk for falling ill as they transition from place to place, often experiencing crowded conditions, poor shelter and sanitation, inadequate water and food, and increased stress.

Nurses, as providers and consumers of healthcare, are in a unique position to provide healthcare services to immigrants and nonimmigrants at all levels of illness prevention. With an increased awareness and understanding of the immigrant's need for preventive care and health promotion, nurses can help ensure that the potential spread of disease due to lack of treatment is minimized. A good place for nurses to start in addressing this matter is by gaining knowledge about the groups they care for, recognizing the diversity among them. An important caveat is to consider each individual unique, while determining whether the individual is newly arrived or a long-standing member of the community who has already acculturated. New immigrants may have untreated health issues that have accompanied them, and all immigrants may have psychologic needs for trauma-informed care due to the hardships of their immigration experiences.

Understanding the patient's history of immigration, the circumstances under which immigration occurred, and the patient's present living conditions in the United States is critical when planning care for members of this population.

Most importantly, the culturally competent nurse recognizes that even undocumented immigrants deserve quality care and to be treated with dignity and respect. With each of these things in mind, the nurse attempts to overcome any language barriers to ensure patients' understanding of their diagnosis and treatment plan, using medical interpreters when needed to ensure effective communication with new immigrants. The nurse also remembers that health education is critical and identifies appropriate resources in language the patient understands to assist the new immigrant in promoting health at all levels of illness prevention. A listing of some important websites to assist nurses in this role is included at the end of this chapter.

SUMMARY

For many Americans, issues of immigration are not only viewed from a practical or political perspective, but also with ethical and humanitarian considerations in mind. Echoing the sentiments of Pope Francis, Zoucha (2015), when reaching out to transcultural nurses, reminded us that today globally "there are mass movements of people from Central and Latin America, Asia, Africa, and the Middle East seeking peace, justice, and hope" (p. 449) Further, he notes, "[w]e are all connected and the pain of some is our pain" (Zoucha, 2015, p. 449). As others observe, "the impact of premigration losses, traumatic events, adapting to differences in weather, religion, language, clothing, legal principles, and financial pressures" seriously impact the mental health of immigrants (Wolf et al., 2016, p. 349). In his 2018 Message on the 104th World Day of Migrants and Refugees, Pope Francis affirmed the need for "all men and women of good will . . . to respond to the many challenges of contemporary migration with generosity, promptness, wisdom, and foresight, each according to their own abilities" (2018, para. 3). Further he encouraged everyone "to welcome, protect, promote, and integrate" immigrants into our society. Today, many of our global neighbors are left homeless and alone through circumstances not of their own making. Americans must somehow individually and collectively ask themselves which approach to immigration best serves not just their personal interests, but the common good, and which model best reflects the kind of global citizen America wishes to be.

IMPORTANT POINTS

- Various push and pull factors explain why so many people migrate from their places of birth.
- In the United States in 2021, there were 331.9 million people; of these, 14.2% or 46.2 million people were foreign born.
- It is projected that by 2050, 19% of the population will have been born outside of the country.
- Most immigrants are lawfully in the United States.
- Migrant farm laborers have made an important contribution to America since the 1940s.
- Most legal permanent residents are eligible for naturalization.
- The five regions from which immigrants currently come to America are Asia, Africa, Europe, Latin America, and Oceania, a group of Pacific islands.
- The six countries from which the majority of new immigrants come are Mexico, the Philippines, China, Cuba, India, and the Dominican Republic.
- Despite a commitment by the U.S. government to increase the numbers of U.S. asylum seekers admitted to the country, a huge backlog makes this goal difficult to achieve.
- The states with the most new immigrants are California, New York, Florida, Texas, and New Jersey.
- The CDC reports that immigrants generally enjoy better health on arrival than their U.S. counterparts, yet become increasingly less healthy the longer they stay in America.
- Rates of smoking, hypertension, and heart disease are greatest among U.S.-born adults.
- Some countries from which emigrants leave for the United States, including Haiti and some African nations, have limited health resources and a high prevalence of diseases like tuberculosis (TB) and HIV.
- The terrorist attacks of September 11, 2001, led to mixed attitudes and some confusion about immigration among greater numbers of Americans.
- The various groups of immigrants that come to America are diverse in their cultural attitudes and healthcare beliefs.
- All immigrants and especially asylum seekers and children are at risk for posttraumatic stress disorder (PTSD) because of the lengthy and arduous process and therefore require trauma-informed care.
- Language barriers are one of the biggest problems influencing immigrants' ability to access quality healthcare; there may be a need for a medically trained interpreter.
- Nurses enjoy a critical position from which they can prevent illness and promote health in immigrant populations through patient education.
- Nurses can begin to address barriers to healthcare by gaining knowledge about the immigrant groups for whom they provide care.
- Regardless of immigration status, all patients deserve healthcare, dignity and respect.

SELECTED IMMIGRANT GROUPS

Because of the large numbers of immigrant groups that come to America each year, it is impossible to include each in this chapter. The section that follows will describe some of the health-related issues of selected Asian, Arab, Black, and Latinx immigrants who currently reside either temporarily or permanently in the United States.

Asian Immigrants

According to the U.S. Census Bureau and Pew Research Center, one quarter of foreign-born individuals living in America come to the United States from Asia. In 2019, Asians were the fastest growing ethnic group (72%), with 22.4 million people. Asians are predicted to reach 48.6 million by 2060 and become the largest minority in the United States, outpacing Hispanics. Asians now make up about 6% to 7% of the U.S. population, but are expected to make up 36% of all U.S. immigrants. As one researcher noted, "while great heterogeneity exists between Asian subgroups, they are usually homogenized into an 'Asian'" collective (Xiao et al., 2020, p. 711). Unfortunately, since the emergence of the COVID-19 pandemic, there has been an increase in anti-Asian hate crimes in 16 of America's largest cities (Guillermo, 2021). Reported incidents included verbal harassment (68.1%), shunning (20.5%), physical assault (11.1%) and other civil rights violations, and "the mass killing of eight people, including six Asian women, in Atlanta [that was fueled by anti-Asian-American] hateful speech and rhetoric that have become common at the highest levels of our government, as well as in society at large" (Stewart, 2021, paras. 2 & 9). Such incidents promote ignorance and fear and make it difficult for new and older Asian immigrants to reach out and seek healthcare from American healthcare providers. Nurses can make a positive difference by building their knowledge and understanding of the various Asian cultural groups that have lived and worked in America for several generations and those who have newly arrived.

The large collective of people referred to as Asian/Pacific Islanders represents 47 countries and includes more than 20 specific ethnic groups. The largest number of Asian immigrants to America come from China, with 5.4 million; India, with 4.6 million; the Philippines, 4.2 million, Vietnam with 2.2 million, Korea with 1.9 million, and Japan with 1.5 million. Nearly half of U.S. Asians live in the West (45%). Asian populations are concentrated in Hawaii, California, New York, Texas, New Jersey, Nevada, Washington, and in metropolitan areas such as Los Angeles, California; New York, New York; and San Francisco, California (Lopez & Patten, 2017). Asians enjoy the highest citizenship rates among the foreign-born living in America, "More than half of Asians age 25 and older 54% have a bachelor's degree or more education as compared with 33% of the U.S. population at the same age" (Budiman & Ruiz 2021). In 2019, 95% of all U.S.-born Asians were proficient in English (Budiman & Ruiz, 2021). Fifty-four percent of all Asians have a bachelor's degree, as compared to 33% of all Americans. Indian Asians have the highest rate of bachelor's degrees (75%); some Asian groups with lower percentages of bachelor's degrees include Cambodians, Hmong, Laotians, and Bhutanese. Asians also enjoy the highest annual income ($73,000, as compared to $53,600 among native Americans) and are more likely to be employed in managerial or professional positions than either native or all other foreign-born workers. They are also the least likely, as a group, to love in poverty compared to all Americans. Fifty-two percent have health insurance coverage at a similar rate to natives.

Asian Religions

As a reflection of the wide variety of ethnic groups coming from the various Asian countries, religious practices among Asians also vary. Today, among the 10.5 million unauthorized immigrants in America, 14% are Asians from four countries: India (525,000), China (375,000), the Philippines (160,000), and South Korea (150,000; Budiman & Ruiz, 2021). With the exception of China and Vietnam, for which data about religious affiliations are not readily available, one can assume that the religions "within an Asian country are similar to that within its community in the U.S." (Le, n.d., para. 10). Thus, Asian immigrants from India are more likely to be Hindu, Muslim, Buddhist, or Sikh as compared to Asians from the Philippines, who are more likely to be Roman Catholic or Protestant Christians. Muslims represented 8% of the Asian population. Other groups, including Scientologists, Pagans, Druids, Rastafarians, and others, comprised 2% of the Asian population. Several researchers examined the impact of religious practices and spirituality of Asian immigrants (Chen & Park, 2019; Kim & Kim-Godwin, 2019; Stroop et al., 2022). Kim and Kim-Goodwin studied the cultural context of family religiosity and spirituality among Korean American families and how it changed with immigration to the United States. These researchers found that the religiosity/spirituality of the participants was influenced by traditional family values, which were shaped by Korean culture. Findings revealed a strong desire by Koreans who practiced Shamanism, Buddhism, and Confucianism in Asia to pass their religion on to their children and to maintain traditions and routines with all family members' participation. Koreans view this participation as vital to family unity and health; emphasized family harmony, obedience, and self-sacrifice; and are motivated by family norms, goals, and needs. In this study, the Korean church provided a significant support in the absence of extended family after immigration to the United States. Church members became a supportive social network. The authors reminded nurses of the importance of assessing these beliefs and practices in their patients, especially older adult, first-generation immigrants who may be socially isolated from their cultural traditions. Further, the researchers suggest healthcare professionals working "with Korean ethnic churches to develop culturally tailored interventions" (Kim & Kim-Godwin, 2019, p. 62). Stroop and colleagues (2022) in a large study of religious group involvement among Asians found that group prayer involvement was positively associated with self-rated health and mental health functioning.

In a study that sought to determine the impact of differing Asian cultures and attitudes on cancer-screening rates, researchers found differences among Cambodian, Chinese, Vietnamese, and Korean Americans on their tendencies to get screenings for various types of cancer (Nguyen-Truong et al., 2012) studied Vietnamese women's Pap smear adherence. However, another important finding in the study was the high number of participants across all four groups who reported never being screened for prostate, colorectal, or hepatitis B (HBV). The researchers believed that this study provided evidence of the need for preventive health services in the Asian communities and gave some direction to healthcare providers as to where to focus their efforts. The American Heart Association reported that Asian immigrants were more likely to experience ischemic strokes. To address early detection in Asian communities, the researcher suggested a range of cultural and language-sensitive interventions to stress the need for education and access to preventive care.

Asians and Health

Xiao and colleagues (2020) examined differences between Korean and Vietnamese immigrants. Their findings suggest that although Asian immigrants are labeled as an aggregate, there were significant differences between them in demographics like age; citizenship; time in the United States; education; marital status; English proficiency; health insurance; and utilization of health services including Pap smear, colorectal screening, and mammogram screening. Koreans tended to be newer immigrants who were less acculturated than Vietnamese, had less time in the United States, lower levels of English proficiency, higher education, and were more likely to visit doctors and seek health screenings than Vietnamese. Seo and colleagues (2019) identified language barriers, low finances, discrimination, and an unfamiliar health system among the hardships facing new Asian immigrants. These researchers found having health insurance was the most significant predictor of health utilization. The findings of this study suggest that, in assisting Korean patients, a multifront approach to improve health literacy through language classes, opportunities for formal education, and assistance with health insurance would be helpful. Vietnam immigrants would benefit by improving language/English proficiency.

In another study in 2022, Shafeek Amin and Driver compared Middle Easterners to Asian and Hispanic patients and found that Asian patients are less likely to use healthcare than Middle Easterners. They stated that Asian immigrants may often combine traditional or alternative medicine with Western medicine in their health-seeking behavior. Members of these groups, although sharing some common health beliefs, differ in their tendency to practice cultural traditions. For example, among Chinese and Vietnamese, practices like coining, cupping, and the belief in the relevance of maintaining the internal balance of hot and cold forces in the body are a part of the health belief system. Even within the same ethnic group, some members may place more value than others on folk healers, herbal remedies, or other practices.

Gautam and colleagues (2018) studied older Bhutanese adults to explore their experiences and adjustment to life in the United States. Following life in refugee camps in Nepal for 15 to 20 years, 84,000 Bhutanese refugees have resettled in the United States since 2007. These researchers observed that the psychologic adjustment period can have a profound effect on the health of Bhutanese older adults.

Prior to resettlement in the United States, many of the refugees were found to have serious mental illness, such as depression, anxiety, and PTSD (Gautam et al., 2018). Cultural challenges like language differences, unemployment, social stress, and declining physical health, placed them at high risk for suicide. Family separation, the language barrier, and the need to maintain Bhutanese/Nepali culture in the United States created loneliness and isolation. Also, for older immigrants, the language barrier made it difficult to pass the civics test, creating a major challenge to becoming a citizen. In addition, refugees are ineligible for Social Security benefits after being in the country beyond 7 years; limiting access to benefits as they age results in poorer health outcomes. The researchers recommended that nurses advocate for a community venue for elders to gather, and for policy changes to support citizenship programs, language classes, and resources to address mental health and physical needs of these citizens.

IMPORTANT POINTS

- The large collective of people referred to as Asian/Pacific Islanders represents 47 countries and includes more than 20 specific ethnic groups. The largest number of Asian immigrants to America come from China, with 5.4 million (24%), India, with 4.6 million (21%), the Philippines, 4.2 million (19%), Vietnam with 2.2 million, Korea with 1.9 million, and Japan with 1.5 million (Budiman & Ruiz, 2021).
- Anti-Asian hate rhetoric and hate crimes that grew out of the 2019 COVID-19 pandemic sparked fear and ignorance that make it difficult for many Asian immigrants to reach out to American healthcare professionals.
- Asian immigrants tend to live in large metropolitan areas like Los Angeles, California; New York, New York; and San Francisco, California.
- Asian immigrants have the highest level of U.S. citizenship.
- More than half of all Asian immigrants to the United States have a bachelor's degree and the rate among Indian Asians is 72%, compared to 30% of all Americans.
- Seventy-three percent of all adult Asians in the United States are foreign born. Among Bhutanese, 92% are foreign born, but only 27% of Japanese are foreign born.
- Asian immigrants are more likely to be employed in management or professional positions, and to enjoy higher incomes, than are other foreign-born people employed in the United States; however, much variation exists between Asian groups.
- Asian immigrants to the United States identify with a diverse range of religious faiths, including Buddhism, Hinduism, Islam, Sikhism, Roman Catholicism, and other Christian religions.
- Asians vary in language, communication styles, and their use of folk practices such as coining, cupping, and the use of healers, even among the same ethnic group. Sixty-eight percent of Asians in the United States speak a language other than English in the home, but 55% of the foreign-born Asians speak English proficiently.
- Thirteen percent of Asian immigrants in the United States are unauthorized immigrants from four countries: India, China, the Philippines, and South Korea.
- Family solidarity and the concept of "saving face" ranked high among cultural values.

Black Immigrants

In the past, immigrants coming to the United States from Africa typically came from the west and east coasts of sub-Saharan Africa (Wilhelm et al., 2021). As a result, immigrants from Ghana and Nigeria on the west, Ethiopia and Somalia on the east, and South Africa represent the largest number of sub-Saharan African immigrants living in the United States. Today, due to civil wars and limited economic opportunities throughout the continent, corrupt and oppressive regimes, and a more relaxed U.S. diversity policy toward African immigrants, a more diverse population of Africans are attracted to America; however, many Subsaharan Africans (63%) lived elsewhere in the region, like the Côte d'Ivoire, South Africa, Uganda, Sudan, and Nigeria (Lorenzi & Batalova, 2022). In 2019, the large majority, approximately 90%, of the 46.8 million individuals (or 14% of the U.S. population) who self-identify as Black or African American were born in this country (Pew Research Center, 2020). However, the Black immigrant populations come to the United States from around the world: Africa, Europe, South America, the Caribbean, and the West Indies. Although one third of Black immigrants speak a foreign language, the majority of them speak English fluently. Thus, most Black immigrants are bilingual.

In 2019, more than 4.6 million Black or African American people in the United States were born outside the country, representing 10% of the Black population (Tamir, 2022). These numbers have increased at a rate of 71% since 1980. Africans account for 42% of the overall Black foreign-born. Among the top five countries of origin are Nigeria, Ethiopia, Ghana, Jamaica, and Haiti. Other Black immigrants come from Latin America and smaller numbers come to the U.S. from Europe, Asia, and North America; 46% are from the Caribbean, including Jamaica (760,000) and Haiti (700,000; Tamir, 2022). Although the United States is the top destination for sub-Saharan Africans, large numbers have also migrated to the United Kingdom, (1.4 million), France (1.1 million), Italy (524,000), and Canada (435,000; Lorenzi & Batalova, 2022).

Black immigrants are more likely to be naturalized and speak English well as compared to other immigrant groups. Among Black immigrants ages 25 and older, 31% had at least a bachelor's degree in 2019, up from 21% in 2000. Immigrants from Africa are more likely than U.S. citizens or American-born Blacks to have a college degree (Tamir & Anderson, 2022). African immigrants are more likely to hold an advanced degree than the U.S.-born population (Boundless, 2022). However, there are variations among Africans regarding their educational status: 59% of immigrants from Nigeria have a college degree, compared to 10% among Somalian immigrants. In 2019, the median age of Black people in the United States was 32; 58% of the U.S. Black population was age 38 or younger, and 35% was 22 years or younger. Black immigrants tend to be older, with a median age of 42, similar to the age of all U.S. immigrants (Boundless, 2022). In 2019, many sub-Saharan African immigrants were either refugees or came seeking asylum (25%).

The foreign-born Black population is less likely than U.S. immigrants overall to be unauthorized. According to the Migration Policy Institute (Lorenzi & Batalova, 2022), as of December 2021, approximately 3,300 unauthorized immigrants from sub-Saharan Africa actively participated in the DACA program, which provides temporary relief from deportation and work authorization. The DACA participants represented individuals from Nigeria (840), Kenya, (550), and Ghana (380), a total of about 1% of all the DACA participants.

Black immigrants tend to migrate to the most concentrated regions of the country, such as New York (856,272), Florida (713,236), Texas (276,326), New Jersey (223,189), Maryland (225,190), Massachusetts (187,691), and California (179,426). (See Table 10.4).

Since hypertension is a major health problem among native Black Americans, Cole and colleagues (2018) studied immigrants' awareness of having high blood pressure and found that one in five hypertensive U.S. adults are unaware that they have hypertension. In this study, there were differences in hypertension death rates between non-Hispanic middle-aged and older Black men (47.1 per 100,000) and non-Hispanic White men (17.6 per 100,000) due in part to inequities in blood pressure control. These researchers found that foreign-born participants were less likely to be aware of having hypertension than their native-born participants, which may lead to an increase in the burden of hypertension outcomes that result in uncontrolled high blood pressure. The researchers also discussed other immigrant studies that documented "distinct health advantages among foreign-born Blacks," which included, having a low body mass index (BMI), lower rates of diabetes, and self-reports of high blood pressure as compared to their U.S.-born counterparts (Cole et al., 2018). The findings of this study indicate that foreign-born Black men were overall less

TABLE 10.4 ■ TOP METRO AREAS OF AFRICAN IMMIGRATION (2015–2019)

METROPOLITAN AREA	IMMIGRANTS FROM SUB-SAHARAN AFRICA
New York-Newark-Jersey City, NY-NJ-PA Metro Areas	194,000
Washington-Arlington-Alexandria	192,000
Dallas-Fort Worth-Arlington, Texas Metro Area	99,000
Minneapolis-St. Paul- Bloomington-MN-WI Metro Area	95,000
Atlanta-Sandy Springs-Alpharetta, GA Metro	90,000
Houston-The Woodlands-Sugar Land, TX Metro Area	88,000
Boston-Cambridge-Newton, MA-NH Metro Area	66,000
Philadelphia-Camden-Wilmington- PA-NJ-DE-MD	56,000
Seattle-Tacoma-Bellevue, WA Metro Area	53,000
Los Angeles-Long Beach Anaheim, CA Metro	52,000

Source: Lorenzi, J., & Batalova, J. (2022, May 11). *Sub-Saharan African immigrants in the United States.* Migration Policy Institute. https://www.migrationpolicy.org/article/sub-saharan-african-immigrants-united-states-2019

likely than U.S.-born Black men to be aware of having high blood pressure. Further, they remind us that Blacks are erroneously considered a homogeneous racial group, despite diversity by nativity, ethnicity, and experiences of social determinants of health. In most of the countries in Africa, food- and waterborne diseases like typhoid, hepatitis A bacterial diarrhea, and meningitis are among some of the health risks most Africans encounter. Across the continent, too, severe poverty and the HIV virus have taken a devastating toll on the lives of children and adults. In 2020, 350,000 people in Ghana were living with HIV, and 620,000 were impacted in Ethiopia. Considering the poverty, waterborne diseases, and high prevalence of HIV, it is not surprising that the life expectancy is 71 years for a female and 67.7 years for a male in Ethiopia, and in Ghana it is 66 years for a male and 70.4 years for a female (Central Intelligence Agency [CIA], 2022).

In two other studies on Black immigration, researchers noted many socioeconomic differences between Black immigrants and native-born African Americans that are important to include here. First, the Bureau of Labor Statistics (BLS; 2022) reported that Black immigrants have a slightly lower employment rate than all other U.S. immigrants (93% vs. 95%, respectively); second, a significant percentage of Black immigrants work in healthcare (nearly 28%). Of that group, 10% work as nursing assistants, 6% as personal care aides, and 4% as registered nurses. The median income of Black immigrants is $57,700 compared to $63,000 for all immigrants. Sub-Saharan African-born immigrants were more likely than U.S.-born citizens to be uninsured at 16% versus 8%; however, they were less likely to be uninsured than other immigrants at 20%. Most Black immigrants are less likely to own their own homes when compared to other immigrants (42% vs. 53%), but their home ownership is not much different from U.S.-born Black Americans (42% vs. 41%). Based on the 2020 Census, the top three states where Black immigrants have lived for several years are New York, Florida, and Texas. However, "Black immigrant populations in the Dakotas and Minnesota are the largest in the country when measured as a percentage of the state's total immigrant population" (Boundless, 2022, "Where Black Immigrants Call Home"). For example, the percent of the immigrant population in North Dakota that is Black is 28.1% (8,450 Black immigrants of a total 30,036 immigrants in the state). Other states where large numbers of Black immigrants can be found include New Jersey, Maryland, Massachusetts, and California.

Despite the fact that "African born immigrants are often highly educated professionals when they arrive in America, they must seek employment where less skills and education are required. This happens because in America, Black immigrants are forced to confront some of the same stereotypes and prejudices often associated with their African American counterparts" (Foner, 2016, p. 63). As Nteta and Rice (2021) observed, "blacks who strongly believe in linked fate may perceive a sense of commonality with new immigrants based on their similar status in the racial hierarchy" (p. 74). Otusanya and Bell (2018) discussed communication struggles between African Americans and West African immigrants. Kusow and colleagues (2014) explored socioeconomic and educational attainment of African immigrants based on the region of their home countries to determine intracultural differences between the groups. The researchers found that the sending region is an important determinant of hourly wages, with earnings of males and Whites higher than females and Blacks; South Africans fared better than North, East, and West African counterparts. Also important to African immigrant success is English fluency and education, although education for immigrants from East and West African regions did not translate into higher earnings. These researchers concluded that the sending region of origin was the most important factor in socioeconomic attainment and recommended studies that further explore regional differences between the groups. Because there is wide diversity among Africans in their native languages, religions, and cultural values and beliefs, the authors caution against the treatment of African immigrants as one homogeneous group. Therefore, it is important for nurses to keep these differences in mind when attempting to identify African patients' cultural or spiritual needs.

Afro-Caribbean Immigrants From Haiti

Haiti is said to be "the poorest country in the Western Hemisphere, which has been plagued by political violence for most of its history" (CIA, 2017). In 2010, a catastrophic earthquake displaced more than 1.5 million people from Haiti. Following the earthquake that devastated the country and its infrastructure, thousands of Haitian refugees migrated to the United States and were given 4 years of TPS (Somilleda, 2021). With that status, Haitian immigrants were granted work authorization. During the time these Haitians lived in the United States, many children were born to them. Unfortunately, as their temporary status designation ended, the U.S. government gave them 18 months to return to Haiti. In response, several thousands of Haitians migrated illegally to Montreal, Ontario, seeking asylum in Canada. Others remained in America, fearfully awaiting their change in status in 2019.

In 2021, the secretary of homeland security announced a new 18-month designation of Haiti for TPS. This determination was made based on the fact that current conditions that include: "social unrest, an increase in human rights abuses, crippling poverty, and lack of basic resources, which are exacerbated by the COVID-19 pandemic" (Mayorkis as cited in DHS, 2021, para. 2) pandemic in Haiti made it difficult for Haitians to return safely to their country (Quarshie & Anderson, 2021). This designation enabled Haitian nationals residing in the United States as of May 21, 2021, to file an application for TPS status if they met the requirements.

The native languages of Haiti are French and Creole. Because of poor health conditions, the people of Haiti are exposed to major infectious diseases including HIV, food- and water-borne diseases such as hepatitis A and E, and typhoid fever, as well as vector-borne diseases like malaria. Like many African Americans, Haitians are at high risk for several health problems and diseases. For example, one study indicated 26% of Haitians smoked and 67% were overweight (although Haitians consider obesity a sign of good health). In Haiti, some common diseases include malnutrition, sexually transmitted infections (due partially to a belief in polygamous practices), TB, malaria, typhoid, and hypertension. According to the WHO, life expectancy in Haiti is reported to be 64.7 years in 2022.

Immigrants from Haiti qualify for a family-sponsored or employment-based immigrant visa or can stay in America through temporary or **asylee** visas. The five states with the largest number of foreign-born Haitians are Florida (487,632), New York (182,316), Massachusetts (81,050), New Jersey (73,757), and Georgia (30,664; World Population Review, n.d.-b). Some African Caribbean groups, while sharing physical traits like skin color and facial features with African Americans, do not identify culturally with them. Although many Haitians do speak fluent English. Haitian immigrants are predominantly Roman Catholic (80%); however, many Protestant religions are also represented among them (16%). Protestant groups include Baptist (10%), Pentecostal (4%), Adventist (1%), and other (1%). Only 1% of Haitians claim to practice no religion, while approximately half of the population practices voodoo (World Atlas, 2017).

IMPORTANT POINTS

- There is much cultural and language diversity among Black immigrants.
- The majority of African- and Caribbean-born Blacks are bilingual and speak fluent English.
- Most immigrant Blacks arrive in America in a better state of health than their African American counterparts.
- African immigrants, despite being highly educated professionals, usually find employment where fewer skills and less education are required.
- Black immigrants experience the same stereotypes and prejudices as African Americans.
- Haitians are among the poorest Black immigrants, and many come to America as refugees.
- Afro-Caribbean groups do not identify culturally with African Americans.
- Life expectancy for Haitians is 64.7 years. Obesity is high among Haitians, but is considered a sign of good health.
- U.S.-born Blacks disproportionately experience coronary heart disease (CHD), higher intake of calories from fat, low infant birth weight, and worse cardiovascular (CV) and mental health outcomes then both African- and Caribbean-born immigrants.

CASE SCENARIO 1

Chinaza Okonkwo, a 62-year-old Nigerian woman, came to America after her daughter and her husband were selected by lottery. Cecelia, Chinaza's daughter, was fearful that her mother would die before she could bring her to the United States, because they lived in a small rural town in which there was little to eat. Food was obtained through farming and women had to walk several miles before reaching a place where they might harvest something substantial to eat. In this town, there was only one general doctor who took care of everything from childbirth to more serious health problems. As soon as Chinaza's daughter was eligible, she applied for a green card for her mother, a recent widow, to join her in America. All of Chinaza's other children remained in the small village in eastern Nigeria. When Cecelia met Chinaza at the airport, she could not believe her eyes. Chinaza, at 5 feet 8 inches, weighed only 108 pounds. That night Chinaza told her daughter that she was having burning on urination, difficulty passing her urine, and itching around the perineal area. Mrs. Okonkwo told her daughter that her urine had had a foul odor for the past several days. Cecelia took her mother to the medical clinic to visit her gynecologist. During the interview, the doctor attempted to get a health history from Chinaza, but to each question he asked, Chinaza had no answer. This was Chinaza's first visit to any doctor in her entire life. She was terrified when the tall, young, White doctor entered the room with a female nurse accompanying him. Chinaza spoke some English, but needed to rely on Cecelia to translate for her. The doctor became more and more upset as Chinaza answered no to each of his questions. "When was your last Pap smear?" "No," she replied. "Your last breast examination?" "No," said Chianza. "Your last vaginal examination?" the doctor asked. "No," Chianza replied. "No means never," said Cecelia. The doctor was so upset on learning that Chinaza had seven children but had never once seen a doctor before or after her deliveries that he left the room and asked the nurse to complete the interview. He did return later to perform the physical. The nurse remained with Chinaza and attempted to comfort her throughout the procedure.

WHAT NURSES NEED TO KNOW ABOUT THEMSELVES

Application of the Staircase Self-Assessment Model: Self-Reflection Questions

1. How prepared would you be to care for this patient? How many encounters have you had with patients from this background?
2. Where would you place yourself on the staircase with regard to this patient?
3. What steps could you take to move to the next level? (See Chapter 1.)
4. If you were the nurse, what attitudes and feelings would you have about this patient or her situation?
5. How would you have managed this situation if you were the nurse?
6. What skills do you need when caring for this patient?
7. What do you need to know about this patient to deliver culturally relevant care?

Responses to Self-Reflection Questions 5 and 7

Response: How would you have managed this situation if you were the nurse?

Clearly, healthcare providers in this situation need good cultural assessment and communication skills to determine how the patient who is unable to speak English well is feeling about the visit. Because the patient has an adult daughter with her, the nurse may be able to get some information through her. It would be advisable to use a medical interpreter, if one is available, to explain the doctor's findings and/or to ask questions as needed. Because there are a variety of dialects spoken in Nigeria, it might be difficult to find someone to interpret for Chinaza. It would be helpful for the provider to communicate nonverbally in a way that is assuring and comforting when the patient is stressed.

Response: What do you need to know about this patient to deliver culturally relevant care?

Knowledge of this patient's cultural history would be helpful, but as the patient admits, there have been no medical assessments or treatments by a doctor in the past. Knowing Chinaza's attitudes and beliefs and usual methods of caring for her illnesses would also be useful. Are there folk practices that Chinaza has used in the past to manage infections or other illnesses? Is Chinaza likely to follow the doctor's orders to take the medication he prescribes? A cultural assessment is needed to comprehensively determine this patient's needs. The nurse selects an appropriate model and proceeds using the model as guidance.

Hispanic/Latinx Immigrants

The Hispanic/Latinx American population includes any person of Cuban, Mexican, Puerto Rican, South or Central American, or other Spanish culture or origin, regardless of race (Office of Minority Health [OMH], n.d.). According to the 2020 Census, the Hispanic or Latinx population of any race included 62 million people or 19% of the U.S. population (Peña et al., 2023). In 2016, the Hispanic population became the largest ethnic group in America, comprising 57.5 million people, or almost 18% of the U.S. population (U.S. Census Bureau, 2017). As the Pew Research Center reported, however, the growth rate has flattened from 2016 to 2017 as compared to the Asian population, which is rapidly increasing (Krogstad, 2017). Spanish-speaking people from around the world share an ethnic identity and a common language, but may be of any race (Taylor et al., 2012). Although the term *Hispanic* generally refers to persons who can trace their heritage and lineage from Spain (Purnell, 2013), Latinos and Latinas are persons living in America who come from Latin American countries where both Spanish and Portuguese are spoken. However, the terms *Hispanic and Latinx* (*Latino/a*) are used interchangeably throughout the literature to describe members of any of the three groups. The term *Hispanic* is used in this chapter to refer to members of any one of the three groups.

Hispanic immigrants come to America from more than 21 different Spanish-speaking nations (World Population Review, n.d.-c). The federal government considers race and Hispanic origin to be two separate and distinct concepts and categorizes an individual's ethnicity as Hispanic or non-Hispanic irrespective of their race. The number of Latinx who identify as multiracial has increased from 3 million to more than 27 million. Four out of five Latinx or 80% are U.S. citizens, because they were born in the United States or one of its territories; born abroad to American citizens; or are naturalized citizens (Krogstad et al., 2023). People who are born in Puerto Rico are U.S. citizens at birth. Many Hispanics prefer to be referred to by their place of origin rather than a more collective term. For example, many Puerto Ricans self-identify as Puerto Ricans, not Latinx or Hispanic, just as Mexicans living in America might prefer the term *Chicano* or *Mexican* (World Population Review, 2022). The largest subgroups of Hispanic immigrants include Mexicans (58.9%); Puerto Ricans (9.3%); Central Americans (10.8%, includes El Salvador, Honduras, and Guatemala); Cubans (3.8%); Dominicans (3.8%), and South Americans (approximately 6.5%; Krogstad et al., 2023). The fastest population growth among U.S. Latinx was seen in populations coming from Venezuela, Guatemala, and Honduras, while people from Mexico made up 62% of the Hispanic population.

The Hispanic population is younger than the overall U.S. national average. In 2019, 30.8% were younger than 18 years as compared to only 19% of Whites (DHHS, 2021). The median age for Hispanics is 30.7 years as compared to 39, the median age of the overall U.S. population (United States Census, 2023). In 2019, states with the largest Hispanic populations were California, Texas, Florida, New York, Arizona, Illinois, New Jersey, Colorado, Georgia, and New Mexico, although North and South Dakota have seen the fastest growth in their Hispanic population (Krogstad, 2020).

As a group, educational attainment for Hispanics has been increasing; in addition, the number of Latinx enrolled in college has also increased from 2010 to 2022 from 2.9 million to 4.2 million (Krogstad et al., 2023). Their high school dropout rate has decreased from 11.6% in 1995 to 5.1% in 2022 (Korhonen, 2023). According to the 2019 U.S. Census Report, 71.8% of Hispanics had a high school diploma or higher, as compared to 94.6% of non-Hispanic Whites; 18.8% of Hispanics had a bachelor degree or higher, as compared to 40.1% of non-Hispanic Whites; and 5.7% of Hispanics held advanced professional degrees, as compared to 15.1% of non-Hispanic Whites (OMH, n.d.). Most Hispanics stated that the need to support family was the reason for not enrolling in a 4-year program; 21% of Hispanics versus 28% of Blacks, 61% of Asians, and 42% of Whites hold 4-year degrees (Pew Research Center, 2022). As a result of this education gap, Hispanic immigrants are employed largely within service, construction and maintenance, production, and transport jobs, as compared to others living in America. Consequently, the income for most Hispanics falls below that of the general population. In 2022, median income for Hispanics of all races was $62,800, as compared to $81,060 for White non-Hispanics (Statista, 2023). In 2019, the CDC reported that Hispanics have the highest uninsured rates, with only 51% of Hispanics having private insurance coverage as compared to 74.7 non-Hispanic Whites. However, there were variations between Hispanic groups, with Mexicans (47.9%) and Central Americans (41.7%) having the lowest coverage. In 2019, Hispanics had the highest uninsurance rates of any racial or ethnic group. As the Robert Wood Johnson Foundation (RWJF) reported, low income and limited access to health insurance make it more difficult for immigrants to navigate the health care system. In addition, those who are undocumented and who may have limited English proficiency (LEP) will be less willing to seek care and to be satisfied with the quality of care they ultimately receive (RWJF, 2020).

English language fluency varies among the Hispanic population, with 71.1% of Hispanics speaking a language other than English in the home. In addition, 70.4% of Mexicans, 58.8%

of Puerto Ricans, 77% of Cubans, 86.2% of Central Americans, and nearly one third of Hispanics state they are not fluent in English (OMH, n.d.). However, 72% of Latinx age 5 and older spoke English proficiently as of 2019 (Treisman, 2021). Among expressed concerns, Moslimani (2022) reported that four in 10 Latinx in the United States worry that they or someone close to them might be deported. This was an even greater fear among Latinx immigrants without a green card.

According to the CDC, chronic illnesses among older Hispanics include heart disease, stroke, diabetes, obesity, liver disease, pneumonia, influenza, and cervical cancer, but these diseases vary in morbidity among subgroups. The DHHS (2021) reports that asthma, chronic obstructive pulmonary disease (COPD), HIV/AIDS, obesity, suicide, liver disease, and infant mortality disproportionately impact Hispanics. While birth weight is lower for all Hispanics compared to Whites, Puerto Ricans have a low-birth-weight rate double that of non-Hispanic Whites. Puerto Ricans also suffer disproportionately from asthma, HIV, and infant mortality. Mexicans have higher rates of diabetes (DHHS, 2021). Johnson and Farquharson (2019) discussed the rich traditions and religious foundation that often guide healthcare beliefs and practices in the homes of Hispanic people. Further, these authors emphasize the value Hispanics place on human life, family, privacy among women, and on the use of folk medicine and herbs, home remedies, and lay "healers" as well as traditional Western medicine. As Hispanics grow older, family members feel an obligation to "care for their own" and they find it difficult to relinquish the responsibility of caring for one's older adults, despite having work and parenting responsibilities. Spirituality is essential in Hispanic people's lives and serves as a strong source of support for them, particularly during times of crisis. The researchers suggested that nurses utilize good listening and observation skills, emphasize the importance of a balanced diet and daily exercise, and make use of interprofessional collaboration and continuing education to address the needs of all Hispanic clients.

Selected Hispanic Groups

Mexicans

Mexican Americans have been discussed in the previous section on the migrant farm workers; however, it is important to note that Mexicans, despite their declining numbers as immigrants, remain the largest group of Hispanic immigrants currently living in the United States.

Like other Hispanic people, Mexicans place a high value on family, friends, and sustaining close personal relationships. *Respeto* (giving and receiving respect in communications with others) is an important consideration among Mexicans as well as other Hispanics. According to a Centers for Disease Control and Prevention (CDC, n.d.) report, health considerations of particular significance to Mexicans living in America today include the high rate of cigarette smoking, which for men is at 14.3% and for women is at 6.4%; obesity, which is at 49.5% for men and 50.9% for women; and hypertension, at 45.3% for men taking antihypertensive medications and 34.2% for women taking antihypertensive medication. With all of these risk factors for heart disease, 31.3% of Mexican immigrants are without health insurance (CDC, n.d.).

Puerto Ricans

Puerto Ricans represent the second largest Hispanic group living in the United States (5.6 million, or 10% of the U.S. Hispanic population, Noe-Bustamante et al., 2019). As a result of the Spanish American War, Puerto Rico became a commonwealth of the United States and Puerto Ricans are full U.S. citizens (CIA, 2022). Most Hispanics who can trace their lineage to Puerto Rico were born within the continental United States. According to the Pew Hispanic Center, only about one third of all Puerto Ricans (1.6 million) were actually born there. Those born outside of either the United States or Puerto Rico and who were not citizens by birth are considered foreign born (Noe-Bustamante et al., 2019). Today, races among Puerto Ricans include White Spanish (76.2%), Black (12.4%), Asian (0.5%), and Amerindian (0.2%). Puerto Ricans who self-identify as mixed-race account for over 122,000 people. Puerto Ricans migrate most often to large urban areas and are dispersed throughout the country, but are more concentrated in the Northeast. States with the largest population of Puerto Ricans are New York, New Jersey, Pennsylvania, Illinois, Florida, and California. According to the Pew Research Center, Puerto Ricans (39%) are less likely to be married than all Hispanics (46%). The median age of Puerto Ricans is 31 as compared to 29.5 for all Hispanics (Moslimani et al., 2023).

Puerto Ricans share many of the cultural values of other Hispanic groups; for example, they are family oriented, value interpersonal interactions and respect for adults (especially older people), and hold a relativistic view of time (Purnell, 2013). Like other Hispanics, Puerto Ricans speak Spanish and English, although many (83%) report speaking English with greater fluency than do other Hispanics (72%). Sixty-seven percent of Hispanic adults are English proficient, while 80% of Puerto Ricans are English proficient (Moslimani et al., 2023).

About 24% of Puerto Ricans as compared to 20% of all Hispanics age 25 and older have obtained at least a bachelor's degree. Among U.S. Hispanics, the median personal earnings were $30,000, compared to $34,000 for Puerto Ricans; however, among Puerto Ricans living in the United States and District of Columbia, 21% and 18% of Hispanics, respectively, live in poverty (Moslimani et al., 2023).

In September 2017, Puerto Rico was hit by Hurricane Maria, a Category 4 hurricane storm with 150 MPH winds that devastated the island, destroying the infrastructure and leaving its 3.4 million U.S. citizens without water for drinking, bathing, or toileting; light or electricity; and cellular service, and left them with limited food. Many villagers were cut off from communication with others on the island, some schools closed, and some hospitals were not able to provide services (Resnick & Barclay, 2017). As many houses were destroyed, thousands of people were displaced. Because of Puerto Rico's location in the Caribbean Sea, rescuers from the U.S. mainland had a difficult time reaching people who lived in remote villages on the island. Many were without power and water for several months. The United States sent supplies, and the Navy's *USNS Comfort* was sent to provide healthcare and other support. Over 200,000 people left for the U.S. mainland for refuge. According to news reports, on April 18, 2018, Puerto Rico suffered an island-wide blackout that left many without power for as long as 11 months after the hurricane. The initial official report noted 64 deaths due to the hurricane, but subsequent reports noted that more than 4,600 people in Puerto Rico lost their lives due to the hurricane (BBC, 2018). At this writing, some Puerto Ricans still require the use of backup generators or candles when night falls and are still struggling to survive after the devastation. The Centers for Medicare and Medicaid Services (CMS, 2018) compared Puerto Rican's health status, access to care, and satisfaction with care to their U.S. mainland counterparts before Hurricane Maria. Puerto Ricans on the island had lower ratings than the mainland-dwelling groups regarding having a usual source of care, such as having a flu or pneumonia shot for those age 65 or over. In another study (Mattei et al., 2018), the researchers found that adults living in Puerto Rico have multiple lifestyle risk factors and high prevalence of chronic cardiometabolic and psychologic conditions as compared to Puerto Ricans living on the U.S. mainland. Puerto Ricans living in the mainland United States stated that they have poor health behaviors and chronic conditions as compared to other Hispanics. In comparison, those on the mainland tended to have higher household incomes and rates of health insurance, employment, and educational attainment than other Hispanics, but lower rates than the general U.S. population (Mattei et al., 2018). Nurses caring for Puerto Rican patients should determine their health histories in light of the impact of this devastating natural disaster on their physical and psychologic health.

IMPORTANT POINTS

- In 2022, Hispanics accounted for more than 62 million people and represented 19% of the U.S. population.
- The terms *Hispanic* and *Latinx* (*Latino/a*) are often used interchangeably.
- Most Hispanics prefer references to their nation of origin.
- Hispanics come to America from more than 23 Spanish-speaking countries.
- Most Hispanics immigrate to America from Mexico; others come from Puerto Rico, Cuba, El Salvador, Guatemala, the Dominican Republic, and Columbia.
- People born in Puerto Rico are citizens at birth.
- Half of all Hispanics live in California and Texas; there are also significant Hispanic populations in Florida, New York, and Illinois.
- Chronic illness among Hispanics includes diabetes, hypertension, obesity, CV disease, liver disease, and HIV.
- The population of Hispanic immigrants is on average younger than that of native-born Americans.
- This is true of immigrants and native-born Hispanics; the majority are Catholics; however, there are also Protestants and other religions among them.
- Hispanics place a high value on family and close relationships.
- The high school dropout rate is declining among Hispanics and college enrollment is increasing at 2- and 4-year colleges.
- Unemployment is higher and median income and health insurance coverage are lower among Hispanic immigrants than native-born Americans and some other minorities.
- Hispanics vary in the use of folk practices and use of herbal remedies.
- Cultural variations may be based on immigration status.

In one study, the researchers found that adults living in Puerto Rico have multiple lifestyle risk factors and high prevalence of chronic cardiometabolic and psychologic conditions. They also described multiple studies of Puerto Ricans living in the mainland United States and found that they have poor health behaviors and chronic conditions as compared to other Hispanics. In comparison, those on the mainland tended to have higher household incomes and rates of health insurance, employment, and educational attainment than other Hispanics, but lower rates than the general U.S. population (Mattei et al., 2018). In this study, the findings reveal many social and health disadvantages for Puerto Ricans living on the island. These disadvantages include a median income lower $20,000; high unemployment, despite relatively high educational attainment; and multiple chronic health conditions. Health conditions include a higher prevalence for hypertension on the island versus the mainland (42% in Puerto Rico compared to 31% on the mainland); 39% versus 36% for high cholesterol; 16% versus 10% for DM; and 9% versus 6% for coronary artery disease (CAD); in addition, 66% of those on the island reported having a BMI indicating overweight or obesity. As the authors noted, since Hurricane Maria, the island remains in an "economic crisis" (BBC, 2018). Following the hurricane, illness and death ensued because of "interruptions in medical care by power cuts and broken road links" and widespread devastation (BBC, 2018, para. 1).

So, for Puerto Ricans who live on the island or who migrated to the U.S. mainland, much of the physical and psychologic stress that they endured as a result of "Maria" and the socioeconomic problems that followed will influence their health and well-being for years to come. Nurses caring for Puerto Rican patients should determine their health histories in light of the impact of this devastating natural disaster on their physical and psychologic health.

Arab Immigrants

The U.S. government defines persons of Arab heritage as those who can trace one or more ancestries to an Arab-speaking country or region such as the Middle East or Northern Africa (Global Perspectives, n.d.). There are 22 Arab countries, including Palestine, which are members of the Arab League and share a common history, language, and culture. Although current American attitudes are more positive than in the past, attitudes toward Arabs and Muslims have vacillated between fear and anger since September 11, 2001. Therefore, this ethnic group is discussed here as a silent vulnerable population living in America. It is estimated that 3.7 million Americans trace their roots to an Arab country. The majority of Arab Americans are native born (63%), and nearly 82% of Arabs living in America are citizens. Advocacy groups have requested that the Census include another category for people of Middle Eastern or North African (MENA) descent to better reflect their racial and ethnic makeup and provide information that would assist in identifying the needs of this heterogeneous population (American-Arab Anti-Discrimination Committee, 2015; Chebli et al., 2021; see www.adc.org.) Historically, the first of three waves of Arab immigrants were Christians from Lebanon and Syria who immigrated to New York and to Boston between 1887 and 1913 with the intention of improving their life circumstances and one day returning home. Many members of this first wave were unskilled workers, along with some poets and writers, who became permanent residents and whose descendants are now natives. A second wave of Arab immigration included displaced Palestinians and other Muslims after the United Nations Partition Plan for Palestine opened the way to the creation of the Jewish state of Israel in 1948. This wave included many more refugees fleeing war, among them many professionals and people seeking academic degrees (Little, 2022). A third wave in the mid-1960s brought more professionals and entrepreneurs who fled ongoing political unrest and war in the Middle East. Arabs who came during this wave were more educated and affluent, and many became U.S. citizens (Little, 2022). Thus, Arab people have been a significant part of American life for several generations.

The primary way Arabs identify themselves is based on their place of origin.

Culture and Religion

The majority of Arabs in America have ancestral ties to Lebanon, Syria, Palestine, Egypt, and Iraq, while the Arab population can trace its roots to every Arab country (Arab American Institute [AAI], 2021). Among Arab populations, there are several ethnic categories and 17 religious sects. Muslims (59.7%), which include Shias, Sunni, Ismaelites, Druze, and Nusayr, constitute the largest group. Muslims comprise diverse ethnic groups including one third Arab and one third South Asian; one fifth are U.S.-born Black Muslims. Thus, not all Muslims are Arab, nor are all Arabs Muslim. Like other religious groups, there are also variations among Muslims regarding their degree of religiosity (Arab America, n.d.). Therefore, one cannot assume the degree to which religion plays a role in a particular Muslim's life. Many Muslims are very devout, whereas others are less influenced by their religion. A second group of Arabs, about 39%, are Christians, which include Maronite, Greek Orthodox, Armenian, Syrian Catholic, Armenian Catholic, Roman Catholic, and Protestant (CIA, 2017). Muslim groups tend to be more traditional than their non-Muslim peers and are also more likely to have an Arab spouse and believe in *inerrancy*, the belief that the Qur'an is completely without error. Among women, the degree of attachment to the Arab community is a significant factor influencing their beliefs about gender roles. Consequently, as in other cultural groups, the problem of domestic violence exists between Arab men and women and lies in the cultural values and norms abusers have to coerce and abuse their victims in the Arab community (Abuelezam et al., 2018). Women in this community experience domestic violence at a much higher rate than men based on Arab American views about family unity and keeping it intact to maintain the family's honor and reputation, despite situations of abuse, belief in a patriarchal and patrilineal family, use of the immediate and extended family as a support system, the difficulties and social stigma around divorce, and a lack of females' financial independence. Because of the cultural values and beliefs that make it difficult for women to extricate themselves from abusive relationships, nurses caring for patients from Arab/Muslim communities should consider the possibility of domestic violence when indications present themselves during patient care encounters and determine strategies for offering support.

Attitudes Toward Arabs and Muslims

Unfortunately, since the terrorist attacks of September 11, 2001, increased racial and ethnic animosity has left Arabs, other Middle Easterners, Muslims, and those that bear physical resemblance to members of these groups, fearful. As Faheid (2021) observed, Arab Americans are twice as likely to commit suicide because of the discrimination and stigma they encounter. This is a reciprocal fear as members of this group fear retaliation for the events of 9/11 and some individuals outside the group look on the group members with suspicion and, at times, misplaced anger and mistrust. "Feelings of discrimination and societal stigma post 2001 increased for Arab Americans seeking health care" (Kundrik & Saoud, 2020, p. 444). There is also a partisan divide in Americans' approval of banning Muslim immigrants, or in justifying law enforcements' profiling of Arab and Muslim Americans based on appearance.

Demographics

According to the Arab American Institute (2021), Americans of Arab and North African descent live in all 50 states, but more than two thirds of them live in just 10 states: California, Michigan, New York, Florida, Texas, New Jersey, Illinois, Ohio, Pennsylvania, and Virginia. Pennsylvania has one of the fastest growing Arab populations in the country. Arab Americans in Pennsylvania reside in all 67 counties of the state. One third of the Arab population lives in metropolitan Los Angeles, Detroit, and New York. Ethnic enclaves where many Arabs live include Dearborn, Michigan, and El Cajon, a city on the east side of San Diego.

Arab Americans are among the most highly educated and skilled workers in the nation; 89% hold a high school diploma or better. More than 45% of Arab Americans have a bachelor's degree, compared to 30% of other Americans. Nearly twice as many Arabs hold postgraduate degrees (18%) as do other Americans. Among Americans from the Middle East and North Africa, Egyptians are the most highly educated, at 94% with high school diplomas or better and 64% with a bachelor's degree or higher, compared to Iraqis, at 73% with a high school education and above and only 36% with bachelor's degrees. As a result, Egyptians are more likely (51%) to work in professional and management positions. Seventy-three percent of working Arabs are employed in managerial, professional, technical, sales, or administrative fields. Only 5% are unemployed. As a result, Arabs living in the United States generally enjoy higher incomes than most other Americans. According to Arab America (n.d.), approximately 30% of Arabs have an annual income of more than $75,000, compared to 22% of all households in the United States. The average income of Arab Americans is 22% higher than the U.S. national average. However, a $10,000 earning gap exists between male and female Arabs, with men earning significantly higher pay. These differences may reflect the educational differences between men and women and that less emphasis is placed by the culture on females working outside the home.

Arabs/Muslims and Health

Past community-based studies of Arab Americans' health point to significant health problems among this immigrant population. In 2018, Abuelezam and colleagues reviewed the findings on health of Arab Americans in the United States in an updated comprehensive literature review. In this study, researchers found that Arab Americans had lower estimated rates of recommended vaccinations (flu and pneumonia) than non-Hispanic Whites, as well as a high prevalence of diabetes and higher odds of diabetes when compared to non-Arab, non-Hispanic Whites. Arab Americans also commonly had vitamin D insufficiencies, which were linked to insulin resistance, metabolic syndrome, and glucose intolerance in Arab men. Further, the authors noted that "[a] number of studies found a lack of appropriate diabetes education tools for Arab Americans" and "[c]ultural and linguistic deficiencies in the existing educational literature," (para. 16) preventing Arab Americans from understanding their risks for DM. **Acculturation** was found to influence diabetes control differently for men than for women, with negative associations found between acculturation and diabetes risk in Arab men; for women, however, acculturation was associated with diabetic risk. In this study, Ramadan was found to pose a potential barrier to diabetes control in the Arab population.

As Chebli and colleagues (2021), Kundrik Leh and Saoud (2020), and Abuelezam and colleagues (2018) observed, "relatively little has been published about the health status of this population" (Kundrik Leh & Saoud, 2020, p. 444). The paucity of health information about this group is probably because Arabs are not considered among the U.S. minority groups, and because of "their racial/ethnic misclassifications as Whites" (p. 5915). However, in 2020 Chebli and colleagues found that participants emphasized five major themes that Arab Americans faced: cancer stigma leading to concealment of diagnosis, aversion to support groups, economic barriers to cancer treatment, language barriers in healthcare, and limited cancer support and assistance resources. The researchers identified several strategies to address each of the themes in their findings. Establishing peer mentorship programs will address cancer stigma leading to concealment of diagnosis outside of Arab Americans' families and provide a means of support. A hospital-based navigation plan would address the economic barriers to cancer treatment. Increased workforce diversity in healthcare could address the language barrier. Further, the authors suggested community coalitions to lobby for recognizing Arab Americans as an ethnic group to increase cancer assistance support. Abuelezam and colleagues (2018), based on a comprehensive review of the literature, found that Arab women with higher levels of education and who had lived in the United States for longer times were more likely to get screened for breast cancer

According to Abuelezam and colleagues, mental health research studies revealed an estimated 14% of Arab American adolescents were diagnosed with depression. Another study found 50% of Arab Americans met that criteria. Studies of Iraqi refugees found they were at high risk for PTSD. In a 2022 study, Abuelezam and colleagues found Arab Americans were also at greater risk of testing positive for SARS-CoV-2 than non-Hispanic Whites and Blacks, but had a lower risk of hospital admission or mortality.

In a study of Somali immigrants (Wolf et al., 2016), researchers discovered the significance of Islamic practice on mental health among this population. Somalis viewed practicing Islam and reading the Qur'an as essential treatments for illness. Tribal connectedness, cultural history, and the use of a stimulant/substance from a tree, called Khat, that was placed under Somali men's tongues also influenced their mental health. Somalis greatly respected their imams, religious leaders of their mosques, and Sheiks and made time for prayer, meditation, reading, and spending time with family and friends. Therefore, it is important for nurses and caregivers to allow time for these activities when caring for members of this population.

In understanding the sociocultural context in which the individual experiences physical and mental illness, the nurse is more likely to be able to identify appropriate strategies for providing Arab or Muslim patients with culturally competent healthcare. Each immigrant population comes to America under a particular set of circumstances, bringing with them their own value systems, goals, and aspirations for life in America. As we have discussed throughout this chapter, many factors influence immigrants' ability to live healthy and productive lives in a foreign land: immigration status, a family support system, ability to speak the English language, economic resources, and receptiveness of the host community. As nurses, we are most concerned about the factors that influence immigrants' health and access to healthcare, irrespective of their country of origin or immigration status. Providing culturally competent care requires that we maximize the time we spend with patients during each encounter with them. Learning as much as we can about the cultural needs of the individuals we serve ensures that we will be able to make informed decisions about how best to care for them. For more information about Arab Americans, go to www.aaiusa.org. Another excellent resource is Arab American Stories on YouTube at www.youtube.com/results?search_query=arab+american+stories.

IMPORTANT POINTS

- It is estimated that 3.7 million Americans trace their roots to an Arab country. This figure is likely an underestimate.
- Some underreporting of data about Arabs may be due to mistrust about how information may be used considering the current attitudes toward the Arab population in the United States and misclassification of Arabs as non-ethnic group members.
- Among Arabs in the United States, the majority (63%) is native born, and 82% of Arabs living in America are citizens.
- Arab Americans are ethnically, religiously, and politically diverse.
- The earliest Arabs came to the United States from Lebanon and Syria.
- Most Arabs come to the United States from Lebanon, Egypt, Syria, Palestine, Jordan, Morocco, and Iraq.
- The largest, most recent groups of Muslim immigrants come from Iraq, Somalia, and Egypt.
- There are two major sects within the Arab immigrants: Shias and Sunni.
- Among Muslims, there are Arabs, South Asians, Blacks, and increasing numbers of Hispanics.
- Arabs live in all 50 states in the United States; two thirds of Arabs live in 10 states: California, Michigan, New York, Florida, Texas, New Jersey, Illinois, Ohio, Pennsylvania, and Virginia. One third of Arab Americans live in metropolitan Los Angeles; Detroit; Texas; New York; Dearborn, Michigan; and El Cajon, near east San Diego. Pennsylvania has the fastest growing Arab population.
- Arabs are among the most highly educated ethnic group in the United States, with more than 45% having bachelor's degrees compared to 30% of other Americans. Compared to other Americans, twice as many Arabs (18%) have postgraduate degrees.
- Arabs are more likely to work in higher-paying management jobs.
- Not all Arabs are Muslim; there are Catholics and Protestants among them as well.
- Many Muslims are deeply devout.
- Gender roles are influenced by the attachment to the Arab community. Domestic violence toward women in the Arab community is linked to cultural values and beliefs related to the patriarchal family.
- Since the terrorist attacks of September 11, 2001, there has been an increase in ambivalence as well as in some anger and hostility toward Arabs. However, since 2017, despite the continuation of hate crimes toward Arabs and Muslims, favorable opinions by Americans are increasing.
- There is limited health research about the Arab population. However, some reports indicate Arab Americans suffer higher rates of common noncommunicable diseases including obesity, diabetes, and CV issues.
- Because of their exposure to traumatic preimmigration conditions, as well as hostility, ambivalence, and religious discrimination, reports of anti-Arab hate crimes place some Arab Americans at risk for depression and PTSD.
- Violence is a major concern in the Arab community. Arab males are six times more likely to die of homicide than their White U.S. counterparts.

CASE SCENARIO 2

Hasim Amad is a merchant who was born and raised in an urban area in Beirut. Mr. Amad struggled all his life to earn a modest income to support his family. He always wanted his son Youseff to become a physician and enjoy a better life in America. Mr. Amad made sure that each of his six children learned English, as well as both classical Arabic and the Arabic dialect spoken in his region. Youseff honored his father's wishes, studied English as well as classical Arabic, and received excellent grades in school. He applied to many universities in America. After being accepted to medical school, Youseff came to America with the intention of ultimately returning home. Following his residency, Youseff returned home and married Raja, age 16, the daughter of a family friend, and brought her to America. Today, Youseff and his wife have three children, Nour, Naseem, and Nizir. Raja is expecting her fourth child and is 38 weeks' pregnant. They have lived in America for 5 years. Raja has learned to speak English, but has trouble reading it. As Muslims, Youseff and Raja practice Islam and live a quiet life in Dearborn, Michigan, within a large Arab community. Youseff practices as a physician at a local clinic, while Raja cares for their children at their modest home near the clinic where Youseff works. She sometimes socializes with the women of her community, but spends most of her time at home. One morning as Raja is returning home from taking the children to school, she is involved in a car accident. Although Raja experiences no critical injuries, the accident causes her to go into premature labor and she is rushed to a nearby hospital. On Raja's arrival in the labor room, Sarah, the nurse, determines that Raja is very upset, but is limited in her ability to provide information in English. After performing a brief assessment, she notifies the physician on call that Raja is in labor and needs to be examined immediately. She also contacts Dr. Hassan, an Arab doctor on staff, who she knows is on duty today. She explains that she needs an interpreter to assist in communicating with Raja. Dr. Hassan says that he will be happy to assist, but warns that not all people of Arab heritage speak the same dialect. Dr. Hassan tells Sarah that they will need to have a female physician and nurses, if possible, if the patient is Muslim. Raja is taken to the labor room and her husband is notified. The nurse shares her conversation with the other staff members. Raja's contractions are occurring every 15 minutes. Although Raja is pain free, Cindy, the nurse in the labor room, decides to learn more about Raja and utilizes Purnell's cultural assessment (Purnell, 2013). This model includes considerations of patients' country of origin, communication, family roles and organization, workforce issues, biocultural ecology, high-risk behaviors, nutrition, pregnancy and childbearing practices, death rituals, spirituality, healthcare practices, and healthcare practitioners (Purnell, 2014). By considering these areas, Cindy is able to learn much about Raja and to determine the best approach for her care. Despite the fact that Raja appears to be about Cindy's age, the nurse begins by asking the patient what she prefers the nurses to call her. Raja states that she prefers being called by her first name, rather than Mrs. Amad. Cindy is also unsure about whether it is appropriate to touch Raja. When assisting her patients in labor, Cindy likes to hold their hand or rub their backs, but she has never cared for an Arab patient before. She learns from Raja that touching is permitted between members of the same gender. She is relieved to know that she can comfort Raja in her usual way throughout her labor. Between labor contractions, Raja is offered but refuses ice chips to her lips. Many Arabs believe that receiving cold or icy beverages during the morning or during illness is inappropriate. Despite being offered comfort measures, Raja moans and screams out as contractions occur. Some staff members are annoyed by Raja's screaming. "All that screaming is not necessary," one nurse comments. Cindy recognizes that this behavior is an acceptable cultural norm for many Arab women and other ethnic groups. When Raja's contractions are 3 minutes apart, Raja's husband arrives in the delivery room; his sister accompanies him. Youseff asks Raja's uncles and two brothers to wait in the reception room. On entering the room, Youseff asks to speak with the physician in charge and is pleased when Dr. Joy Kim approaches him. The doctor introduces herself and tells him, "Your baby is coming early, but baby and mom are doing well." Youseff asks the nurses to give Raja something for pain. He also tells his sister to put something cool over Raja's head. The nurses explain that Raja received an epidural anesthetic before he arrived. Cindy realizes that it is the role of Arab family members to speak to the healthcare professionals on behalf of the patient and to actively participate in their care. She provides Raja's sister-in-law with a cool cloth to place on Raja's head. Typically, the male is not supposed to participate in the actual birth; however, because Youseff is a physician, albeit not an obstetrician, he chooses to remain with Raja. Raja's contractions occur closer and closer together and are now 2 minutes apart. Youseff frowns each time a male nurse or doctor stands at the door to speak with one of the individuals in the room. "That is our way," he says. "There should be no males in the room except me." As the staff prepares to take Raja into the delivery room, Cindy reassures Youseff that the nurses will do their best to adhere to the Amads' traditional practices. She further explains that there will be a need to have a pediatrician in the room once the baby is born and there is no female pediatrician on call today. Youseff states that he understands and together with the staff anxiously awaits the birth of his child.

WHAT NURSES NEED TO KNOW ABOUT THEMSELVES

Application of the Staircase Self-Assessment Model: Self-Reflection Questions

1. What feelings and attitudes would you have toward the Amads?
2. Where are you on the Cultural Competency Staircase when caring for Arab patients?
3. How will you progress to the next step?
4. What skills are needed when caring for the Amads?
5. If you were the nurse, what would you and the other staff members need to know to provide culturally competent care to the Amads?

Responses to Self-Reflection Questions

Response: What feelings and attitudes would you have toward the Amads?

Your personal attitudes and feelings will depend on the number of clinical or personal encounters you have had with Arab patients and the nature of those experiences. As you gain more knowledge about this cultural group and understand their values, norms, and health needs, you will feel more comfortable caring for Arab patients. Both of the nurses assigned to care for Raja in this case example demonstrate an awareness of the possible influences cultural differences may have on this patient's hospital experience. As examples, the first nurse seeks an interpreter and raises the awareness of others by informing the labor room nurses that the patient is Muslim, so that some of the patient's known cultural needs may be anticipated. The second nurse demonstrates an understanding of her own preference for calling the patient by her first name because she is about the same age. The nurse also recognizes her tendency to hold patients' hands as a way of showing support. However, in both these instances, the nurse understands that in some cultures these behaviors may be offensive and decides to speak with the patient first before acting on assumptions or misperceptions. Both nurses remain nonjudgmental and responsive to the patient's cultural needs. The nurses who express resentment of Raja's screaming during labor consider this behavior inappropriate because it is culturally incongruent with their own values and attitudes. These nurses lack cultural understanding and respect for cultural differences.

Response: Where are you on the Cultural Competency Staircase when caring for Arab patients?

Response: How will you progress to the next step?

From the moment the nurse first meets the patient and throughout each subsequent meeting, the nurse must utilize skills in cultural assessment to identify and prioritize the patient's cultural needs. Each encounter between the patient and the nurse is also an opportunity to identify the nursing behaviors that are most likely to positively affect patient care outcomes. Since a patient–nurse encounter may take many forms, these opportunities can occur even before the nurse actually meets the patient. For example, when receiving documentation or a verbal report about the patient of Arab heritage, the nurse may begin to collect data about potential cultural issues that can impact care. Culturally competent nurses proactively explore potential areas of cultural conflicts between the medical staff and the patient. By doing so, they are able to anticipate potential problems and address them before they occur. Despite cultural differences that might exist, the nurse consistently strives to demonstrate respect and caring to the patient and family, even when the patient's views are incongruent with the nurse's own values and beliefs. By exploring cultural differences, the nurse is able to build on previous cultural knowledge. When caring for Arab patients, nurses should explore gender roles and determine to what extent a female patient might wish to defer to her husband in healthcare decision-making. Because family relationships are important to Arab patients, family members should be considered when planning care. Speaking with the family's designated spokesperson, asking appropriate questions, and explaining technical information will enable the nurse to establish a positive working relationship with the patient and the family. When time permits, speaking with other members of the Arab community through formal (continuing education, staff development) or informal means to gain insight about the health issues and concerns of this cultural group helps prepare the nurse for future encounters with Arab patients. All of these behaviors enable the nurse to build skill and confidence to progress to the next step in cultural competency.

Response: What skills are needed when caring for the Amads?

The nurses in this case, and nurses during any encounter with patients, need to have skills in cultural assessment. Being skilled involves having several cultural assessment models in one's repertoire from which to choose the one that best fits the clinical situation and time frame (see earlier in this chapter). One model that might be useful is Purnell's *Twelve Domains of Culture,* which includes considerations of patients' (a) country of origin, (b) communication, (c) family roles and organization, (d) workforce issues, (e) biocultural ecology, (f) high-risk behaviors, (g) nutrition, (h) pregnancy and childbearing practices, (i) death rituals, (j) spirituality, (k) healthcare practices, and (l) healthcare practitioners (Purnell, 2013). When conducting the cultural assessment, the nurse must have the ability to listen actively to determine the most effective approach for care. Communication skills that incorporate the use of an interpreter are also needed should the patient or the nurse have difficulty exchanging information. Fortunately, in this case there is a doctor on staff who may be able to assist. However, in some cases, the nurse will need to be skilled at recognizing and utilizing nonverbal cues, body language, or other strategies to communicate effectively with the patient who speaks no English or English as a second language.

Response: If you were the nurse, what would you and the other staff members need to know to provide culturally competent care to the Amads?

When caring for the Amads or any other Arab patients, the nurses need an *understanding* of the Arab culture. This knowledge includes the recognition that Arab cultures are diverse and that even language may vary between Arab groups, although most Arabs are fluent in English. Differences between groups are influenced by the geographical origins of a particular group, length of time in the United States, and other variables such as age, socioeconomic status, education, and language ability. Because many Arabs practice Islam, nurses need some knowledge of what that means in terms of patients' dietary restrictions, religious practices or spirituality needs, health beliefs, and lifestyle. However, not all Arabs are Muslim, so the nurse must acquire knowledge of the patient's specific religion and determine what relevance it has in the patient's life. In this case, knowledge of cultural attitudes about labor and delivery is helpful; however, in other situations, cultural beliefs and attitudes around death and dying may be more relevant. Having knowledge of these things enables the nurse to work with the patient in establishing meaningful healthcare goals and implementing culturally appropriate interventions. Knowledge of other resources such as interpreters, language banks, or reference texts that offer detailed information about the culture is also useful for nurses who are attempting to communicate with people from culturally diverse groups. As in this case, the patient's and family's acknowledgment of the nurse's respect for their cultural values and beliefs is demonstrated by their expressions of satisfaction with the care they receive.

SUMMARY

Despite current policies and attitudes toward immigration, America remains a refuge for thousands of immigrants each year. Each new group of immigrants comes with the hope of experiencing a welcoming social environment, decent housing, employment, and superior healthcare services. Culturally competent nurses appreciate the need to partner with their patients in determining culturally relevant healthcare goals and interventions. The health and well-being of immigrants, whether legal or unauthorized, impacts the health of the communities in which they live. The more nurses and other healthcare workers can do to ensure culturally competent, preventive, and supportive care, the more they are able to minimize disease and illness and promote health in their communities.

NCLEX®-TYPE QUESTIONS

1. The staff development nurse conducts a workshop on the care of new immigrants. The nurse states that according to the U.S. Census, 46.2 million people, or 14.2% of the population, are:
   A. Citizens
   B. Residing in the country illegally
   C. Lawful permanent residents (LPR)
   D. Foreign born

2. The newly admitted patient explains to the nurse that he recently immigrated to the United States and holds a green card. The nurse understands that this means:
   A. The patient must at some point return to his native land
   B. The patient has citizenship
   C. The patient has a legal right to reside permanently in the United States
   D. The patient is a foreign national

3. A Mexican migrant farmworker is seen in the ED for a work-related injury. During the intake interview, the patient reveals that she is worried about being treated because she has no health insurance. The nurse's best response is:
   A. Only citizens are eligible to receive hospital care.
   B. All persons who live and work in America are entitled to emergency care.
   C. Green card holders may receive only hospital care.
   D. There is a fee that must be paid by those without health insurance.

4. The nurses on a busy hospital unit in an urban metropolitan area observed a sudden influx of Hispanic patients from Puerto Rico and Mexico over the past several months. Which statement by the staff is accurate about current demographics and Hispanic populations? *Select all that apply.*
   A. Hispanics currently represent more than 16% of the population with a projection of 19% by 2050.
   B. Current trends suggest a decrease in the number of Hispanics coming to America.
   C. The largest group of Hispanic immigrants come from Mexico.
   D. Hispanics are typically younger than their U.S. counterparts.

5. A new graduate nurse relocates to California in search of employment and is to begin working in a busy medical–surgical unit in San Diego. What statement by the nurse indicates a good understanding of the diversity of patient populations in California?
   A. According to the 2020 Census, California had the largest immigrant population in the United States.
   B. California is second only to Texas in having the largest numbers of immigrants.
   C. Largely Asian immigrants migrate to California.
   D. There is limited cultural and ethnic diversity in California.

6. The nurse reads the chart of a newly admitted recent immigrant to the United States. The patient's chart reads that the patient was admitted to the country due to a fear of returning to her country of origin because of the danger of political persecution. Based on this information, the patient is best described as:
   A. An alien
   B. An asylee
   C. A lawful permanent resident (LPR)
   D. An illegal

7. The culturally competent nurse recognizes that the majority of new immigrants come to the United States from what regions around the world?
   A. Oceania and Europe
   B. Africa and Asia
   C. Asia and Oceania
   D. Latin America and Asia

8. The greatest barrier to healthcare access for new and older immigrants is:
   A. Problems in communication due to language issues
   B. Religious and value differences
   C. Gender and family role variations
   D. Gaining access to hospitals due to transportation problems

9. When nurses are caring for new immigrants, one of their most important roles is:
   A. Learning a foreign language
   B. Teaching foreign patients to speak English
   C. Learning illness prevention and health promotion
   D. Providing acute care for those who arrive in an illness state

10. What statement(s) are true about the healthcare needs of immigrants in the United States? *Select all that apply.*
    A. Some immigrants require healthcare as soon as they arrive in the country.
    B. Immigrants' health on arrival to the United States is usually better than their U.S. counterparts.

C. Obesity and other illnesses among immigrants increase with time spent in the United States.

D. Hypertension and heart disease are experienced more by U.S.-born adults than foreign-born adults.

11. According to the research, what factors best explain how American citizens are divided in their attitudes toward immigrants?
    A. The division is based on differences in religious beliefs.
    B. The division is based on language diversity and communication problems.
    C. The division is based on partisan, political misunderstandings and value differences.
    D. The division is due to socioeconomic differences.

12. When initiating care for new immigrants, nurses should be guided by what important principle?
    A. The patient's culture determines values, attitudes, and beliefs.
    B. The patient is a unique individual with cultural attitudes, values, and beliefs.
    C. The patient's religion will determine values and behavior.
    D. Members of the same cultural group share similar attitudes and ideals.

13. The nurse performs a cultural assessment for a Puerto Rican patient using the Giger and Davidhizar model. When considering the biologic variations of members of this group, the nurse realizes that among Puerto Ricans:
    A. There is a high incidence of asthma, hypertension, and diabetes
    B. There is a high susceptibility to gastrointestinal disorders
    C. Arthritis and lupus are prevalent
    D. Neurologic and hematologic illnesses are common

14. The ED nurse gives a report to the receiving nurse on a medical–surgical unit. She explains that the unit will receive Mr. G., a 45-year-old Arab patient. The receiving nurse expresses concern about what important consideration impacting this admission?
    A. There is an all-female staff on the unit.
    B. The nursing staff is uncertain about the correct pronunciation of the patient's name.
    C. The nurse assumes the patient will not like the food.
    D. The nurse is confused about the patient's attitudes toward American nurses and doctors.

ANSWERS TO NCLEX-TYPE QUESTIONS

1. D	6. B	11. C
2. C	7. D	12. B
3. B	8. A	13. A
4. A, C, and D	9. C	14. A
5. A	10. A, B, C, and D	

AMERICAN ASSOCIATION OF COLLEGES OF NURSING COMPETENCIES ADDRESSED IN THIS CHAPTER

1. Apply knowledge of social and cultural factors that affect nursing and healthcare across multiple contexts.
2. Use relevant data sources and best evidence in providing culturally competent care.
3. Promote achievement of safe and quality outcomes of care for diverse populations.
4. Advocate for social justice, including commitment to the health of vulnerable populations and the elimination of healthcare disparities.
5. Participate in continuous cultural competence development.

REFERENCES

Abuelezam, N. N., El-Sayed, A. M., & Galea, S. (2018). The health of Arab Americans in the United States: An updated comprehensive literature review. *Frontiers in Public Health, 6,* 262. https://doi.org/10.3389/fpubh.2018.00262

Abuelezam, N. N., Greenwood, K. L., Galea, S., & Al-Naser, R. (2022). Differential COVID-19 testing, admissions, and mortality for Arab Americans in Southern California. *PLoS One, 17*(4), e0267116. https://doi.org/10.1371/journal.pone.0267116

Abu El-Haj, T. R. (2007). I was born here, but my home, it's not here: Educating for democratic citizenship in an era of transnational migration and global conflict. *Harvard Educational Review, 77*(3), 285–316. https://doi.org/10.17763/haer.77.3.412l7m737q114h5m

America: The Jesuit Review. (2017, December 27). *The editors: What we owe the American farmworkers.* https://www.americamagazine.org/politics-society/2017/12/27/editors-what-we-owe-americas-farmworkers

American-Arab Anti-Discrimination Committee. (2015). *2014-2015 recap report.* https://adc.org/wp-content/uploads/2015/08/ADC_Annual_Report_2015.pdf

Arab America. (n.d.). *Arab Americans.* Retrieved October 18, 2023, from https://www.arabamerica.com/arab-americans

Arab American Institute. (2021). *National Arab American demographics.* https://www.aaiusa.org/demographics

Asylum Access. (2021, July 24). *What is the 1951 Refugee Convention—and how does it support human rights?* https://asylumaccess.org/what-is-the-1951-refugee-convention-and-how-does-it-support-human-rights

Baker, B. (2021). *Estimates of the unauthorized immigrant population residing in the U.S. January 2015–January 2018.* U.S. Department of Homeland Security. https://www.dhs.gov/sites/default/files/publications/immigration-statistics/Pop_Estimate/UnauthImmigrant/unauthorized_immigrant_population_estimates_2015_-_2018.pdf

BBC. (2018, May 29). *Hurricane Maria "killed 4,600 in Puerto Rico."* https://www.bbc.com/news/world-us-canada-44294366

Boundless. (2022). *Black immigrants in the United States: Status, challenges, and impacts. Newsletter.* https://www.boundless.com/research/black-immigrants-in-the-united-states-status-challenges-and-impacts

Budiman, A. (2020, August 20). *Key findings about U.S. immigrants.* Pew Research Center. https://www.pewresearch.org/short-reads/2020/08/20/key-findings-about-u-s-immigrants

Budiman, A., & Ruiz, N. G. (2021, April 29). *Key facts about Asian Americans, a diverse and growing population.* Pew Research Center. https://www.pewresearch.org/short-reads/2021/04/29/key-facts-about-asian-americans

Bureau of Labor Statistics. U.S. Department of Labor. News Release. (2022). *Foreign-born workers: Labor force characteristics—2022.* https://www.bls.gov/news.release/pdf/forbrn.pdf

Camarota, S. A., & Zeigler, K. (2021). *Immigration population hits record 46.2 million in November 2021.* Center for Immigration Studies. https://cis.org/Camarota/Immigrant-Population-Hits-Record-462-Million-November-2021

Centers for Disease Control and Prevention. (n.d.). *Health of Mexican American population.* Retrieved October 17, 2023, from https://www.cdc.gov/nchs/fastats/mexican-health.htm

Center for Immigration Studies. (2017). *Immigration data portal.* https://cis.org/Immigration-Statistics-Data-Portal

Central Intelligence Agency. (2017). *World fact book 2017.* https://www.cia.gov/library/publica tions/the-world-factbook/docs/notesanddefs.html?fieldkey = 2122&term = Religions

Central Intelligence Agency. (2022). *The world factbook.* https://www.cia.gov/the-world-factbook/about/archives/2022

Chebli, P., Reyes, K., Muramatsu, N., Watson, K., Fitzgibbon, M., Abboud, S., & Molina, Y. (2021). Perspectives of multisectorial community stakeholders on Arab American cancer patient's needs and suggested interventions. *Supportive Care in Cancer, 29,* 5915–5925. https://doi.org/10.1007/s00520-021-06169-x

Chen, C., & Park, J. Z. (2019). Pathways of religious assimilation: Second generation Asian Americans' religious retention and religiosity. *Journal for the Scientific Study of Religion, 58*(3), 666–688. https://doi.org/10.1111/jssr.12612

Children's Defense Fund. (2021). The State of America's Children® 2021. https://www.childrensdefense.org/state-of-americas-children/soac-2021-immigrant-children

Centers for Medicare and Medicaid Services Office of Minority Health. (2018, October). Comparing Puerto Rican's health status, access to care, satisfaction with care to their mainland counterparts prior to Hurricane Maria (Data Highlight. No. 13). https://www.cms.gov/About-CMS/Agency-Information/OMH/Downloads/CMS-OMH-October2018-Puerto-Rico-Data-Highlight.pdf

Cole, H. V. S., Reed, H. E., Tannis, C., Trinh-Shevrin, C., & Ravenell, J. E. (2018). Awareness of high blood pressure by nativity among black men: Implications for interpreting the immigrant health paradox. *Preventing Chronic Disease, 15,* E21. https://doi.org/10.5888/pcd15.170570

DHHS. Office of Minority Health. (2021). *Profile: Hispanic/Latino Americans.* https://www.minorityhealth.hhs.gov/hispaniclatino-health

Faheid, D. (2021, August 10). *American Muslims are 2 times more likely to have attempted suicide than other groups.* NPR. https://www.npr.org/2021/08/10/1025430083/muslims-suicide-attempts-study-religion-american

Fakhouri, M., Dallo, F., Templin, T., Khoury, R., & Fakhouri, H. (2008). Disparities in self-reported diabetes mellitus among Arab, Chaldean, and Black Americans in Southeast Michigan. *Journal of Immigrant and Minority Health, 10*(5), 397–405. https://doi.org/10.1007/s10903-007-9108-0

Fleuriet, K. J. (2013). *Online book review.* [Review of the book *Fresh fruit, broken bodies: Migrant farmworkers in the United States* by S. M. Holmes]. University of California Press. https://www.nyjournalofbooks.com/book-review/fresh-fruit-broken-bodies-migrant-farmworkers-united-states-california-series-public

Foner, N. (2016). Black immigrants and the realities of racism: Comments and questions. *Journal of American Ethnic History, 36*(1), 63–69. https://doi.org/10.5406/jamerethnhist.36.1.0063

Gautam, R., Mawn, B. E., & Beehler, S. (2018). Bhutanese older adult refugees recently resettled in the United States: A better life with little sorrows. *Journal of Transcultural Nursing, 29*(2), 165–171. https://doi.org/10.1177/1043659617696975

Global Perspectives. (n.d.). *The Middle East: Peoples.* http://www.cotf.edu/earthinfo/meast/mepeo.html

Guillermo, E. (2021, March 15). *What can we do to stop anti-Asian hate crimes.* Diverse. https://www.diverseeducation.com/demographics/asian-american-pacific-islander/article/15108803/what-can-we-do-to-stop-anti-asian-hate-crimes

Johnson, M. J., & Farquharson, H. R. (2019). Hispanic culture and healthcare in the United States: One person's perspective. *Journal of Nursing Research and Practice, 3*(4), 1–2. https://doi.org/10.37532/jnrp.2019.3(4).1-2

Kanno-Youngs, Z. (2019, June 8). Death on the Rio Grande: A look at a perilous migrant route. *The New York Times.* https://www.nytimes.com/2019/06/08/us/politics/migrants-drown-rio-grande.html

Kim, S.-S., & Kim-Godwin, Y. S. (2019). Cultural context of family religiosity/spirituality among Korean-American elderly families. *Journal of Cross-Cultural Gerontology, 34*(1), 51–65. https://doi.org/10.1007/s10823-019-09363-x

Korhonen, V. (2023). *High school dropout rate of Hispanic students in the U.S. from 1975 to 2022.* https://www.statista.com/statistics/260345/high-school-dropout-rate-of-hispanic-students-in-the-us/#:~:text=In%202022%2C%20about%205.1%20percent,of%2011.6%20percent%20in

Krogstad, J. M. (2016, July 28). *5 facts about Latinos and education.* Pew Research Center. https://www.pewresearch.org/short-reads/2016/07/28/5-facts-about-latinos-and-education

Krogstad, J. M. (2017, August 3). *U.S. Hispanic population growth has leveled off.* Pew Research Center. https://www.pewresearch.org/short-reads/2017/08/03/u-s-hispanic-population-growth-has-leveled-off

Krogstad, J. M. (2020). *Hispanics have accounted for more than half of the total U.S. population growth since 2010.* https://www.pewresearch.org/short-reads/2020/07/10/hispanics-have-accounted-for-more-than-half-of-total-u-s-population-growth-since-2010/#:~:text=In%20fact%2C%20the%20two%20states,of%20U.S.%20Hispanics%20in%202019.

Krogstad, J. M., Passel, J. S., Moslimani, M., & Noe-Bustamante, L. (2023, September 22). *Key facts about U.S. Latinos for National Hispanic Heritage Month.* Pew Research Center. https://www.pewresearch.org/short-reads/2023/09/22/key-facts-about-us-latinos-for-national-hispanic-heritage-month

Kundrik Leh, S., & Saoud, S. (2020). Using community-based participatory research to explore health care perceptions of a select group of Arab Americans. *Journal of Transcultural Nursing, 31*(5), 444–450. https://doi.org/10.1177/1043659619875181

Kusow, A. M., Kimuna, S. R., & Corra, M. (2014). Socioeconomic diversity among African immigrants in the United States: An intra-African immigrant comparison. *Journal of International Migration and Integration, 17*, 115–130. https://doi.org/10.1007/s12134-014-0377-x

Lauzardo, M., Kovacevich, N., Myers, D. A., Flocks, J., & Morris, J. G. (2021). An outbreak of COVID 19 among H-2A temporary agricultural workers. *American Journal of Public Health, 111*(4), 571–573. https://doi.org/10.2105/AJPH.2020.306082

Le, N. (n.d.). *Religion, spirituality, and faith.* Asian-Nation. Retrieved October 18, 2023, from https://www.asian-nation.org/religion.shtml

Little, B. (2022). *History stories: Arab immigration to the United States: Timeline.* https://www.history.com/news/arab-american-immigration-timeline

Lopez, G., & Patten, E. (2017). *Key facts about Asian Americans, a diverse and growing population.* Pew Research Center Fact Tank. http://www.pewresearch.org/fact-tank/2017/09/08/key-facts-about-asian-americans

Lorenzi, J., & Batalova, J. (2022). *Sub-Saharan African immigrants in the United States.* Migration Policy Institute. https://www.migrationpolicy.org/article/sub-saharan-african-immigrants-united-states-2019

Martin, P., & Rutledge, Z. (2021). Proposed changes to the H-2A program would affect labor costs in the United States and California. *California Agriculture, 75*(3), 135–141. https://doi.org/10.3733/ca.2021a0020

Mattei, J., Tamez, M., Ríos-Bedoya, C. F., Xiao, R. S., Tucker, K. L., & Rodríguez-Orengo, J. F. (2018). Health conditions and lifestyle risk factors of adults living in Puerto Rico: A cross-sectional study. *BMC Public Health, 18*(1), 491. https://doi.org/10.1186/s12889-018-5359-z

McQueen, M. (2021). *Pew Research finds nearly 60 percent of Americans oppose giving citizenship to illegal aliens.* Immigration Reform.com. https://www.immigrationreform.com/2021/05/06/pew-americans-disapprove-border-policy-immigrationreform-com

Meeks, S. (2021). *Fiscal year 2020 U.S. nonimmigrant admissions annual flow report.* U.S. Department of Homeland Security: Office of Immigration Statistics. https://www.dhs.gov/sites/default/files/2022-01/21_1004_plcy_nonimmigrant_fy2020.pdf

Monin, K., Batalova, J., & Lai, T. (2021). *Refugees and asylees in the United States.* Migration Information Source. https://www.migrationpolicy.org/article/refugees-and-asylees-united-states-2021

Moslimani, M. (2022). *Around four-in-ten Latinos in U.S. worry that they or someone close to them could be deported.* Pew Research Center. https://www.pewresearch.org/fact-tank/2022/02/14

Moslimani, M., Noe-Bustamante, L, & Shah, S. (2023, August 16). *Facts on Hispanics of Puerto Rican origin in the United States, 2021.* Pew Research Center. https://www.pewresearch.org/hispanic/fact-sheet/us-hispanics-facts-on-puerto-rican-origin-latinos

Moyce, S. C., & Schenker, M. (2018). Migrant workers and their occupational health and safety. *Annual Review of Public Health, 39*(1), 351–365. https://doi.org/10.1146/annurev[1]publhealth-040617-013714

National Center for Farmworker Health. (2018). *Agricultural worker factsheet.* http://www.ncfh.org/uploads/3/8/6/8/38685499/fs-facts_about_ag_workers_2018.pdf

National Immigration Forum. (2019, April 17). *Polling update: American attitudes on immigration steady, but showing more partisan divides.* https://immigrationforum.org/article/american-attitudes-on-immigration-steady-but-showing-more-partisan-divides

National Immigration Forum. (2021). *Fact sheet: Immigration detention in the United States.* https://immigrationforum.org/article/fact-sheet-immigration-detention-in-the-united-states/

Nguyen-Truong, C. K. Y., Lee-Lin, F., Leo, M. C., Gedaly-Duff, V., Nail, L. M., Wang, P., & Tran, T. (2012). A community-based participatory research approach to understanding Pap testing adherence among Vietnamese American immigrants. *JOGNN: Journal of Obstetric, Gynecologic & Neonatal Nursing, 41*(6), E26–E40. https://doi.org/10.1111/j.1552-6909.2012.01414.x

Noe-Bustamante, L., Flores, A., & Shah, S. (2019). *Facts on Hispanics of Puerto Rican origin in the United States, 2017.* Pew Research Center. https://www.pewresearch.org/hispanic/fact-sheet/us-hispanics-facts-on-puerto-rican-origin-latinos

Nteta, T. M., & Rice, D. (2021). Driving a wedge? Republicans, immigration, and the impact of substantive appeals on African American vote choice. *Political Research Quarterly, 74*(1), 228–242. https://doi.org/10.1177/1065912919900012

Office of Minority Health. (n.d.). *Hispanic/Latino health.* https://minorityhealth.hhs.gov/hispaniclatino-health

Otusanya, A. D., & Bell, G. C. (2018). *"I thought I'd have more trouble with White people!": Exploring racial microaggressions between West African immigrants and African Americans.* https://web-p-ebscohost-com.ezproxy.sju.edu/ehost/pdfviewer/pdfviewer?vid=4&sid=16ca08cb-83fb-4434-98ae-56903b5207bc%40redis

Paat, Y.-F., Saucedo, C. M., Rojas, R., Muñoz, L., Molina, A. A., Yoshimoto, M., Sanchez, S., Gonzalez, A. M., & De La Hoya Roto, R. (2022). Living in limbo: Aspiration-attainment gap, occupational health risks, and intergenerational mobility of Mexican origin migrant farm workers in El Paso, Texas. *Journal of Poverty, 26*(1), 73–91. https://doi.org/10.1080/10875549.2021.1890666

Peña, J. E., Lowe Jr., R. H., & Ríos-Vargas, M. (2023, September 26). *Colombian and Honduran populations surpassed a million for first time; Venezuelan population grew the fastest of all Hispanic groups since 2010.* U.S. Census Bureau. https://www.census.gov/library/stories/2023/09/2020-census-dhc-a-hispanic-population.html

Pew Research Center. (2022). *10 facts about today's college graduates.* https://www.pewresearch.org/short-reads/2022/04/12/10-facts-about-todays-college-graduates/#:~:text=Among%20adults%20ages%2025%20and%20older%2C%2061%25%20of,adults%2C%20according%20to%202021%20Current%20Population%20Survey%20data.

Pope Francis. (2018). *Message of his holiness Pope Francis for the 104th World Day of migrants and refugees 2018.* http://w2.vatican.va/content/francesco/en/messages/migration/documents/papa-francesco_20170815_world-migrants-day-2018.html

Purnell, L. D. (2013). *Transcultural health care: A culturally competent approach* (4th ed.). F. A. Davis.

Quarshie, M., & Anderson, J. (2021, September 21). Del Rio migrant crisis: How did so many Haitians end up at the southern U.S. border? *USA Today.* https://www.usatoday.com/story/news/politics/2021/09/21/what-led-haitian-nationals-migrating-u-s-southern-border/8419170002

Read, J. G., Amick, B., & Donato, K. M. (2005). Arab immigrants: A new case for ethnicity and health? *Social Science & Medicine, 61*(1), 77–82. https://doi.org/10.1016/j.socscimed.2004.11.054

Resnick, B., & Barclay, E. (2017). What every American needs to know about Puerto Rico's hurricane disaster. *Vox.* https://www.vox.com/science-and-health/2017/9/26/16365994/hurricane-maria-2017-puerto-rico-san-juan-humanitarian-disaster-electricty-fuel-flights-facts

Robert Wood Johnson Foundation. (2020). *Research review: Achieving a cohesive culture for health equity for Latino and all communities.* https://salud-america.org/wp-content/uploads/2020/09/Research-Review-Achieving-a-Cohesive-Culture-for-Health-Equity-in-Latino-and-All-Communities-9-15-20.pdf

Robertson, L. (2018, January 22). *The facts on DACA.* FactCheck.org. https://www.factcheck.org/2018/01/the-facts-on-daca

Roos, M., & Rouhandeh, A. J. (2021). With nearly half of U.S. farmworkers undocumented, ending illegal immigration could devastate economy. *Newsweek.* https://www.newsweek.com/nearly-half-us-farmworkers-undocumented-ending-illegal-immigration-could-devastate-economy-1585202

Rosenbloom, R. (2023). *A profile of undocumented agricultural workers in the United States.* Center for Migration Studies. https://cmsny.org/agricultural-workers-rosenbloom-083022/

Saldanha, K. (2021). Making labor visible in the food movement: Outreach to farmworkers in Michigan. *Qualitative Social Work, 20*(5), 1297–1316. https://doi.org/10.1177/1473325020973265

Scuglik, D. L., Alarcon, R., Lapeyre, A. C., Williams, M. D., & Logan, K. M. (2007). When the poetry no longer rhymes: Mental health issues among Somali immigrants in the U.S.A. *Transcultural Psychiatry, 44*, 581–595. https://doi.org/10.1177/1363461507083899

Seo, J. Y., Kuerban, A., Bae, S. H., & Strauss, S. M. (2019). Disparities in health care utilization between Asian immigrant women and non-Hispanic White women in the United States. *Journal of Women's Health, 28*(10), 1368–1375. https://doi.org/10.1089/jwh.2018.7532

Shafeek Amin, N., & Driver, N. (2022). Health care utilization among Middle Eastern, Hispanic/Latino, and Asian immigrants in the United States: An application of Anderson's behavioral model. *Ethnicity & Health, 27*(4), 858–876. https://doi.org/10.1080/13557858.2020.1830034

Somilleda, J. (2021). *The Haitian immigration crisis.* Galeo. https://galeo.org/2021/10/the-haitian-immigration-crisis%EF%BF%BC/

Song, S., & Teichholtz, S. (2020). *Mental health facts on refugees, asylum-seekers, & survivors of forced displacement.* American Psychiatric Association. https://www.psychiatry.org/File%20Library/Psychiatrists/Cultural-Competency/Mental-Health-Disparities/Mental-Health-Facts-for-Refugees.pdf

Statista. (2023). *Median household Income in U.S. in 2022 by race & Ethnicity.* Accessed at https://www.statista.com/statistics/233324/median-household-income-in-the-united-states-by-race-or-ethnic-group/

Stewart, P. (2021, May 10). *Scholars call for academia to address anti-Asian bias with structural change.* Diverse. https://www.diverseeducation.com/demographics/asian-american-pacific-islander/article/15109186/scholars-call-for-academia-to-address-anti-asian-bias-with-structural-change

Stroop, S., Kent, B. V., Zhang, Y., Spiegelman, D., Kandula, N., Schachter, A. B., Kanaya, A., & Shields, A. E. (2022). Mental health and self-rated health among U.S. South Asians: The role of religious group involvement. *Ethnicity & Health, 27*(2), 388–406. https://web-p-ebscohost-com.ezproxy.sju.edu/ehost/pdfviewer/pdfviewer?vid=4&sid=7c98b326-82e3-4f38-b8e2-d90e6c4c0f2b%40redis

Tamir, C. (2022, January 27). *Key findings about Black immigrants in the U.S.* Pew Research Center. https://www.pewresearch.org/short-reads/2022/01/27/key-findings-about-black-immigrants-in-the-u-sr

Tamir, C., & Anderson, M. (2022, January 20). *One-in-ten Black people living in the U.S. are immigrants.* Pew Research Center. https://www.pewresearch.org/race-ethnicity/2022/01/20/one-in-ten-black-people-living-in-the-u-s-are-immigrants/

Taylor, P., Lopez, M. H., Martínez, J., & Velasco, G. (2012, April 4). *When labels don't fit: Hispanics and their views of identity.* Pew Research Center. https://www.pewresearch.org/hispanic/2012/04/04/when-labels-dont-fit-hispanics-and-their-views-of-identity

Treisman, R. (2021). *Key facts about the U.S. Latino population to kick off Hispanic heritage month.* https://www.kpbs.org/news/2021/09/15/key-facts-about-the-us-latino-population-to-kick

UNHCR. (2022). *The U.S. Refugee Resettlement Program explained.* https://www.unrefugees.org/news/the-us-refugee-resettlement-program-explained/#:~:text=In%202021%2C%20the%20number%20of%20refugees%20who%20resettled,the%20Con

UN Refugee Agency. (n.d.). *Refugees in America.* Retrieved October 17, 2023, from https://www.unrefugees.org/refugee-facts/usa

United States Citizenship and Immigration Services. (2019). *Immigration and Nationality Act 1952.* https://www.uscis.gov/laws-and-policy/legislation/immigration-and-nationality-act

USA Facts. (n.d.). How is the population changing and growning. Retrieved October 11, 2023, from https://usafacts.org/state-of-the-union-2022/population

U.S. Census Bureau. (2017). *Facts for features: Hispanic heritage month 2017.* https://www.census.gov/newsroom/facts-for-features/2017/hispanic-heritage.html

United States Census. (2023). *Hispanic Heritage Month: 2023.* https://www.census.gov/newsroom/facts-for-features/2023/hispanic-heritage-month.html

U.S. Citizenship and Immigration Services. (2021). *Consideration of deferred action for childhood arrivals (DACA). DACA decision in state of Texas, et al., v. United States of America et al.1:18 CV-00068, (S.D. Texas July 16, 2021) ("Texas II").* https://www.uscis.gov/humanitarian/consideration-of-deferred-action-for-childhood-arrivals-daca/additional-information-daca-decision-in-state-of-texas-et-al-v-united-states-of-america-et-al-118-cv

U.S. Department of Agriculture, Economic Research Service. (2023). *Farm labor.* https://www.ers.usda.gov/topics/farm-economy/farm-labor

U.S. Department of Homeland Security. (2016). *U.S. lawful permanent residents: 2016.* https://www.dhs.gov/sites/default/files/publications/immigration-statistics/fy16_lawful-permanent-residents.pdf

U.S. Department of Homeland Security. (2019). *Annual flow report.* https://www.dhs.gov/sites/default/files/publications/Refugees_Asylees_2017.pdf

U.S. Department of Homeland Security. (2021). *Secretary Mayorkas designates Haiti for temporary protected status for 18 months.* https://www.dhs.gov/news/2021/05/22/secretary-mayorkas-designates-haiti-temporary-protected-status-18-months

U.S. World Population Review. (2022). U.S. immigration by country. https://worldpopulationreview.com/country-rankings/us-immigration-by-country

Wilhelm, A. K., McRee, A.-L., Bonilla, Z. E., & Eisenberg, M. E. (2021). Mental health in Somali youth in the United States: The role of protective factors in preventing depressive symptoms, suicidality, and self-injury. *Ethnicity & Health, 26*(4), 530–553. https://doi.org/10.1080/13557858.2018.1514451

Wolf, K. M., Zoucha, R., McFarland, M., Salman, K., Dagne, A., & Hashi, N. (2016). Somali immigrant perceptions of mental health and illness: An ethnonursing study. *Journal of Transcultural Nursing, 27*(4), 349–358. https://doi.org/10.1177/1043659614550487

World Atlas. (2017, April). *Religious beliefs in Haiti.* https://www.worldatlas.com/articles/religious-beliefs-in-haiti.html#:~:text=Religious%20Beliefs%20In%20Haiti%20%20%20%20Rank,Eastern%20Re%20...%20%20%20%20%203%25%20

World Health Organization. (2019). *10 things to know about the health of refugees and migrants.* https://www.who.int/news-room/feature-stories/detail/10-things-to-know-about-the-health-of-refugees-and-migrants

World Population Review. (n.d.-a). *U.S. immigration by country 2024.* Retrieved February 29, 2024, from https://worldpopulationreview.com/country-rankings/us-immigration-by-country

World Population Review. (n.d.-b). *Haitian population by state 2024.* Retrieved February 29, 2024, from https://worldpopulationreview.com/state-rankings/haitian-population-by-state

World Population Review. (n.d.-c). *Latin American countries 2024.* Retrieved February 29, 2024, from https://worldpopulationreview.com/country-rankings/latin-american-countries

World Population Review. (2024). *U.S. immigration by country 2024.* https://worldpopulationreview.com/country-rankings/us-immigration-by-country

Xiao, Z., Lee, J., & Liu, W. (2020). Korean and Vietnamese immigrants are not the same: Health literacy, health status, and quality of life. *Journal of Human Behavior in the Social Environment, 30*(6), 711–729. https://doi.org/10.1080/10911359.2020.1740852

Zoucha, R. (2015). Global refugees and the long road. Their hope and our role! *Journal of Transcultural Nursing, 26*(5), 449. https://doi.org/10.1177/1043659615611766

IMPORTANT WEBSITES

Central Intelligence Agency World Fact Book. Retrieved from www.cia.gov/the-world-factbook/

Department of Homeland Security: Yearbook of Immigration Statistics 2022. Retrieved from www.dhs.gov/immigration-statistics/yearbook/2022

Hispanic Americans by the Numbers. Retrieved from www.infoplease.com/history/hispanic-heritage/hispanic-americans-by-the-numbers

Office of Refugee Resettlement 2021. Retrieved from www.acf.hhs.gov/orr

Pew Research Center: Striking Findings From 2022. Retrieved from www.pewresearch.org/short-reads/2022/12/13/striking-findings-from-2022

VIISTA—Villanova Interdisciplinary Immigration Studies Training for Advocates. Retrieved from www1.villanova.edu/university/professional-studies/academics/professional-education/viista.html

Cultural Considerations When Caring for the Poor and Uninsured

Gloria Kersey-Matusiak

If the world seems cold to you, kindle fires to warm it.

—LUCY LAROM

LEARNING OBJECTIVES

After this chapter, the reader will be able to
1. Examine the socioeconomic factors that impact healthcare decision-making and outcomes.
2. Discuss poverty in the United States and its relationship to healthcare disparities.
3. Describe health-related problems encountered by the poor and uninsured.
4. Examine homelessness and its impact on health.
5. Discuss the intersection of cultural differences, language barriers, and poverty and their impacts on healthcare access.

KEY TERMS

Barrier	Poverty
Healthcare disparities	Poverty threshold
Indigent	Socioeconomic status
Limited English proficiency	Tuskegee study

OVERVIEW

Throughout this text, the authors have focused on clinical situations in which nurses experience various differences between themselves and their patients. These differences may be based on race, ethnicity, religion, culture, or other attributes that reflect the wide range of human diversity. This chapter focuses on yet another area of human diversity, socioeconomic class, and, more specifically, it examines **poverty** and its impact on health. This topic is included here because **socioeconomic status** has been identified as one of the major determinants of health (World Health Organization [WHO], 2023). WHO (2023) defines social determinants of health (SDOH) as the conditions in which people are born, live, work, grow and age. Therefore, nurses and other healthcare providers must attempt to find ways to minimize the impact of low income on healthcare access to reduce **healthcare disparities** in the United States. Despite nurses' desire to give optimum care to all patients, the socioeconomic status of the patient can sometimes interfere with nurses' and other healthcare workers' best efforts to positively influence the quality of healthcare the patient receives.

SOCIOECONOMIC CLASS AND HEALTHCARE

Indicators of socioeconomic class include income, completed education, net worth, and private health insurance (Benson et al., 2023a, 2023b; Creamer et al., 2021; Keisler-Starkey & Bunch, 2021). Research indicates that there is a positive relationship between these indicators of socioeconomic status and health (Bennett et al., 2022; Creamer et al., 2021; Office of Disease Prevention and Health Promotion, n.d.; Samuel et al., 2021). In the United States, variations exist between racial and ethnic groups on each of these indicators. For example, research illustrates that life experiences of Blacks and Whites in the United States have been characterized by different patterns of education, economic success, and employment which have led to differences in access to affordable housing and healthcare (Jones, 2021). Blacks and other people of color including Hispanics, American Indians, and Alaskan Natives, as well as foreign-born noncitizens compared to foreign-born citizens, are less advantaged in terms of income, wealth, and access to care (Bennett et al., 2022; Keisler-Starkey & Bunch, 2021; Zaidi & Sederstrom, 2018). Often, race has been thought of as a factor influencing one's health; however, when socioeconomic factors were controlled for, the influence of race became less significant. The Pew Research Center (2020) reported that most Americans believe that people are poor because they have faced more obstacles than others.

Persons who are poor, irrespective of their race or ethnicity, experience health and healthcare differently from their wealthier counterparts in society. Hartz and Wright (2019) described the plight of healthcare workers who themselves could not afford health insurance for their families. Poverty, then, acts as a **barrier** to quality healthcare. For this reason, patients who are poor are in need of care that focuses on identifying ways to help them overcome its impact on their healthcare outcomes (Blacksher & Valles, 2021; Haarbauer-Krupa et al., 2023; Wray, 2018).

Poverty in the United States

According to the U.S. Census Bureau report for 2021, 11.6% of the population (37.9 million people) lived in poverty. The official rates decreased for people under the age of 18, but increased for people 65 or over (Creamer et al., 2021).

There were no significant differences in the rate or number between 2020 and 2021. Among Blacks, 19.5% lived in poverty, as did 17.1% of Hispanics and 24.3% of American Indians and Alaskan Natives in 2021. Although the percentage of the White (non-Hispanic) population living in poverty is much lower (8.1%), the numbers of White (non-Hispanic) persons living in poverty is 15,805,000 compared to 8,583,000 Black Americans (Creamer et al., 2021).

While Whites had a median income of $77,999 in 2021, Black Americans have consistently had the lowest median income ($48,297), while Asians ($101,418) had the highest (which is typically around double that of Black Americans; U.S. Census Bureau, 2022). As the statistics illustrate, you are much more likely to live in poverty if your income is low.

The U.S. Census Bureau defines **poverty** based on predetermined thresholds for cash income relative to family size. That threshold is set by the current value of [t]hree times the cost of a minimum food diet in 1963, adjusted by family composition (Creamer et al.,

TABLE 11.1 ■ TOP 10 U.S. STATES IN TERMS OF POVERTY RATES

STATE	STATE POPULATION (2021)	PERCENTAGE OF POPULATION LIVING IN POVERTY
1. Mississippi	2.94 million	18.1
2. Louisiana	4.59 million	17.2
3. New Mexico	2.11 million	16.7
4. Kentucky	4.5 million	14.6
5. West Virginia	1.78 million	15
6. Arkansas	3.04 million	15.1
7. Alabama	5.07 million	14.6
8. Arizona	7.36 million	11.2
9. Oklahoma	4.01 million	13.8
10. Georgia	10.91 million	13.1

Number & Percentage of People by State Using 3-year average
Source: Creamer, J., Shrider, E. A., Burns, K., & Chen, F. (2021). *Poverty in the United States: 2021* (P60-277). U.S. Census Bureau. https://www.census.gov/content/dam/Census/library/publications/2022/demo/p60-277.pdf

2021; p. 2), or, one could say, the dollar amount a family needs to meet its needs (World Atlas, 2017). The 2021 median household income was $77,999, which was an increase from $59,039 in 2016.

An individual or family is considered poor if their pretax income falls below the **poverty threshold** (U.S. Census Bureau, 2023). For example, in 2022 the threshold for a single-parent family with two children was $23,578. A single mother whose total cash income was $19,000 or less would be considered poor. National Center for Children in Poverty (NCCP, 2021) reported that while children represented 23% of the population, they make up 32% of all people in poverty, as stated in the Important Points. In that same year, the poverty threshold for a family of four with two adults and two children was $29,678. The highest poverty rates are found among families headed by single women (27.9%), especially among those who are Black or Hispanic. In contrast, in 2021 only 4.8% of married couples lived in poverty. There are also disparities in poverty rates between the native born and foreign-born living in the United States.

For patients who are poor and who speak English as a second language (ESL), their problems are compounded. Without a clear understanding of the medical terms and jargon used by healthcare personnel, it becomes even more difficult for people to negotiate the healthcare system or to utilize available resources.

According to the U.S. Department of Agriculture, in 2021, 12.8% of children live in households considered food insecure (Economic Research Service, 2023). Consequently, children who experienced chronic poverty were those who were more likely to develop persistent asthma, and moving out of poverty had a protective effect on children (Thomas et al., 2019). For very young children, the impact of asthma can have a detrimental effect on their school achievement throughout their lives (Bread for the World, 2019; Thomas et al., 2019). Being poor in America often means less access to quality care, and higher morbidity and mortality rates, despite living in one of the wealthiest nations in the world. There are also differences among states in the percentages of the population who live in poverty (see Table 11.1). For example, it is important to note that in Louisiana in 2021, 17.2% of the population lived below the poverty level; however, 8.5% of those who are poor live below one-half the poverty threshold. The states of Vermont, Connecticut, and New Hampshire were at the opposite end of the poverty scale, with poverty rates in 2021 of 8.2%, 9.2%, and 5.6%, respectively (Creamer et al., 2021). Among those who live in poverty, many also find themselves homeless.

Homelessness

As the United States Interagency Council on Homelessness (USICH, 2022) reminds us, there are many faces of homelessness (Iscoe, 2023). The face with which we are most familiar is that of the person sleeping on the street; however, there are many other forms of homelessness that are just as likely to make a significant impact on a person's health. Whether temporarily or chronically experiencing the loss of physical shelter, sharing living space with family or friends, or living in an abandoned building, one's car, or other crowded spaces, homelessness challenges the physical and psychologic well-being of its victims (Koh, 2020).

For many, the United States is a country of great wealth; and, in the words of President Obama, "It is simply unacceptable for individuals, children, families, and our nation's Veterans to be faced with homelessness in this country" (as cited in Sullivan, 2009, para. 3). On a single night in 2021 more than 326,000 people experienced sheltered homelessness in the U.S. In 2021, in a sample of 138 communities that conducted unsheltered counts, 15% were unsheltered individuals, and 3% were people in families with children. In this report, the number of unsheltered remained unchanged from 2020 (U.S. Department of Housing and Urban Development [HUD], 2022b). Forty percent of the homeless population at the 2022 point of contact were unsheltered, sleeping in cars, streets, or encampments (de Sousa et al., 2022).

HUD's (2022a) Annual Homeless Assessment Report (AHAR) to Congress revealed that 76% of all people experiencing homelessness were adults 25 or older (444,041 people), whereas 17% were children under 18 (98,244). Seven percent of the homeless were 18 to 24 years of age (40,177 young adults; de Sousa et al., 2022).

In that same year, COVID-19 stressors and dramatic increases in rental costs drove homelessness upward, and 582,462 people experienced homelessness in January that year. There was a slight increase of 0.3% since 2020. Two of every five people experiencing homelessness (233,832 people) were living in unsheltered situations. The number of families with children that were homeless decreased to 50,767 in 2022, which was down 6%, marking a decline in unsheltered homelessness among families. Veteran homelessness also declined that year, with 33,129 veterans experiencing homelessness (de Sousa et al., 2022).

African Americans represented a disproportionate share of people experiencing homelessness. While African Americans accounted for 12% of the U.S. population in 2022, they represented 37% of the total homeless population that year. Homeless individuals who identified as Hispanic or Latinx increased by 8% between 2020 and 2022. Unsheltered homelessness increased by 16% among Hispanic people (8,513 people) during that period (de Sousa et al., 2022).

The HUD report also revealed a decline in homelessness among youth. There were 30,090 unaccompanied youth experiencing homelessness that year, a decrease since 2020. Children who experienced homelessness were either in families or on their own, and most often stayed in sheltered locations (90%), although 10,284 children were in unsheltered sites (de Sousa et al., 2022). Consequences of homelessness for children include having poor health that is exacerbated by hunger and poor nutrition after becoming homeless and an increased likelihood of having asthma and receiving sporadic care. Homeless children are also more likely than nonhomeless children to encounter domestic and community violence and to be educationally and socially deprived. Because of the social conditions associated with homelessness, homeless children are more likely to develop a negative self-image, drop out of school, and get in trouble with the law. Besides these problems typically associated with homelessness, during the time frame of this HUD report, the United States and the world was also coping with the COVID-19 pandemic. Hodwitz and colleagues (2022) explored the unique challenges posed by the COVID-19 pandemic on homeless persons and frontline healthcare workers. The researchers identified three major themes: (1) A collective feeling of "navigating the unknown." Workers were challenged by having to respond to continuously evolving public health guidelines, while patients felt uncertain about testing and isolation protocols and having limited options due to their homelessness. (2) A sense of placelessness, a feeling of having nowhere to go in the pandemic either because of awaiting test results or having tested positive. In these situations, patients needed to stay in impromptu spaces in the ED and/or needing to stay in encampment spaces. (3) A sense of powerlessness was experienced by both patients and healthcare workers. Patients lacked control due to placelessness and care workers lacked control on the care they could provide.

Problems of the Uninsured

Not surprisingly, those who live in poverty are also those who are most likely to be uninsured. In 2020, 8.6% of the population (28 million people) did not have health insurance. In 2021, 27.5 million people were uninsured and were non-older adults in working families with low incomes. Six in 10 were people of color. Hispanic and White people comprised the largest share of the non-older adult uninsured population at 39%. Most of the people who are uninsured live in the South or the West (nearly three quarters) and have been without coverage for a long time. Seven in 10 had at least one full-time worker. More than 80% of uninsured people had incomes below 400% the federal poverty level (FPL). Most of the uninsured (77.1%) were U.S. citizens, while 22.9% were noncitizens (Tolbert et al., 2022). Those who had coverage for all or part of that year represented 91.4% of the population. Private health insurance was the most common type, supported mostly by employment-based insurance (54.4%), then Medicare (18.4%), Medicaid (17.8%), and direct purchase (9.9%; Keisler-Starkey & Bunch, 2021). In 2020, those who worked full-time year around were more likely to be covered by private insurance compared to part-time workers. More children under the age of 19 who lived in poverty were uninsured in 2020 compared to 2018.

Research by the Henry J. Kaiser Family Foundation revealed that the Affordable Care Act (ACA) led to historic gains in health insurance coverage by extending Medicaid to many low-income individuals and providing marketplace subsidies for individuals below 400% of poverty. The ACA was able to reduce the number of uninsured (non-older adult) from 44.4 million in 2013 to 25.6 million by 2022. The most notable gains in health insurance were found in the states that expanded Medicaid. However, despite these findings, there are still 28 million Americans who remain uninsured. In 2021, 69.6% of the uninsured give high cost as the reason for not being insured, especially in states that did not expand Medicaid (Tolbert et al., 2023). Some of the people living in those states may not be eligible for financial assistance under ACA, and others may not be aware of their eligibility. Undocumented immigrants are ineligible for Medicaid or marketplace coverage (Tolbert et al., 2022). Ironically, low-income families with at least one worker represent the most uninsured people. As a result of being uninsured, "one in five adults went without needed medical care due to cost and they are least likely than the insured to receive preventive care and services for major health conditions and chronic diseases" (Tolbert et al., 2023). Because the uninsured have low incomes and hardly any savings, medical care, when it is sought, results in high cost and ultimately medical debt for the uninsured. Additionally, to avoid cost, many uninsured do not obtain health providers' recommended care (Grossman & Mayne-Jarman, 2016). Because of less frequent outpatient visits, the uninsured are more likely to be hospitalized for "avoidable" health problems, to be more seriously ill, and have higher mortality rates than those who are insured (Tolbert et al., 2023).

During the previous Trump administration, there was much partisan debate over the ACA. Many expressed concerns about being mandated to purchase health insurance. In

2023, only five states have a tax penalty for not having health insurance: Massachusetts, California, Rhode Island, New Jersey, and Vermont. According to Smart Financial (Majidi, 2022), the demographics that are the most uninsured are people with a high school education or less, Hispanics, younger adults, residents in rural areas, and people without internet access. Obviously, individuals who are unemployed or who are living in poverty would have considerable hardship in making high-cost insurance premiums. The poverty level for 2023 is $13,590 for individuals and $27,750 for a family of four. People with poverty level incomes may be able to get subsidized health insurance plans costing $10 or less a month. Other subsidies are available for premium assistance that are income-based (Majidi, 2022). In addition, in 2022 the U.S. Department of Health and Human Services (DHHS) announced a new policy to make coverage more accessible and affordable for millions of Americans in 2023. The plan includes new standardized plan options on Healthcare.gov to make it easier for consumers to compare quality and value across healthcare plans. Despite the controversial enactment and implementation of the ACA, as DHHS Secretary Xavier Becerra stated, "The Affordable Care Act has successfully expanded coverage and provided hundreds of health plans for consumers to choose from" (DHHS, 2022 a, para. 2).

The debate about healthcare in the United States has become a very partisan one, with Democrats and Republicans holding very different views on how quality healthcare for all might best be achieved.

Regardless of one's political party affiliation, the need for quality healthcare for all remains. Just as one's economic status is tied to homelessness, both measures are inextricably linked to the acquisition of health insurance. Every one of these measures is a social determinant of one's healthcare access and ultimately one's health outcomes. For this reason, it is important for nurses to stay informed about the issues, be engaged in the discourse, and participate in the democratic process of voting based on one's beliefs. Most importantly, nurses must consider each of these indicators—poverty, homelessness, and health insurance—as part of the context when assessing their patients' needs for care.

THE ROLE OF THE NURSE

Nurses, like physicians, have an opportunity and a responsibility to ensure quality care, especially by strengthening their interpersonal skills and by helping to facilitate access to care for patients who are poor. By developing skills at the interpersonal level, nurses can enhance communication between themselves and other healthcare providers and with patients to have a positive influence on their healthcare outcomes. Moreover, advocating for the poor can take many forms, but nurses start by establishing relationships with those who are empowered to make a difference in the life of the poor such as hospital administrators, community activists, local and federal politicians, and social networks and organizations.

Although nurses may be generally aware of patients' socioeconomic status, they seldom focus their attention on it. Thus, it is unlikely that they set out to provide a different kind of care to those who are poor. Yet, the literature attests to differences in the quality of care that patients who are **indigent** receive Often these differences can be attributed to institutional or patient–physician dynamics that inadvertently create barriers to the provision of comprehensive or culturally competent care. For example, racial/ethnic differences in levels of mistrust toward physicians in the United States exist especially among Blacks and Hispanics and other persons of color due to long-standing practices and publicized events that have shaken some minority patients' confidence in the medical profession. These events have affected Black, Hispanic, Asian, Native American, women, disabled, and LGBTQ people who have been vulnerable to medical mistreatment (Asamoah & Evans, 2022). The **Tuskegee Study**, for example, enrolled 66 Black males who were left untreated for syphilis, many of whom died as a result of being uninformed and untreated with penicillin when it became available after 1943. Forced sterilization of people deemed "unfit to reproduce" is another example of mistreatment of immigrants, Black people, Native Americans, poor Whites, and people with disabilities by medical professionals. According to 1950 data from North Carolina, more than three times as many Black were sterilized as White women (Asamoah & Evans, 2022). Other research that explored physician and medical student–patient relationships found that most healthcare providers had some level of implicit bias, with positive attitudes toward White people and negative attitudes toward Black people. Other studies revealed medical students rated pain scores lower in Black patients and had misconceptions about physiologic differences between Black and White patients (Asamoah & Evans, 2022).

These dynamics are often beyond the control of the nurse. However, as the largest group of healthcare providers, nurses can do much to provide the missing link between the poor patient and the healthcare system. By addressing some of the problems that the poor or uninsured patient encounters during healthcare experiences, nurses can enhance the care provided to them. These problems include variations in access, perceived ED overuse, cultural differences, communication barriers, inadequate time for sharing information with the physician, limited trust in healthcare providers, and decreased patient satisfaction. Nurses can assist in minimizing these long-held feelings of mistrust by patients who feel oppressed by the healthcare system. Placing more emphasis on the patient's own attitudes and beliefs enables the nurse to plan care that is more culturally appropriate and effective in meeting the patient's healthcare goals. By working collaboratively with social service organizations, the hospital social worker, and other agents of support within the community, the nurse can apprise the patient of ways to obtain needed resources or services that may be available but unknown to them.

ACCESS TO CARE

Research shows that certain groups have limited access to health services because of discrimination based on their social class, race, ethnicity, or sexual orientation. However, access to care is often directly related to one's ability to pay for medical services, and the poor are often those most in need of care. People without health insurance have the worst access to care and face unaffordable bills when they do seek care. In 2021, one in five uninsured adults went without care due to cost (Tolbert et al., 2023). Throughout the United States, many who live in areas of extreme poverty, such as those found in some parts of the South, the Mexican border states, Appalachia, Native American territories, and impoverished urban areas, experience neglected chronic and debilitating health problems at greater rates than others in the United States. Such untreated problems have a long-lasting and undetected negative effect on children, expectant mothers, and workers in impoverished communities that increase their morbidity and mortality.

In other situations, many patients who may have obtained a prescription from a physician in the ED or clinic may never get it filled because of a lack of funds or insurance to pay for such medications. Middle-class young adults who are no longer young enough to be covered under their parents' health insurance may be in low-paying jobs and lack health benefits. Consequently, these individuals find healthcare unaffordable. This age group, especially males, is still within the high-risk population for trauma injury and these injuries often necessitate extensive, prolonged, and costly hospital care. Patients who believe they will be asked to pay amounts for care they cannot afford will delay or avoid seeking healthcare until they are seriously ill. Those who are underinsured often face similar problems, as their healthcare needs increase. These behaviors increase the need for more extensive use of healthcare services in the future.

Patients who are either uninsured or underinsured are least likely to seek preventive care, such as annual physicals, dental checkups, regular vision screenings, and mammograms. Consequently, they are more likely to be diagnosed with later-stage cancers and to die when hospitalized with serious conditions like heart attacks and strokes (Institute of Medicine, 2009; Minemyer, 2017).

EMERGENCY DEPARTMENT OVERUSE

There is a popular belief that the poor and underinsured use the ED indiscriminately in place of primary care physicians or urgent care centers. The Emergency Medical Treatment Active Labor Act (EMTALA) is a federal statute that was passed into law in 1986 to ensure emergency services to the indigent. This law enables care to persons irrespective of their citizenship, insurance, or employment status. However, uninsured patients often do not realize that hospitals receiving Medicare funding have an obligation to treat all patients' emergent needs when they cannot afford to pay. As a result, many patients who are indigent delay seeking treatment until they are seriously ill for fear of being turned away. As a result, patients who are poor often wait so long to be treated that by the time they are seen in the ED by a physician, they are seriously ill.

Minemyer (2017) discussed the results of a study that analyzed data on over 41,000 adults from 2013 that revealed uninsured patients visit the ED about as frequently as the insured, 12.2% compared to 13.7%. In fact, the uninsured were less likely than those on Medicaid (29.3%) to go to the ED. Moreover, only 3% of the study participants who were uninsured were hospitalized. More recent studies indicate the uninsured were less likely to seek outpatient care elsewhere because of fears of being refused care due to an inability to pay, may lack access to other settings and may feel stigmatized, or may not fully understand how insurance coverage works (Minemyer, 2017). Additionally, some patients lack knowledge of special programs or other supportive services. For example, some pharmaceutical companies offer assistance through programs that provide prescription medications to medically needy patients. To address the increasing need of patients who live in poverty, there are more than 1,400 free clinics in the United States (National Association of Free and Charitable Clinics [NAFC]). The working poor and uninsured patients who utilize them receive primary care and pharmacy services that would otherwise be unavailable to them and thereby avoid ED overuse. Additionally, parish nurses and other community health nurses offer healthcare information through church bulletins and flyers that describe free services or those offered at nominal cost that are available to eligible members of the community to support the growing needs of the poor.

Zhou and colleagues (2017) discussed the common view of the overuse of the ED by the uninsured and its impact on the healthcare system. In their study, the researchers found that insurance coverage increased ED use instead of decreasing it. The study also found that both insured and uninsured used the ED in very similar circumstances; insured and uninsured adults use the ED at very similar rates, but the uninsured use the ED substantially less than the Medicaid population. In this study, the authors also observed that the uninsured do use other types of care much less than the insured.

POVERTY, CULTURAL DIFFERENCES, AND LANGUAGE BARRIERS

The combination of poverty, cultural differences, and language barriers makes achieving healthcare services even more difficult for patients who are poor, especially when there is **Limited English Proficiency,** or the ability to speak and understand English well.

Patients from culturally diverse backgrounds who live in poverty are more likely than dominant group members to use folk practices as a remedy for certain illnesses and diseases. Because of limited economic resources, these cultural practices, which may include herbal medicine, teas, or the use of folk healers, are sought before the patient considers going to a physician. Sometimes herbal medicines or folk remedies used by the patient, while being treated for an illness with Western medicine, are incompatible with those that are later administered by healthcare providers. When there is a trusting relationship between the patient and the nurse, the patient feels free to discuss any home remedies or treatments without fear of being judged by the nurse. Nurses who demonstrate caring and respect for their patients' beliefs and values can establish trust and maintain an open and honest working relationship. In such relationships, nurses avoid receiving misinformation or limited information that may compromise care. Sharing critical information is particularly difficult when a language barrier exists between the patient and the nurse.

Moreover, the language of the healthcare system is particularly difficult for someone who speaks a second language. However, conducting a cultural assessment that identifies the patient's language abilities and communication style or pattern enables the nurse to select the appropriate resources to strengthen communication between them. It is helpful for the nurse to communicate in clear, simple language, avoiding the use of medical jargon. Ideally, information about procedures and treatments should be provided in the patient's own language. If an interpreter is needed, the nurse makes sure that, when possible, the interpreter is age- and gender-appropriate and is knowledgeable of medical terminology. In all situations, when speaking with the patient, the nurse places attention on the patient, not the interpreter.

INADEQUATE TIME WITH PRIMARY CARE PROVIDERS

In clinical situations where physicians are forced to see large numbers of patients, they are naturally compelled to limit the time of each visit. Consequently, the time needed to provide adequate explanations about the patient's illness, test results, or treatment is limited. Moreover, patients may sense the physician's hurried demeanor and be reluctant to ask relevant questions pertaining to their care. Although this situation is not unique to minority or disadvantaged patients, patients who are poor are more likely to be less educated and less able to understand medical terminology used by physicians. Immigrants, for example, are more likely to follow traditional healthcare practices that deviate from those of Western medicine, have more difficulty understanding medical jargon, have language barriers, like having **limited English Proficiency** and have fewer opportunities to meet with primary care physicians due to limited health insurance. Additionally, social and cultural differences between White middle-class physicians and poor minority patients may result in some communication problems due to differences in language usage and styles of communication.

In settings where there are advance practice nurses, they can be used as resources for all staff personnel to provide medical information to patients, and to support the staff in using the nursing process to overcome barriers to access care for patients who are poor. When nurses sense that patients are confused or lack knowledge or understanding of their illness or treatment, they are in a prime position to offer support. The culturally competent nurse is sensitive to an indigent patient's feelings of inadequacy, particularly in disadvantaged groups when there is a language barrier. Information is provided in simple language and the nurse makes the time to encourage questions about issues of concern to the patient. The nurse also remains nonjudgmental in listening to the patient's own beliefs and ideas about the causes and impact of illness as well as the patient's preferred methods of treatment.

LACK OF CONFIDENCE IN THE HEALTHCARE SYSTEM

Moreover, it is often the values and healthcare beliefs of the healthcare provider that are emphasized when care is being provided. Sometimes these values conflict with those of patients from different cultures. For example, being given intimate care by a member of the opposite gender may be considered an indignity by members of some cultural groups. Lack of privacy for prayers or for getting washed and dressed is among some patients' concerns about avoidable breaches of privacy in hospital care. Because of the mistrust of healthcare providers by some cultural groups, some patients who are poor may feel they are just being used as guinea pigs. Patients who are poor may also believe that they will be turned away because of an inability to pay, even when they are seriously ill. When culture, race, and poverty intersect, these problems can become even more challenging for the patient. For this reason, many persons of color are distrustful of the healthcare system because their perception, accurate or not, is that they will be discriminated against because of their race or a lack of ability to pay.

Nurses can assist in minimizing these long-held feelings of mistrust by patients who feel oppressed by the healthcare system. Placing more emphasis on the patient's own attitudes and beliefs enables the nurse to plan care that is more culturally appropriate and effective in meeting the patient's healthcare goals. By working collaboratively with social service organizations, the hospital social worker, and other agents of support within the community, the nurse can apprise the patient of ways to obtain needed resources or services that may be available but unknown to them. The nurse can gain new insights to assist patients by partnering with Black and other churches and community resources to gain an understanding of the cultural needs of the populations they serve and to allay patients' feelings of fears and mistrust toward (Stafford et al., 2023) the medical community.

DECREASED PATIENT SATISFACTION

Because nurses often have more frequent encounters with the patient and are knowledgeable of significant clinical information, they can share that information with patients and families in a manner that incorporates ethical standards of practice. The knowledgeable, skilled, and culturally competent nurse intervenes on the patient's behalf by providing the requested information clearly and honestly. This approach helps allay the fears of patients and families, enables them to make appropriate healthcare decisions, and fosters greater patient satisfaction with the healthcare experience.

WHAT NURSES CAN DO

Nurses who are knowledgeable about the Patients' Bill of Rights and their hospital's policies regarding the care of the poor can help explain these policies to patients who lack this information. By exploring the local city or county websites, local newspapers, or hospital and church bulletins, nurses can locate services that are available to people in their communities who are indigent or lack health insurance. This information enables nurses to educate the community about free or nominal-cost services offered by local organizations, hospitals, nurse-managed clinics, and health centers. Opportunities for sharing health information exist at community health fairs, church functions, and civic gatherings, as well as during encounters with patients in tertiary care facilities. Individual nurses and nursing organizations, such as the American Nurses Association (ANA) and the National League for Nursing (NLN), can affect healthcare policy by encouraging legislators to respond to the health needs of the poor both nationally and locally. All these efforts enable nurses to influence access to care for those who are indigent.

Culturally competent nurses can be effective advocates for patients who are poor. To address uninsured patients' health goals, nurses must be knowledgeable about available health services and resources so they can direct needy patients to them (DHHS, 2022b). Although individual nurses can do much within their communities, nurses are even stronger as a united body.

Nurse educators play a role in assisting the poor when they expose students to learning situations that enable them to observe and experience the health-related issues of the poor and witness the effectiveness of strategies used to achieve health outcomes. These experiences prepare students for their future roles in promoting health and advocating for patients from vulnerable populations.

Advocacy for the uninsured and disadvantaged can be facilitated through nursing organizations and social service group efforts. Over the past 20 years, the ANA has fought for the adoption of healthcare reform to provide health insurance for the uninsured and the underinsured.

Regardless of the patient's power, status, or wealth, culturally competent nurses, despite external pressures, find ways to establish themselves as powerful and professional patient allies. These nurses strive to maintain their professional integrity by carefully determining and prioritizing the immediate needs of all those under their care.

Poor Americans experience poorer outcomes and higher morbidity and mortality than those who are wealthier. According to Tiase et al. (2022), nurses play a critical role in collecting patients' social determinants of health (SDOH) data and finding appropriate resources to address the patient needs they identify. Also, health complications multiply the lower you are on the income scale. In this chapter, nurses are asked to consider some of the obstacles they may encounter when caring for the uninsured or patients living in poverty. When caring for members of this group, nurses are challenged to find creative ways to overcome the circumstantial barriers that inhibit effective nurse–patient interactions and to develop strategies for addressing the social determinants of health that contribute to poor health outcomes, ensuring the provision of culturally competent care to both the uninsured and indigent patient.

IMPORTANT POINTS

- Research indicates a relationship between socioeconomic status, private health insurance, and access to quality healthcare.
- Life experiences of Americans that impact healthcare differ along racial lines.
- Among members of culturally diverse groups, Blacks, Hispanics, and single mothers have the highest poverty rates.
- Poverty more than race alone impacts healthcare access.
- Poor patients experience multiple healthcare problems that include variations in access, cultural differences, communication barriers, inadequate time for sharing health information, limited trust in healthcare providers, and decreased patient satisfaction.
- Those who are poor are most likely to be uninsured.
- Middle-class young adults represent a large percentage of the medically uninsured.
- Homelessness is a barrier to healthcare.
- Healthcare disparities are differences between groups in morbidity and/or mortality rates.
- Children living in America experience the most disproportionate share of poverty in that they represent 25% of the total population, but 35% of the poor population.
- Culturally diverse patients who live in poverty are more likely than dominant-group members to use folk practices as a remedy for illnesses and diseases.
- The combination of poverty, cultural differences, and language barriers further impedes healthcare access for the poor.
- The Emergency Medical Treatment Act of 1986 ensures emergency services to those who are unable to pay.
- Nurses can address the problems of poverty, limited access, and healthcare disparities by providing health education to those who are poor and by determining institutional and community resources to assist them.
- Nurses can also advocate for the poor individually through their legislators or collectively through their nursing organizations.

CASE SCENARIO

Mabel Tucker is a 56-year-old African American widow. She lives in a small, three-bedroom home in a federally subsidized housing development. Mabel has asthma and has been experiencing more frequent asthma attacks. Mabel works as a cook at a nearby housing facility, where she earns $9 an hour. On two recent occasions, she had to leave work early because of breathing difficulties. Mabel has also been having more difficulty managing her hypertension, but takes her medication only when she feels ill. Despite her medical problems, Mabel finds it difficult to give up cigarette smoking and smokes one to two packs a day. She says smoking helps her relax. Mabel also struggles with her weight. At 5 feet 4 inches tall, she weighs 190 pounds. She has no healthcare benefits.

Mabel shares her home with her 28-year-old daughter, Cherise, and three grandchildren, Charlie, 8; Carey, 6; and Cala, 2. Together, Mabel and Cherise share household chores and expenses and Mabel cares for the children when Cherise, a clerk typist, attends classes in the evening at a community college.

Mabel worries daily about the stressors of her work environment, being able to make ends meet, and the increasing crime in the neighborhood. Her anxiety often exacerbates her symptoms.

Today Mabel awakens with a severe headache, which signals a need to take her blood pressure medicine. Mabel is worried about the cost of an ED visit and does not wish to go to the hospital. She also feels that some of the ED staff members have treated her unkindly in the past. To Mabel, doctors and nurses always seem rushed and annoyed. On her last visit, after examining Mabel, the doctor advised her to lose weight and stop smoking. He wrote a prescription for an antihypertensive treatment and asked her to follow up with her medical doctor. Mabel could not bring herself to admit to the ED doctor that she did not have a private doctor and could not afford one. Mabel feels guilty about not attempting to lose weight, give up smoking, or follow up with another doctor as the ED doctor suggested. As Mabel's headache worsens, she reluctantly decides to go to the ED. Upon her arrival, the triage nurse takes Mabel's blood pressure and finds it is 192/100. After the physical examination and review of lab studies, the physician admits Mabel to a medical–surgical unit. Mabel is extremely anxious and concerned about leaving her grandchildren and the possibility of missing work and losing her job.

WHAT NURSES NEED TO KNOW ABOUT THEMSELVES

Applying the Staircase Self-Assessment Model: Self-Reflection Questions

1. How comfortable are you caring for this patient?
2. Where do you see yourself on the Cultural Competency Staircase?
3. How would you progress to the next level? (See Chapter 1.)
4. Do you have any biases or prejudices toward, or have you made any assumptions about, patients from this cultural background? Are your preconceived notions or attitudes likely to impact the kind of care you can provide?
5. What information do you and other nurses need about this patient to provide her with quality care?
6. What nurse behaviors and resources do you need to provide culturally competent care for this patient?

Responses to Self-Reflection Questions

Response: How comfortable are you caring for this patient?

Your experience or number of encounters communicating with female African American patients from this socioeconomic background will determine your level of comfort working with members of this cultural group. Although there is probably no language barrier, as English is the shared language, there may be cultural differences between the nurse and the patient in language usage or communication style. This is an important difference. For this reason, during the initial interview, the nurse should make an effort to project courtesy and respect without becoming too familiar, especially with an older patient like Mabel.

Response: Where do you see yourself on the Cultural Competency Staircase?

First go to Chapter 1 and review the Cultural Competency Staircase table. Place yourself at the level that best describes you when working with patients from this cultural group.

Response: How will you progress to the next level?

Examine the area of the table in Chapter 1 that describes the ways to progress from where you are to the next level.

Response: Do you have any biases or prejudices toward, or have you made any assumptions about, patients from this cultural background? Are your preconceived notions or attitudes likely to impact the kind of care you can provide?

Today, despite our best efforts, it is difficult for any nurse to escape the impact of racism and ethnocentrism on our psyche. Consider any long-held assumptions you have made about members of this cultural group. Are these assumptions or generalizations evidence-based or are they derived from personal opinions related to experiences with a few representatives from this group? In either case, consider this patient and all others as unique individuals from which you might gain some knowledge or insights about the groups they represent. However, that knowledge cannot ever be used to predict an individual's values, attitudes, and beliefs. Care planning should be specific to the assessed needs of the individual.

WHAT NURSES NEED TO KNOW ABOUT THE PATIENT

Selecting a Cultural Assessment Model

Response: What information do you and other nurses need about this patient to provide her with quality care?

The nurse must evaluate patients by considering the entire circumstances surrounding their illness. The patient's social history is important in this case, as many environmental factors may be influencing this patient's healthcare situation. Having knowledge of the socioeconomic conditions under which this patient lives daily is essential to planning effective care. Having knowledge of the patient's cultural background, lifestyle, health beliefs, and values is equally important for the nurse to gain insight into the patient's healthcare needs. The nurse also needs to know appropriate health resources in the institution or the community that will be useful in addressing the patient's health-related issues.

Response: What nurse behaviors and resources do you need to provide culturally competent care for this patient?

To gain an understanding of the cultural needs of this patient, the nurse begins by selecting a cultural assessment model. In this chapter, the author recommends using the ETHNIC assessment model, as described in Chapter 2. The mnemonic ETHNIC stands for *explanation, treatment, healers, negotiation, intervention*, and *collaboration*. The ETHNIC model affords a collaboration between the nurse and the client in planning culturally appropriate care. By using this model, the nurse is reminded to place emphasis on determining the patient's health concerns from her perspective. In this case, the nurse aims to establish a relaxed, supportive rapport with the patient, and tries to convey empathy and respect. These behaviors facilitate the patient's sharing of her concerns about her asthma, hypertension, and obesity, and factors such as cigarette smoking and stress that may be contributing to them.

During the initial meeting with the patient, the nurse uses the time to build trust, gather pertinent information, and assist the patient in planning a new approach to managing her health problems. The nurse also explores the patient's current home situation and looks for clues about stressors that might be impacting the patient's health.

Some examples of questions the nurse might ask when using this approach are the following:

- "Why do you believe you have hypertension and how do you usually treat it?"
- "Do you have people other than nurses and doctors to whom you go for medical advice, or use herbal medicine or other folk practices?"

Using this model, the nurse speaks to the patient using clear, simple language the patient can understand, avoiding any medical jargon, if possible. The nurse offers to answer any questions or concerns, which enables the patient to identify areas of interest that the nurse may not have considered. During the interaction, the nurse listens reflectively to the patient to determine what the client expects to happen during the illness based on that person's healthcare beliefs and attitudes.

It is also important for the nurse to determine why Mabel has neglected to take her medications regularly, which is likely to be linked to Mabel's understanding about its significance and her ability to pay for it. While Mabel describes her personal concerns, the nurse listens attentively and identifies any factors that may be causing stress in Mabel's life. The nurse collaborates with social services to discuss any socioeconomic concerns and to ensure Mabel's utilization of any available hospital or community resources for patients who need financial support. At this point, the nurse might describe controllable and uncontrollable factors influencing hypertension, such as diet, exercise, and efforts to manage stress. It is important that the nurse remains attentive and nonjudgmental as Mabel shares her thoughts and feelings about her asthma attacks, hypertension, and practice of taking her medication only when she feels ill. Considering all the factors that may be influencing Mabel's health, the nurse identifies several important issues of concern.

Problems and Concerns

Considering Mabel's ethnic background, stressful lifestyle, poor dietary habits, and cigarette smoking, the nurse recognizes that these factors place her at high risk for cardiovascular and cerebrovascular complications. In addition, Mabel's lack of understanding about the management of asthma and hypertension, and her limited financial resources, interfere with her access to care.

Planning Care

Using lay terms, the nurse explains the relationship among Mabel's dietary habits, exercise, smoking, asthma, and hypertension and the possible complications that may result (see Table 11.2). The nurse also offers Mabel some literature on managing hypertension that is written in simple, nonmedical jargon terms. Identifying any available pamphlets or other materials that list both free and inexpensive community services and their contact

TABLE 11.2 ■ PLAN OF CARE

GOALS	INTERVENTIONS	EVALUATION
The patient will have an enhanced understanding of her illness, including risk factors, clinical manifestations, treatment, and potential complications. The patient establishes contact with a medical provider on a regular basis. The patient takes medication on a regular basis. The patient will reduce weight and stressors impacting hypertension.	The nurse explains the relationship among diet, exercise, smoking, asthma, and hypertension in lay terms. The nurse provides written information about asthma, hypertension, and obesity and gives Mabel a list of free community workshops and presentations at the local hospitals on these topics. The nurse encourages Mabel to visit a local nurse-run health clinic that charges based on a sliding scale to establish a working relationship with a nurse practitioner and/or physician on a more regular basis. Mabel is given information about a pharmacy-assistance program for patients who are indigent. The nurse encourages Mabel to participate in a local hospital's exercise program as a means of reducing stress and weight.	Mabel takes all prescribed medications regularly and begins to reduce or seek help in reducing her cigarette smoking. Mabel has ongoing monitoring and management of her multiple chronic illnesses. Mabel takes medications regularly and controls hypertension.

information will also be useful. To assist the patient in staying on track with prescribed medications, the nurse can explore pharmacy-assistance programs for which the patient can apply. Such programs, offered by pharmaceutical companies, provide some medications free of charge to those who are unable to afford them. The individual must be ineligible for Medicare and Medicaid and have no other insurance plan. For medications that are needed immediately, the nurse might ask the physician if samples are available that the patient can use while waiting for prescriptions to be filled. The nurse should explain the danger of using others' medication even when the patients share a diagnosis, like hypertension, with a near relative.

Another important nursing strategy in the care of this patient is to identify any support groups in the area for patients with asthma, and/or exercise programs at local hospitals or community centers that the patient might attend. The nurse should explain the benefits of exercise and stress reduction in addressing this patient's health problems.

Finally, the nurse explains to Mabel the benefit of seeing one healthcare provider on a more consistent basis, rather than waiting to go to the ED when she becomes ill. However, it is also important for the patient to understand that when there is a real clinical emergency, patients have a right to be seen in the ED irrespective of their ability to pay.

Because of this patient's socioeconomic issues, the nurse will need to find creative ways to ensure that the patient's identified health goals are met. In many cities, there are medical clinics and nurse-operated health centers where patients who are indigent can be seen and can pay for services based on a sliding scale. Under certain circumstances, some hospitals offer special clinic services where needed tests, laboratory work, or procedures are done at the hospital without charge to the patient. Nurses should explore whether this is an option at their place of employment on behalf of the patients they serve who are unable to afford care.

Caring for patients who are poor or who lack medical insurance is one of the most challenging clinical situations for nurses. Nurses faced with this challenge must have effective cross-cultural skills in communication that allow them to listen attentively so that care can be planned from the patients' perspectives. The culturally competent nurse is also knowledgeable about appropriate cultural assessment tools, and has an arsenal of resources from which to choose to address patients' specific needs. Over time, the culturally competent nurse develops skill in each of these areas and can offer each patient quality care while maintaining their dignity and respect. Ultimately, the nurse empowers the patient who is poor to manage their own health problems in a more effective way.

SUMMARY

Caring for a patient who is indigent or uninsured poses many challenges for the culturally competent nurse. In caring for these patients, the nurse needs to be knowledgeable about the degree to which socioeconomic factors are impacting the patient's access to care. By using an appropriate cultural assessment tool, the nurse gains insight into the patient's cultural perspective on healthcare problems. Understanding cultural influences on the patient's healthcare decision-making will enable the nurse to determine areas for patient teaching. Nurses caring for indigent patients will need to develop knowledge regarding useful community agencies and other resources to assist patients on an emergency basis until more permanent support can be attained. The problems of limited access, ED overdependence, cultural differences, communication barriers, inadequate time with physicians, limited trust of the healthcare system, and decreased patient satisfaction can be addressed by the knowledgeable, skillful, and culturally sensitive nurse. By working collaboratively with patients who are uninsured, and utilizing available hospital and community resources, culturally competent nurses can assist in removing some of the barriers patients who are uninsured encounter.

NCLEX®-TYPE QUESTIONS

1. Research indicates that _____ is/are among the *most significant* factors in determining healthcare outcomes.
   A. Race and ethnicity
   B. Socioeconomic status
   C. Language skills
   D. Religious beliefs

2. The nurse is planning the discharge of a patient who is unemployed. The nurse realizes that it is important to include what strategies in the patient's discharge planning? *Select all that apply.*
   A. Teach the patient preventive health measures.
   B. Identify community resources.
   C. Provide any medical information in the patient's own language.
   D. Determine the patient's ability to pay for prescriptions.

3. The nurse who works in a busy urban area has frequent encounters with patients from multicultural populations. When working with members of ethnically diverse groups, the nurse understands that the poorest patients are most likely to be found among:
   A. Asian immigrants
   B. Pacific Islanders
   C. Blacks and Hispanics
   D. Ethnic Whites

4. When discussing a patient's eligibility for indigent programs based on U.S. government definitions of poverty, what statement by the nurse demonstrates a good understanding of poverty thresholds?
   A. Thresholds vary based on individual states' determinations.
   B. Thresholds are based on the income of the person designated head of household.
   C. Thresholds are consistent throughout the nation and are based on family size and age of its members.
   D. Thresholds are determined by townships and/or municipalities.

5. A patient explains to the nurse that she delayed coming to the ED after experiencing a severe burn because she did not have any money to pay for the visit. What statement by the culturally competent nurse is most appropriate?
    A. Patients who are unable to pay are guaranteed emergency services by the Civil Rights Act of 1963.
    B. Patients are provided with services through the Patients' Bill of Rights.
    C. Patients are protected by the Equal Opportunities Amendment.
    D. Patients are guaranteed services by the Emergency Medical Treatment Act.

6. According to research, what problems are most often encountered by patients who live in poverty? *Select all that apply.*
    A. Bilingualism
    B. Too little time for sharing information with providers
    C. ED overuse
    D. Mistrust of healthcare providers

7. What statement by the nurse is true regarding the intersection of cultural differences, language barriers, lack of health insurance, and poverty?
    A. The combination of these factors compounds the problem of access for the poor.
    B. There are no differences between those with language barriers and those without in their impact on healthcare access.
    C. Cultural differences have little impact on healthcare access.
    D. All persons who lack private healthcare insurance are eligible for Medicare or Medicaid.

8. Research shows a positive relationship among income, completed education, net worth, and:
    A. Language abilities
    B. Cultural attitudes
    C. Private health insurance
    D. Religious values

9. The nurse admits a patient who is homeless to the unit. When planning care for this patient, what attitude by the nurse is most realistic?
    A. Homelessness poses a serious barrier to healthcare access.
    B. There are many available healthcare services provided by governmental agencies for the homeless.
    C. Quality care is provided to the homeless to the same extent it is provided to others.
    D. Persons who are homeless are aided by government subsidies like Medicaid.

10. The nurse encounters multiple patients from culturally diverse groups who are living in poverty in the hospital's local community. The nurse desires to get involved in attempting to address this problem. The most effective *initial* approach by the nurse is to:
    A. Contact the local council members and other legislators to state some of the problems these patients are experiencing
    B. Study a foreign language to reduce the language barrier that exists between the nurse and at least one ethnic cultural group
    C. Join a nursing organization and advocate for the groups through collective action
    D. Attempt to establish a trusting relationship with each individual patient to identify their specific healthcare needs

ANSWERS TO NCLEX-TYPE QUESTIONS

1. A and B
2. A, B, C, and D
3. C
4. C

5. D
6. B and D
7. A
8. C

9. A
10. D

AMERICAN ASSOCIATION OF COLLEGES OF NURSING COMPETENCIES ADDRESSED IN THIS CHAPTER

1. Apply knowledge of social and cultural factors that affect nursing and healthcare across multiple contexts.
2. Use relevant data sources and best evidence in providing culturally competent care.
3. Promote achievement of safe and quality outcomes of care for diverse populations.
4. Advocate for social justice, including commitment to the health of vulnerable populations and the elimination of healthcare disparities.
5. Participate in continuous cultural competence development.

 A robust set of instructor resources designed to supplement this text is located at http://connect.springerpub.com/content/book/978-0-8261-8302-6. Qualifying instructors may request access by emailing textbook@springerpub.com.

REFERENCES

Asamoah, T., & Evans, A. (2022, May 13). *The origins of medical mistrust in the U.S.* Good RX Health. https://www.goodrx.com/hcp/providers/the-origins-of-medical-mistrust

Bennett, N., Hayes, D., & Sullivan, B. (2022, August 1). *Wealth inequality in the U.S. by household type: 2019 data show baby boomers nearly 9 times wealthier than millennials.* U.S. Census Bureau. https://www.census.gov/library/stories/2022/08/wealth-inequality-by-household-type.html

Benson, C., Bishaw, A., & Glassman, B. (2023a). *Persistent poverty: Identifying areas with long-term high poverty: 341 counties experiencing persistent poverty.* U.S. Census Bureau. https://www.census.gov/library/stories/2023/05/persistent-poverty-areas-with-long-term-high-poverty.html

Benson, C., Bishaw, A., & Glassman, B. (2023b). *Persistent poverty in counties and census tracts.* U.S. Census Bureau. https://www.census.gov/content/dam/Census/library/publications/2023/acs/acs-51%20persistent%20poverty.pdf

Blacksher, E., & Valles, S. A. (2021). White privilege, white poverty: *Reckoning with class and race in America. The Hastings Center Report, 51(Suppl.* 1), S51–S57. https://doi.org/10.1002/hast.1230

Bread for the World. (2019). *2019 hunger report.* https://www.bread.org/article/2019-hunger-report/

Creamer, J., Shrider, E. A., Burns, K., & Chen, F. (2021). *Poverty in the United States: 2021* (P60-277). U.S. Census Bureau. https://www.census.gov/content/dam/Census/library/publications/2022/demo/p60-277.pdf

de Sousa, T., Andrichik, A., Cuellar, M., Marson, J., Prestera, E., & Rush, K. (2022). *2022 annual homelessness report (AHAR) to Congress.* U.S. Department of Housing and Urban Development. https://www.huduser.gov/portal/sites/default/files/pdf/2022-ahar-part-1.pdf

Economic Research Service. (2023, June 20). *Key statistics & graphics: Food security status of U.S. households with children in 2021.* U.S. Department of Agriculture. https://www.ers.usda.gov/topics/food-nutrition-assistance/food-security-in-the-u-s/key-statistics-graphics/#children

Grossman, E., & Mayne-Jarman, T. (2016). *ER overuse: Leveraging analytics to improve care, reduce visits.* Health IT Outcomes: Guest Column. https://www.healthitoutcomes.com/doc/er-overuse-leveraging-analytics-to-improve-care-reduce-visits-0001

Haarbauer-Krupa, J., Eugene, D., Wallace, T., & Johnson, S. (2023). Neurorehabilitation for the uninsured: Georgia rehabilitation services volunteer partnership clinic. *American Journal of Speech-Language Pathology, 32,* 817–826. https://doi.org/10.1044/2022_AJSLP-22-00100

Hartz, M. R., & Wright, M. J. (2019). In demand and undervalued—The plight of American healthcare workers. *American Journal of Public Health, 109*(2), 209–210. https://doi.org/10.2105/AJPH.2018.304867

Hodwitz, K., Das, P., Parsons, J., Rosenthal, S. H., Juando-Prats, C., Kiran, T., Lockwood, J., & Snider, C. (2022). Placeless and powerless: Experiences of patients who are homeless and healthcare workers caring for them during COVID-19. *The Annals of Family Medicine, 20*(Suppl. 1), 2927. https://doi.org/10.1370/afm.20.s1.2927

Iscoe, A. (2023). The revolving door. *New Yorker, 99*(13), 20–26. https://www.magzter.com/stories/culture/The-New-Yorker/THE-REVOLVING-DOOR

Jones, M. L. (2021). The social determinants of COVID-19. *ABNF Journal, 31*(3), 97–101. https://pesquisa.bvsalud.org/global-literature-on-novel-coronavirus-2019-ncov/resource/en/covidwho-972946

Keisler-Starkey, K., & Bunch, L. (2021). *Health insurance coverage in the United States: 2020* (P60-274). U.S. Census Bureau. https://www.census.gov/content/dam/Census/library/publications/2021/demo/p60-274.pdf

Koh, K. A. (2020). Psychiatry on the streets—Caring for homeless patients. *JAMA Psychiatry, 77*(5), 445–446. https://doi.org/10.1001/jamapsychiatry.2019.4706

Majidi, F. (2022). *The state of health insurance 2023: Has the ACA changed?* Smart Financial. https://smartfinancial.com/state-of-health-insurance#health-insurance-2023-faq

Minemyer, P. (2017). *Study debunks idea that uninsured patients overuse the ER.* FierceHealthcare. https://www.fiercehealthcare.com/payer/uninsured-patients-emergency-care-medicaid-outpatient-care-health-affairs

National Center for Children in Poverty. (2021, April). *Basic facts about low income children: Children under 18 years 2019.* https://www.nccp.org/wp-content/uploads/2021/03/NCCP_FactSheets_All-Kids_FINAL-2.pdf

Office of Disease Prevention and Health Promotion. (n.d.). *Social determinants of health.* Retrieved January 4, 2024, from https://health.gov/healthypeople/priority-areas/social-determinants-health

Pew Research Center. (2020). *Most Americans point to circumstances, not work ethic, for why people are rich or poor.* https://www.pewresearch.org/politics/2020/03/02/most-americans-point-to-circumstances-not-work-ethic-as-reasons-people-are-rich-or-poor

Samuel, L. J., Gaskin, D. J., Trujillo, A. J., Szanton, S. L., Samuel, A., & Slade, E. (2021). Race, ethnicity, poverty and the social determinants of the coronavirus divide: U.S. county-level disparities and risk factors. *BMC Public Health, 21*(1), 1250. https://doi.org/10.1186/s12889-021-11205-w

Stafford, K., Morrison, A., & Ma, A. (2023). *Medical racism in history causes health inequalities for Black Americans.* https://projects.apnews.com/features/2023/from-birth-to-death/medical-racism-in-history.html

Sullivan, B. (2009, June 18). Secretaries Shinseki and Donovan host first meeting of the U.S. Interagency Council On Homelessness under the Obama administration. U.S. Department of Housing and Urban Development. https://archives.hud.gov/news/2009/pr09-092.cfm

Thomas, M. M. C., Miller, D. P., & Morrissey, T. W. (2019). Food insecurity and child health. *Pediatrics, 144*(4), e20190397. https://doi.org/10.1542/peds.2019-0397

Tiase, V., Crookston, C. D., Schoenbaum, A., & Valu, M. (2022). Nurses' role in addressing social determinants of health. *Nursing, 52*(4), 32–37. https://doi.org/10.1097/01.NURSE.0000823284.16666.96

Tolbert, J., Drake, P., & Damico, A. (2023). *Key facts about the uninsured population.* KFF. https://www.kff.org/uninsured/issue-brief/key-facts-about-the-uninsured-populatio

U.S. Census Bureau. (2022, September 13). Income, poverty and health insurance coverage in the United States: 2021. https://www.census.gov/newsroom/press-releases/2022/income-poverty-health-insurance-coverage.html

U.S. Census Bureau. (2023, June 15). *How the Census Bureau measures poverty.* https://www.census.gov/topics/income-poverty/guidance/poverty-measures.html

U.S. Department of Health and Human Services. (2022a). *HHS announces new policy to make coverage more accessible and affordable for millions of Americans in 2023.* https://www.hhs.gov/about/news/2022/04/28/hhs-announces-new-policy-make-coverage-more-accessible-affordable-for-millions-americans-in-2023.html

U.S. Department of Health and Human Services. (2022b). *Homelessness resources and programs.* https://www.hhs.gov/programs/social-services/homelessness/resources/index.html

U.S. Department of Housing and Urban Development. (2022a). *2022 Annual Homelessness Report (AHAR) to Congress.* https://www.huduser.gov/portal/sites/default/files/pdf/2022-ahar-part-1.pdf

U.S. Department of Housing and Urban Development. (2022b). *HUD Releases 2021 annual homelessness assessment report Part 1.* https://www.hud.gov/press/press_releases_media_advisories/HUD_No_22_022

U.S. Interagency Council on Homelessness. (2022). *What is the strategic plan?* https://www.usich.gov/federal-strategic-plan/overview

World Atlas. (2017). *US poverty level by state.* https://www.worldatlas.com/articles/us-poverty-rate-by-state.html

World Health Organization. (2023). *Commercial determinants of health.* https://www.who.int/news-room/fact-sheets/detail/commercial-determinants-of-health

Wray, M. (2018). A crisis of identity, a crisis of place. *The American Journal of Bioethics, 18*(10), 23–25. https://doi.org/10.1080/15265161.2018.1516002

Zaidi, D., & Sederstrom, N. (2018). The racist underbelly of health disparities in America. *The American Journal of Bioethics, 18*(10), 25–26. https://doi.org/10.1080/15265161.2018.1513598

Zhou, R. A., Baicker, K., Taubman, S., & Finkelstein, A. N. (2017). The uninsured do not use the emergency department more—They use other care less. *Health Affairs, 36*(12), 2115–2122. https://doi.org/10.1377/hlthaff.2017.0218

IMPORTANT WEBSITES

Alliance for Children & Families. Retrieved from www.alliance1.org
Catholic Charities USA. Retrieved from www.catholiccharitiesusa.org
Center for People in Need. Retrieved from centerforpeopleinneed.org

Coalition on Human Needs: Retrieved from www.chn.org
National Alliance to End Homelessness. Retrieved from https://endhomelessness.org
National Association of Free and Charitable Clinics. Retrieved from www.nafcclinics.org/find-clinic
National Center for Children in Poverty (NCCP). Retrieved from www.nccp.org
National Coalition for the Homeless. Retrieved from https://nationalhomeless.org/
Poverty & Race Research Action Council (PRRAC). Retrieved from www.prrac.org

12

Cultural Considerations When Caring for the Patient Who Is Morbidly Obese

Gloria Kersey-Matusiak

There is no exercise better for the heart than reaching down and lifting people up.

—JOHN ANDREW HOLMER

LEARNING OBJECTIVES

After this chapter, the reader will be able to

1. Explore the problem of obesity as a national and international healthcare epidemic.
2. Discuss the complex causes of morbid obesity as they relate to patients' ability to manage weight control.
3. Describe the physiologic and psychologic challenges experienced by patients who are morbidly obese.
4. Examine nurses' and other healthcare workers' attitudes toward obesity and the impact on the provision of care to patients experiencing morbid obesity.
5. Explain the psychosocial consequences of stigmatization and discrimination to patients in the United States who are seriously obese.
6. Identify the factors that influence the provision of culturally competent care to patients who are seriously obese.
7. Develop strategies to enhance nurses' ability to provide culturally competent care to patients who are obese.

KEY TERMS

Body mass index

Malnutrition

Morbid obesity

Obesity

Stigma

Waist–hip ratio

OBESITY: A GLOBAL CONCERN

The problem of **malnutrition** impacts adults and children around the world each day. In various forms, it includes undernutrition, inadequate vitamins or minerals, overweight, and obesity. Obesity is a chronic, preventable health condition that leads to life-compromising, diet-related consequences, especially noncommunicable diseases like diabetes, strokes, hypertension, and cardiovascular disease. Globally, in 2020, 38.9 million children were overweight or obese. Although 45% of deaths among children under 5 are linked to under-nutrition in low and middle-income countries, rates of childhood overweight and obesity are rising in these same countries (World Health Organization [WHO], 2021).

According to the WHO, the problem of **obesity** is not only escalating, it has also reached epidemic proportions worldwide. Throughout the world, 1.9 billion adults were over-weight while 650 million were obese (WHO, 2021). Low-, middle-, and high-income coun-tries throughout the world, including the United States and those in Europe, North Africa, and the Middle East, share the burden of obesity. However, the United States leads the group, with the prevalence of obesity among adults aged 20 and over (age adjusted) at 41.9%. The prevalence of severe obesity was 9.2%. Among children and adolescents aged 2 to 19, the prevalence of obesity was 19.7% (Stierman et al., 2021). Globally, more people are obese than underweight. According to WHO, most of the world's population live in countries where being overweight or obese kills more people than being underweight, and the risks of increased morbidity and premature deaths rise with increasing levels of obesity (Greenberg, 2013).

The purpose of this chapter is to examine the problem of **morbid obesity**, its causes and consequences, the attitudinal barriers persons who are morbidly obese face, and the implications for nursing care. As the largest group of healthcare providers having the most intimate relationships with patients, nurses have an opportunity to play a major role in meeting the needs of persons for whom obesity is either a primary or secondary diagnosis Unfortunately, healthcare literature suggests that this is frequently a missed opportunity by nurses and other healthcare professionals because of a lack of confidence and preparation for managing the multifaceted physiologic and psychologic challenges people with mor-bid obesity confront daily. With increased knowledge and skill, and a heightened aware-ness of the serious complications this disease poses, nurses can begin to build an arsenal of resources to strengthen their confidence as frontline warriors that can more effectively assist patients in their battle against obesity and its life-threatening complications.

The Centers for Disease Control and Prevention (CDC, n.d.-a) defines being overweight as having a **body mass index** (BMI), a measure of weight-to-height, of 25 or greater. At a BMI of 30 or greater, one is considered obese. In the United States, the prevalence of obe-sity differs among men and women and among racial and ethnic groups. According to the CDC, serious or morbid obesity occurs when a BMI is equal or greater than 40, or 35 when it is accompanied by a serious health complication such as diabetes mellitus (DM) or hypertension. Obesity is further categorized into three classes or levels: Class I (BMI 30 to 35); Class II (BMI 35 to 40), also called serious obesity; and Class III (BMI greater than 40), also called severe or extreme obesity (Table 12.1).

Weight Assessment

Some researchers argue that using BMI as an approach to weight assessment is faulty because it does not take muscle mass into consideration and may cause an over- or under-estimation of fat in an individual (Johnson, 2019). Many researchers encourage the use of

TABLE 12.1 ■ CLASSES OF OBESITY

CLASS I	CLASS II	CLASS III
BMI 30 to <35	35 to <40 (Serious)	BMI >40 (Severe or extreme)

BMI, body mass index.
Source: Centers for Disease Control and Prevention. (n.d.). *Defining adult overweight & obesity.* Retrieved October 11, 2023, from https://www.cdc.gov/obesity/basics/adult-defining.html

another measure of body fat, the **waist–hip ratio** or waist circumference assessment, and believe that these measurements offer a better indicator of health risks than BMI. One can measure abdominal fat by placing a tape measure around the waist and determining its size in inches. A measurement of over 40 inches in men and 30.5 inches in women is an indicator of excessive abdominal fat and increased health risk (National Heart, Lung, and Blood Institute, 2022).

In addition, there are four ways one can measure body fat at home: using skin-fold calipers, taking skin-fold measurements from three, seven, or eight body sites; body circumference measures, measuring the neck, waist, or hip and following a specific formula based on gender; body fat scales (often inaccurate); and waist circumference measures. Knowing your waist circumference can provide clues about your risk of developing conditions like heart disease and diabetes, and this approach is probably the easiest to use at home (Kubala, 2023).

Nevertheless, irrespective of the approach one uses to determine obesity, in the United States, monitoring one's level of adipose tissue is a way of monitoring one's health. From 2017 to 2020, the U.S. obesity prevalence increased from 30.5% to 41.9%, and severe obesity increased from 4.7% to 9.2% (CDC, National Health and Nutrition Examination Survey [NHANES], 2021). These statistics indicate that urgent measures are needed to contend with this increasing, life-threatening health problem. According to the CDC, among adults over age 20, 73.6% of the U.S. population is overweight (including those who are obese; CDC, n.d.-b).

Prevalence of Adult Obesity

In the United States, the prevalence of obesity varies based on gender, race, ethnicity, income, and education. There were no differences between men and women overall (41.8%), but there was a higher percent of non-Hispanic Black women as compared to non-Hispanic Black males. Obesity was most common among non-Hispanic Black adults (49.9%), Hispanic (45.6%), non-Hispanic White (41.4%), and non-Hispanic Asian (16.1%). Obesity prevalence was highest among non-Hispanic Black women compared with women of other races and Hispanic origin. Among men, obesity prevalence was lowest among non-Hispanic Asian men (Stierman et al., 2021; Table 12.2). Hollerbach and colleagues (2022) studied obesity among officers in the military and found higher rates of obesity than in previous studies, especially for women.

Obesity was lowest among adults with a family income of more than 350% of the federal poverty level (FPL). Higher levels of obesity were found among those with a high school diploma or some college (46.4%), followed by those with less than a high school diploma (40.1%), than those with a college degree (34.2%). Prevalence based on education differed between men and women. Prevalence among men was highest among those with a high school diploma and some college, while among women, obesity was highest for those with less than a high school diploma. Severe obesity was lowest among those aged 60 and over and a higher percentage of women (11.7%) than men (6.6%) had severe obesity (Stierman et al., 2021; Table 12.2).

TABLE 12.2 ■ AGE AND THE PREVALENCE OF OBESITY 2020

AGE	CHILDREN AND ADOLESCENTS	20–39	40–59	OLDER THAN 65
Percent Obese	19.7%	39.8%	44.3%	41.5%

Source: Stierman, B., Afful, J., Carroll, M. D., Chen, T.-C., Davy, O., Fink, S., Fryar, C. D., Gu, Q., Hales, C. M., Hughes, J. P., Ostchega, Y., Storandt, R. J., & Akinbami, L. J. (2021). *National Health and Nutrition Examination Survey 2017–March 2020 prepandemic data files—Development of files and prevalence estimates for selected health outcomes* (National Health Statistics Reports 158). https://www.cdc.gov/nchs/data/nhsr/nhsr158-508.pdf

Children and Obesity

According to the CDC (Stierman et al., 2021), for children aged 2 to 19, in the years 2017 to 2020, the prevalence of obesity was 19.7%, which translated to about 14.7 million affected children and adolescents. Childhood obesity is more common among some populations by age and ethnicity. Obesity prevalence was 12.7% among 2- to 5-year-olds, 20.7% among 6- to 11-year-olds, and 22% among 12- to 19-year-olds (Table 12.3). Prevalence was highest among Hispanic children at 26.2%, followed by non-Hispanic Black children at 24.8%, non-Hispanic White children at 16.6%, and non-Hispanic Asian children at 9% (Table 12.4). Obesity-related health conditions impacting children include high blood pressure, high cholesterol, type 2 diabetes, asthma, sleep apnea, and joint problems. Among children, socioeconomic status was an important factor influencing the prevalence of obesity. Obesity was highest. (18.9%) in children and adolescents 2 to 19 years old in the lowest (10.9%) income groups and lowest in the highest income groups. See Table 12.3.

Causes of Obesity

Today, most researchers agree that the causes of obesity are multifactorial and include biological, psychosocial, and cultural factors. Cultural factors include food choices made out of necessity due to economic constraints, and /or the inaccessibility of healthy food choices. Also, cultural influences have to do with long-standing family traditions from which many individuals develop food preferences or ways of preparing food that are not always healthy.

According to Boutari and Mantzoros (2022), globally, obesity is concentrated among the rich in low-income countries and the poor in high-income countries. The researchers explain that as income rises people can afford more food and their dietary habits become more westernized. Also, the rich adopt a more sedentary lifestyle and occupation. However, the authors noted that this pattern changes in societies where there is a higher level of income and there is a social stigma of being obese. When there is access to healthy

TABLE 12.3 ■ PREVALENCE OF CHILDHOOD OBESITY 2017 TO 2020

AGE	PREVALENCE
2–5 Years	12.7%
6–11 Years	20.7%
12–19 Years	22%

Source: Stierman, B., Afful, J., Carroll, M. D., Chen, T.-C., Davy, O., Fink, S., Fryar, C. D., Gu, Q., Hales, C. M., Hughes, J. P., Ostchega, Y., Storandt, R. J., & Akinbami, L. J. (2021). *National Health and Nutrition Examination Survey 2017–March 2020 prepandemic data files—Development of files and prevalence estimates for selected health outcomes* (National Health Statistics Reports 158). https://www.cdc.gov/nchs/data/nhsr/nhsr158-508.pdf

TABLE 12.4 ■ CHILDHOOD OBESITY BY ETHNICITY 2017 TO 2020

ETHNICITY	PREVALENCE
Hispanic children	26.2%
Non-Hispanic Black children	24.8%
Non-Hispanic White children	16.6%
Non- Hispanic Asian children	9.0 %

Source: Stierman, B., Afful, J., Carroll, M. D., Chen, T.-C., Davy, O., Fink, S., Fryar, C. D., Gu, Q., Hales, C. M., Hughes, J. P., Ostchega, Y., Storandt, R. J., & Akinbami, L. J. (2021). *National Health and Nutrition Examination Survey 2017–March 2020 prepandemic data files—Development of files and prevalence estimates for selected health outcomes* (National Health Statistics Reports 158). https://www.cdc.gov/nchs/data/nhsr/nhsr158-508.pdf

diets, healthcare, education, and activities that promote weight loss, healthy outcomes are improved.

Consequences of Obesity

Why does being obese versus being overweight matter? For one reason, the psychologic and emotional consequences of obesity often trigger a loss of confidence and self-esteem that is related to body image concerns. In the United States, these concerns are generated by the **stigma** associated with being excessively obese, especially for women (Obesity Society, 2023). However, the real problem with being obese is more than merely cosmetic. Of far greater significance, most scientists and researchers agree, is that serious obesity at its worst negatively alters the quality of life of its victims by promoting cardiovascular disease, DM, kidney failure, and some cancers, resulting in an increased mortality rate among adults (Adams, 2022; CDC, 2022; Cuevas et al., 2022; WHO, 2021b). However, this is not to minimize the impact that loss of confidence and self-esteem can have on one's psyche, which can be devastating to some and lead to deep depression and feelings of isolation and even thoughts of suicide in some cases.

Some Global Efforts to Address Obesity

Because of the global nature of this serious healthcare problem, the author has included articles in this section that reflect perspectives about obesity and its clinical management from various countries and cultures throughout the world including Canada, France, Turkey, Iran, and the United States.

In a Canadian study, Van Stiphout and colleagues (2022) examined healthcare professionals' knowledge, attitudes, and beliefs regarding the treatment of patients with obesity. The authors described obesity as a "chronic, relapsing disease." However, results of this study indicated that many respondents identified overeating, stress, and physical inactivity most frequently as the primary causes of obesity. The researchers discussed the stigmatization associated with obesity and its impact on the mental health and quality of life of patients who are obese, acknowledging that these responses indicate a bias toward prioritizing lifestyle choices. Having such a bias might lead health professionals to focus their counseling of patients living with obesity to "eat less and move more"; however, this may be inappropriate and ineffective advice that is "likely to fail" in assisting these patients (Van Stiphout et al., 2022). Moreover, results of this study indicate that current treatment of patients with obesity is inconsistent with the Canadian Adult Obese Clinical Practice Guidelines (CAOCP). Sixty percent of respondents indicated ambiguity in working with patients living with obesity, and more than 35% felt unprepared to discuss weight with their patients. More than 90% agreed training and educational materials were needed, and protocols would be useful. Findings of this study informed the development of a comprehensive institutional program that supports the changing narrative of obesity and integration of the 2020 CAOCP.

In a qualitative study of 25 adults in France, Dao and colleagues (2020) conducted a study that examined attitudes to food consumption and external pressures that influence eating behaviors and weight management and compared the results with an equivalent study conducted in the United States. The researchers found that France and the United States have very different obesity rates, with France having one of the lowest rates in Europe. In 2019, France was reported at 14% compared to the United States at 40%.

External pressures were described as major factors influencing food consumption in the United States, while in France implicit influences of external pressures through eating-related social interactions were observed. In France, foods considered natural were idealized and juxtaposed against processed and industrial food, which was not a salient aspect in the United States. The study identified both common and divergent attitudes toward food culture and eating behaviors. The author recommended further studies to identify effective interventions to address obesity in different populations.

In a study in Turkey, Akkayaoglu and Celik (2020) explored eating attitudes, perceptions, body image, and quality of life before and after bariatric surgery. In the study, 78% of the respondents were female and 89% were morbidly obese prior to surgery. The authors discussed the daily increase of obesity worldwide and its linkages to aging, DM, hypertension, settlement, place and region, social status, education level, bread consumption, substance use, and widespread use of technology. The researchers attributed the development of obesity to genetic, environmental, biochemical, sociocultural, and psychologic issues. Further, they described consequences of increases in the level of obesity and its association with death rates caused by noninfectious diseases like DM, hypertension, and cardiovascular disease.

Results of this study found that while 80% of the participants were morbidly obese prior to surgery, and 36% remained morbidly obese at the first month after surgery, by the third month after surgery none of the participants were morbidly obese and only 84% were classified as obese. At the sixth postop month, 24% of the patients were obese and 8% had normal weight. It was determined that eating attitudes and behaviors changed significantly after surgery compared to pre-surgery. Body image and quality of life were significantly higher in comparison to preoperative values. Results demonstrated that multidimensional evaluation of patients and implementation of nursing interventions contributed to the success of individuals undergoing bariatric surgery.

In a study that took place in Iran in 2018, Yazdani and colleagues assessed the relationship between body image and psychologic well-being in patients who are morbidly obese. In this study, the researchers described three dimensions of body image: cognitive (related to one's perception of weight, size, and shape), subjective (related to one's satisfaction or concern about appearance), and behavioral (associated with avoidance of exposure or anxiety or discomfort). The authors define body image as "a degree of satisfaction about the appearance (size, shape, and general appearance)" (Yazdani et al., 2018, p. 176). Further, the researchers observe that several studies suggest that perceived differences between appearance and ideal body image can lead to considerable dissatisfaction that may lead to depression.

The researchers found a significant relationship between body image and psychologic well-being on all the psychologic subscales of body image, but no significant difference in relationship to levels of BMI. The researchers concluded that body image defects could negatively impact psychologic well-being in all aspects. People with negative body image are more likely to have an eating disorder, suffer negative emotions, and experience loss of self-confidence and obsession with weight loss. Further, they note that morbid obesity is a stigmatized condition and patients face social exclusion, community judgment, and discrimination in many areas of their lives. The authors suggested preventing and supporting interventions should be performed as an effective method for encountering and coping with psychologic effects of obesity.

Other Costs of Obesity

In addition to the health risks, persons who are obese must also pay the price of higher insurance rates and higher fares on many airlines. Despite the Affordable Care Act's (ACA) mandate to insurers forbidding higher premiums for preexisting conditions, insurance companies are allowed to increase rates for persons whose BMI exceeds 30 by up to 25% and, for those whose BMI exceeds 39, up to 50% (Epstein, 2016). Some airlines have also adjusted their policies regarding obese passengers (Hewitt, 2019). For example, Southwest Airlines (2018) includes guidelines for its "customers of size" stating that "[c] ustomers who encroach upon any part of a neighboring seat(s) may proactively purchase the needed number of seats prior to travel in order to ensure the additional seat(s) is available" (para. 1) Subsequently, Southwest promises to refund all extra seat purchases even if the flight is oversold (Hewitt, 2019). Samoa Airlines in the South Pacific has gone further, providing a new pay-by-your-weight guide when you book a flight. The fare, although calculated based on passengers' stated weight online preflight, is confirmed when passengers are weighed on arrival at the airport. The financial burden of these costs adds to the many other challenges of being obese and the stigma that accompanies those challenges.

OBESITY AND STIGMA

Attitudes toward obesity in the United States reflect the larger societal "obsession with thinness" (Brody, 2017.) It is also the form of discrimination most deeply entrenched (Abrams, 2022). Brody observed that weight bias is widespread, and these attitudes can be traced to early childhood. Popular culture, as projected through the media, encourages dieting, fitness, and other programs aimed at reducing weight. Moreover, those who are obese are portrayed as being undisciplined overeaters who have only to change their life-style to correct the problem. This attitude prevails, despite growing evidence suggesting that the process of weight control is far more complicated, especially for some individuals. Paradoxically, individuals who are the most overweight or obese are often the recipients of disparaging or insensitive remarks that reflect negative assumptions and attitudes toward them based on body size. Consequently, many obese individuals experience feelings of low self-esteem because they have internalized these attitudes. Puhl and colleagues (2016) reported higher rates of depression, anxiety, and social isolation and poorer psychologic adjustment in persons who are obese. These feelings are provoked by attitudes held by professionals as well as members of the community, and at times family members as well. Consequently, as a result of those feelings, people living with obesity will begin disordered eating, decrease physical activity, engage in healthcare avoidance, and gain weight (Abrams, 2022; Lee et al., 2021). One way in which a positive outcome is undermined occurs when a person avoids the gym to avoid stigma or overeats to comfort themselves from stress as a result of stigmatization (Lee et al., 2021). Adults face sizeism at work, at some doctor's offices, and in romantic relationships. For children at school, sizeism is the most common reason for bullying (Abrams, 2022).

Dunagan and colleagues (2016) studied attitudes of prejudice and bias in BSNs. They identified two major themes: (a) bias and prejudice toward individuals who were obese and (b) bias and prejudice toward individuals of a different race. These researchers concluded that acknowledging one's bias is a first step toward gaining cultural competence.

Abrams (2022) described the burden of weight stigma and compared it to other forms of isms and discrimination. The global rise in obesity among adults and children around the world is now attributed, in part, to the sudden rise of another major health problem we all encountered at the same time, COVID-19. During the pandemic, many were compelled to stay home and adopt a more sedentary lifestyle, especially if they were compelled to work from home. In this article, the author described the perceptions and attitudes of many who have experienced weight stigma at some point in their lives. As the author reminds us, "unlike many other forms of bias discrimination based on body size is legal in most states" (Abrams, 2022).

Wakefield and Feo (2017) reported results of several studies of patients who were obese and overweight and "found that weight-bias and discrimination occurred in 69% of interactions with doctors, 46% with nurses, and 37% with dieticians and nutritionists" (p. 29). Further, these authors also observed that studies reveal persons who are obese develop a defense mechanism to protect themselves from this bias by "becoming vigilant" for signs of stigma. The authors acknowledged the challenges all nurses must face in overcoming biases before achieving their goals of providing culturally competent care. They recommended that nurses adopt a patient-centered approach that begins with self-awareness, challenges their own fears of weight, helps eliminate bias, and provides compassionate care that addresses the "individual and unique needs" of patients who are obese (p. 31).

In the summer of 2017, the author surveyed a small sample of nurses who were employed in a local acute care hospital with a bariatric unit. The purpose of the survey was to determine nurses' perceptions about the nature and quality of nursing care delivered to patients who are morbidly obese. While only seven nurses returned surveys for analysis, the results are worth mentioning here. Five of the seven nurses had been practicing for more than 10 years and four of the nurses for more than 15 years. Five of the seven nurses were currently practicing in medical–surgical settings; however, home care or critical care, nursing management, and outpatient clinics were listed among the participants' experiences. Five of the respondents reported caring for patients who were morbidly obese often or very often, while the other two reported caring for them only sometimes. An analysis of this survey revealed that all the nurse respondents believed that psychosocial or behavioral factors contributed to morbid obesity, none believed that there were physiologic factors involved in the development of obesity and only one identified genetics as a plausible cause. Most of the respondents were comfortable or very comfortable caring for patients who were seriously obese; were satisfied with care provision to these patients; and identified managing airway/breathing, drug therapy, diet and nutrition, pre- and postop teaching, and teaching about diagnostics among the priorities of care given to these patients. The respondents reported having adequate staffing, equipment, and training among the top challenges for nurses working with patients who are morbidly obese. Most of the respondents ranked providing culturally sensitive, unbiased, emotionally supportive, and safe care among the top considerations when caring for patients who are morbidly obese.

Nurses and others can assess their obesity bias by taking the Implicit Association Test created by Project Implicit at Harvard University. The link can be found under Important Websites at the end of this chapter.

STRATEGIES FOR CULTURALLY COMPETENT CARE DELIVERY

During nurses' encounters with obese patients, their ability to promote health will largely depend on their attitudes toward obesity and the skills they have acquired to overcome their own biases and fears about the care of patients who are obese. Emphasizing self-acceptance at any weight is a positive first step recommended in healthcare literature when establishing a rapport with patients. When communicating with patients living with obesity, it is important for nurses to be sensitive and cognizant of the verbal and nonverbal language they use in discussing obesity to ensure that they convey a nonjudgmental, accepting, and positive attitude toward the patient. When planning care for patients who are obese, nurses should also consider the patient's cultural background, living situation, and lifestyle, as well as the role food plays in the patient's family life, food preferences, and the availability of nutritious versus fast food in that patient's social environment. In collaboration with the nutrition therapist, the nurse can assist the patient in determining alternative food choices that minimize the intake of high caloric, fat, and sodium choices from among the patient's preferred foods. In addition, nurses can recommend inexpensive ways of increasing the patient's activity level and identify appropriate resources and referrals to support groups or counselors as needed. For example, Ballard and colleagues (2022) evaluated the effects walking had on lipids and lipid proteins in women with overweight and obesity. In this meta-analysis of 21 studies published between 1987 and 2016, the authors investigated changes in lipids and lipid proteins in exclusive walking interventions among women with overweight and obesity. This study revealed that hyperlipidemia is improved by exclusive walking independent of diet or weight loss. The recommended engagement was 150 minutes per week of moderate intensity. Nurses can share the results of studies like this with patients living with obesity and seeking inexpensive methods of health promotion.

Hopefully, these strategies will promote a sustained effort of weight control and afford patients who struggle with obesity the ability to maintain an optimum state of health.

IMPORTANT POINTS

- Obesity is a global and national issue, with 1.9 billion people who are overweight and 650 million who are obese.
- Over 41.9% of the U.S. population is overweight or obese.
- The CDC defines overweight as having a BMI of 25 or greater.
- A person who has a BMI of 30 or greater is considered obese.
- Obesity is classified into three classes: Class I, BMI 30 to 35; Class II, BMI 35 to 40 (serious obesity); and Class III, BMI greater than 40 (extreme or severe obesity).
- The waist–hip ratio or waist circumference is an alternative way of measuring body fat.
- A waist measurement of over 40 in men and over 30.5 in women in inches indicates excessive fat.
- The prevalence of obesity is different based on gender, race, ethnicity, and age.
- Causes of obesity are multifactorial and include biological, psychosocial, and cultural factors.
- Health risks of obesity include cardiovascular disease, DM, kidney failure, and some cancers, as well as reduced self-esteem, anxiety, depression, and suicide ideation.
- Negative societal attitudes, weight bias, and discrimination create a stigma for people who are obese.
- Research indicates that some nurses and other healthcare providers hold negative attitudes toward people who are obese.
- When planning care, nurses should consider personal bias, gain knowledge about obesity, use sensitive language, explore the specific causes of obesity, and develop a culturally competent plan of care.
- Many health professionals recognize the need for training and educational resources to better assist them in their care of people living with obesity.

CASE SCENARIO

Patty M., the day-shift charge nurse on a busy orthopedic surgery unit, receives a report from the ED that she is to admit Mrs. L., a 40-year-old female patient in a diabetic crisis. The patient's last blood sugar was 450 mg/dL. She is being admitted with an infected deep decubitus ulcer of her lower sacrum that occurred due to prolonged immobility following surgery last month for a cholecystectomy. The reporting nurse also indicated that the patient is very lethargic and seems depressed. She has received 12 units of regular humulin insulin in the ED and is expecting to get her lunch tray upon arrival at the unit.

Patty reports all the earlier findings to the others at the nurses' station and adds, sarcastically, "Oh, and by the way, she weighs 600 pounds." "So," she adds, "I think I am going to need a little help." Shortly after, the patient arrives and Kathy, the nurse assigned to care for the patient, and two other nurses approach the stretcher. One nurse whispered, "Well, I guess we've got our work cut out for us." None of the others reply, but exchange glances of affirmation. After assessing the situation, Kathy states, "I am not exactly sure how we're going to do this, I know we can't transfer her with the transfer board that we usually use; we'll have to call for the lift."

Mrs. L.'s stretcher is placed against the wall in the corridor until the lift arrives. While waiting, Kathy begins, "I'll check your vital signs and begin your nursing history." Mrs. L. remarks, "I thought that I was to receive my lunch tray when I arrived on the floor, I am starting to feel a little shaky." One nurse remarked, "I am sure that delaying your lunch until we get you settled won't hurt you a bit." Mrs. L. remained quiet and withdrawn throughout the remainder of the shift.

After taking Mrs. L. to her room and providing her lunch, the nurses met in the conference room to do their charting. One nurse expressed concern about how they would manage the care of Mrs. L. Another announced that she would assist in every way she could, but that her bad back prevented her from assisting with lifting or positioning Mrs. L. Another nurse expressed frustration with people who allowed themselves to get that heavy: "Isn't it sad that all she can seem to focus on is her lunch? She needs to be on a strict diet. She's going to have to work on developing some willpower while she's here. I really hope they put her on a strict diet." "I'll make sure she doesn't have any extra food brought in from the outside," another nurse offered. The charge nurse stated that she believed that everyone should take turns in being assigned to take care of Mrs. L. because with the amount of lifting and moving required, her diabetes, wound care, and need for nutritional management, "it just wouldn't be fair for anyone to be stuck taking care of her all the time."

WHAT NURSES NEED TO KNOW ABOUT THEMSELVES

Applying the Staircase Self-Assessment Model: Self-Reflection Questions

1. How comfortable am I caring for patients who are seriously obese?
2. Where do I see myself on the Cultural Competency Staircase?
3. How would I progress to the next level? (See Chapter 1.)
4. Do I have biases toward members of this group? Do I make assumptions about members of this group that are unfounded? Are my attitudes likely to impact the quality of care I can provide in this situation?
5. What information do I need about this patient to provide her with quality care?
6. What nurse behaviors should I be able to demonstrate to provide this patient with culturally competent care?

Responses to Self-Reflection Questions

Response: How comfortable am I caring for patients who are seriously obese?

The level of comfort a nurse has caring for patients who are morbidly obese depends in part on the number of encounters the nurse has had with other patients who are obese and the nature of those encounters. However, each experience is also dependent on the specific needs of the individual patient. In the earlier scenario, the nurses seem to make assumptions about the patient and verbalize their thoughts and feelings in the patient's presence. Even their discussions with one another suggest an "us versus her" pattern of thinking about this patient. The nurses' attitudes about obesity may be outside of their awareness as well as the effect it is having on their ability to provide compassionate care. But it is our own "socially internalized fear of fatness" that drives our tendency to be uncomfortable with people who are morbidly obese.

Response: Where do I see myself on the Cultural Competency Staircase?

Go to Chapter 1 and review the Cultural Competency Staircase table. Place yourself at the level that best describes you when working with patients from this group.

Response: How would I progress to the next level?

Examine the area in the table in Chapter 1 that describes the ways to progress from where you are to the next level.

Response: Do I have biases toward members of this group? Do I make assumptions about members of this group that are unfounded? Are my attitudes likely to impact the quality of care I can provide in this situation?

From the moment of this patient's anticipated admission to the unit, various nurses expressed a reluctance or lack of desire to care for her. While this attitude was probably not verbally expressed, it was certainly communicated between the members of the staff and, perhaps more subtly, to the patient. Unfortunately, when the prevailing attitude of the nurses toward the patient is that of not wanting to deal with this problem, nurses find excuses to avoid the patient, to limit contact, or to keep an emotional distance from them. The quality of care is compromised when nurses limit the time that they spend with their patients. This is a form of rejection that only compounds the societal rejection that these patients encounter on a regular basis.

The nurses appear to make certain assumptions about Mrs. L's obesity that prohibit them from treating her like they would any other diabetic patient. One of the nurses has expressed concerns about the potential for being injured when caring for patients who are morbidly obese. When this fear is acknowledged, the staff can address them realistically by requesting appropriate equipment and in-service programs on body mechanics, as well as lifting and transfer techniques, that will assist them in caring for patients who are morbidly obese. However, expressions of concern about the nurses' well-being in the presence of the patient are inappropriate and insensitive.

Mrs. L is a member of a cultural group, the seriously obese, that is often maligned and discriminated against in our society. In a society that values being thin and trim, obesity is often looked upon with apprehension and disdain, even though a large percentage of the population is overweight or obese. Nurses caring for patients like Mrs. L. must examine their attitudes to obesity and their ability to provide care that is culturally sensitive. Comments made during the patient's admission suggest that some nurses blame Mrs. L. for her predicament. The charge nurse, nurse manager, or other nurse leaders must also assume some responsibility for ensuring that the patient receives appropriate nursing care based on her clinical diagnoses and care needs. Nurse leaders must be cognizant of the staff's values and attitudes that might have a negative impact on the psychologic well-being of this patient. Even more important is the manager's ability to discourage behaviors that reflect these attitudes. Despite our best intentions, these attitudes often lie deep within our psyche, outside of conscious awareness. Because of these societal attitudes and the feelings and attitudes of healthcare providers, patients who are morbidly obese often suffer the psychologic pain of embarrassment, frustration, and depression when they encounter these attitudes while they are receiving care.

One way of addressing these negative attitudes, which are often based upon false assumptions, is to strengthen nurses' knowledge regarding the facts about morbid obesity.

This could be accomplished informally by having a lunch-hour presentation by one of the nurses, bariatric physicians, or staff development personnel. The information shared should include evidence-based knowledge that strengthens the staff's understanding of the etiology of obesity and the psychologic and physiologic challenges severely obese patients' experience, as well as the current gold standard for treatment and care.

Response: What information do I need about this patient to provide her with quality care?

In this case example, morbid obesity is the secondary diagnosis, yet because of its implications for the nursing staff, it has become the primary focus of their attention.

It would be helpful for the nurses caring for patients who are morbidly obese to know some of the facts about obesity in the United States and the world. The WHO and CDC are excellent sources of current statistics and other information about this serious healthcare concern. Their websites and others may be found at the end of this chapter.

As the literature attests, morbid obesity is not a weakness or choice of lifestyle, but a chronic disease that is responsible for other life-threatening diseases. Life-threatening diseases associated with morbid obesity include coronary artery disease, obstructive sleep apnea, type 2 diabetes, and certain cancers. Another major area of concern is the prevention and/or care of tissue damage that requires aggressive care of the skin and perineal area. Patients who are morbidly obese must often face many other problems that complicate their hospitalization, since they often present with a variety of other challenges to their health. Understanding some of the common problems obese patients face would also assist the nurse in establishing a therapeutic relationship with obese patients. For example, breathlessness on exertion, limited mobility, and difficulty in dressing and performing other activities of daily living are a result of excessive weight and increased intra-abdominal pressure. Gastric reflux disease, gallbladder disease and gallstones, liver disease, osteoarthritis, gout, reproductive problems, urinary and fecal incontinence, and limited mobility are but a few of the diseases encountered by patients experiencing morbid obesity. Together with the multitude of physical ailments that accompany morbid obesity, these patients must also face a considerable amount of prejudice as well as feelings of rejection, shame, and depression. Thus, the psychologic impact of this disease may be the most painful (National Institutes of Health [NIH], 2023).

Response: What nurse behaviors should I be able to demonstrate to provide this patient with culturally competent care?

Perhaps more than any other patient, the patient who is morbidly obese requires the understanding and compassion of a culturally sensitive nurse. Nurses caring for these patients must be willing to identify and address the patient's primary health issues in a way that is sensitive to the patient's feelings about themselves, their obesity, and the way they are being perceived by the staff. While weight control is a desirable future goal, an acute hospital stay—particularly when the patient is in crisis—is not the ideal time to focus on this problem. However, the earlier case example is complicated by the fact that control of this patient's diabetes is inextricably tied to her weight management. Therefore, it is important for the nurse in this situation to discuss the relative importance of nutrition as it relates to weight management and DM in the care of bariatric patients.

Some hospitals now have bariatric units or beds assigned within certain units for the care of patients who are morbidly obese. The term *bariatric* refers to those individuals who are more than twice their ideal body weight (IBW), who exceed 100 pounds over their IBW, or whose BMI is greater than 40. The term *morbidly obese* is used to describe those individuals whose body size restricts their mobility, health, or access to available services.

However, not all hospitals have units that are prepared to adequately address care concerns of obese patients without modifying their plans for care, staffing patterns, and use of necessary equipment to assist patients who are morbidly obese. In these situations, it is necessary for the hospitals to provide members of the staff with in-service workshops that provide information about care issues. Other opportunities should be provided for staff members to openly discuss their personal issues and concerns about caring for severely obese patients.

Culturally competent nurses always conduct a careful assessment of the patient to determine their physical needs based on their presenting problem, as well as their cultural beliefs, values, and practices. This assessment affords the nurse an opportunity to better understand the patient in relation to how the patient perceives and is affected by the illness. It also provides insight into what the patient desires as an outcome.

Nursing literature provides several tools for conducting a cultural assessment. An appropriate choice for this case would be to use Kleinman's (1980) explanatory model in which he asks eight open-ended questions to determine the patient's explanation of their illness:

1. What do you call your problem? What name does it have?
2. What do you think has caused your problem?
3. Why do you think it started when it did?
4. What do you think your sickness does to you?
5. How severe is it? Will it have a short- or long-term course?
6. What do you fear the most about your sickness?
7. What are the chief problems your sickness has caused for you?
8. What kind of treatment do you think you should receive? What are the most important results you hope to receive from this treatment? (p. 106)

In asking these questions to Mrs. L., the nurses will be better able to determine her attitudes and beliefs about DM and, perhaps, her views on obesity as well. Most importantly, it provides a starting point for ongoing communication about her illness to occur between the patient and the nurses that may facilitate the development of an effective and culturally sensitive plan of care for this patient.

Obtaining a cultural assessment requires skill that goes beyond knowing the right questions to ask. Of course, these skills are developed over time. To provide ongoing assessment of the patient's care needs, the nurse will need to develop skills in communication such as active listening to facilitate cross-cultural communication. However, skills in assessment and communication can only be achieved through frequent encounters with the patient.

In addition to having assessment skills, nurses will need to be able to pull from their repertoire of skills the ability to, at some point, identify and discuss with the patient some appropriate resources for the patient to utilize in managing her weight. Some of these resources are listed in the Important Websites list at the end of this chapter. In communicating with this patient, the nurse must demonstrate skill in listening actively to determine what goals the patient has for herself. Planning care for her should be based upon mutually agreed upon goals. Nurses will also need to pay close attention to the patient's nonverbal communication, including facial expressions, gestures, and use of silence, and to seek clarification when uncertain about the patient's intended meaning. These nonverbal clues may be indicators of anxiety, confusion, or depression that may signal a need for further interventions or collaborations between the nurse and other members of the healthcare team, such as clinical specialists, psychologists, and nurse practitioners (NPs).

Today's healthcare environment seldom allows nurses the opportunity for frequent face-to-face encounters with each patient, yet multiple encounters are necessary to ensure the establishment of a positive rapport between the patient and the nurse. Culturally competent nurses strive to visit their patients as often as is possible, even if visits are brief. This allows for the establishment of a positive interpersonal relationship in which the nurse and the patient gain mutual respect.

Because of the patient's primary diagnosis, type 2 DM, and a secondary diagnosis of morbid obesity, the patient's nutritional requirements are somewhat complex. It is imperative for the nursing staff and the patient to work collaboratively with the dietitian or nutrition therapist to establish and maintain a suitable dietary plan. It is equally important for the nurses to assist the patient in managing her diet without criticizing or making insensitive remarks. Sometimes, even a glance between colleagues can inadvertently communicate disrespect to the patient. Therefore, it is important to be mindful of nonverbal behaviors that may be negatively interpreted by the patient. Each patient encounter should give the patient and the nurse an opportunity to strengthen the nurse–patient relationship.

HELPFUL HINTS USING THE PEARLS ASSESSMENT MODEL (SEE CHAPTER 2)

The primary nurse's first encounter with this patient might give rise to

Partnership: In welcoming the patient to the unit, introduce yourself as her nurse, and suggest that they would need to work together, probably with the nutrition therapist, in planning management of her diabetes and other nutritional concerns.

Empathy: Express concern about her level of hyperglycemia and complaints of "shakiness" following the insulin administration. "It must be difficult to feel that your blood sugar is so unstable." Or, "It must be scary to hear that your blood sugar was so high."

Apologize: "I am sorry that you've had to wait for us to get you settled in."

Respect: "So, do you feel that your blood sugar has dropped significantly since you were given the insulin?"

Legitimization: Acknowledge the patient's concerns and include her in any conversations that involve her, particularly in her presence. "We'll get that tray to you right away."

Support: "I'll come back to do your history after you've finished your meal. Please ring your call bell if you need anything in the meantime."

SUMMARY

Because of the U.S. societal preoccupation with being thin, morbidly obese individuals are often ridiculed or ignored and may withdraw from active participation in their care in anticipation of this reaction from nurses and other health professionals. Morbid obesity poses a major health risk that has reached epidemic proportions in our country and the world. Since morbid obesity poses a potential threat to patients' cardiac and other vital organs and systems, these patients require immediate and effective medical and nursing intervention. Most nurses appreciate the life-threatening nature of this disease and treat these patients with compassionate care. Hopefully, other nurses who are less motivated and sympathetic to the plight of the morbidly obese will come to appreciate that this disease touches the lives of people without regard for race, class, or gender. Nurses' desire to assist these patients can be inspired by nurses who model culturally sensitive care. By becoming more knowledgeable about patients who are morbidly obese, being aware of stereotypes and biases that many healthcare professionals have toward this group, and developing assessment, communication, and physical skills to overcome some of the fears associated with caring for these patients, nurses can begin to provide more culturally sensitive care for the patient who is morbidly obese.

NCLEX®-TYPE QUESTIONS

1. According to the Centers for Disease Control and Prevention (CDC), the percentage of U.S. citizens who are obese is:
   A. 10%
   B. 25%
   C. 41%
   D. 60%

2. Researchers generally believe that the cause of obesity is most likely:
   A. Genetic
   B. Overeating
   C. Psychosocial
   D. Multifactorial

3. Patients who are experiencing morbid obesity are often challenged by:
   A. Anxiety, low self-esteem, and stigmatization
   B. Gastric reflux, limited mobility, and sleep apnea
   C. Difficulty performing activities of daily living, frustration, and depression
   D. All of the above

4. Research indicates that nurses' attitudes toward obesity are:
   A. Like those of society
   B. More negative than those of physicians
   C. More positive than those of physicians
   D. More negative than those of society

5. Stigmatization of obesity in society has resulted in:
   A. Vigilance by patients who are obese in anticipation of bias by healthcare workers
   B. Attitudes of increased support and empathy toward obese patients by healthcare workers
   C. Enhanced rapport between nurses and patients who are obese
   D. Increased numbers of persons who are obese

6. Which of these statements describes common psychosocial consequences of stigma in morbid obesity?
   A. Anxiety, depression, and social isolation
   B. Anorexia and excessive weight loss
   C. Increased overeating and weight gain
   D. A and C

7. Factors that influence nurses' ability to provide culturally competent care to patients who are obese include:
   A. Nurses' attitudes toward obesity
   B. The ability of the nurse to control bias and discrimination
   C. The number and nature of nurses' encounters with patients who are morbidly obese
   D. All of the above

8. The primary focus of nursing care for patients who are morbidly obese during the initial meeting with the patient should be to:
   A. Assess the patient's cultural values and beliefs
   B. Establish a positive rapport and partnership to identify the patient's care needs
   C. Develop a plan for weight modification
   D. Teach the patient about the importance of good nutrition

9. To ensure effective communication when caring for patients who are severely obese, nurses should pay close attention to:
    A. Patients' nonverbal communication, including body language and silence
    B. The level of the patient's active participation in their care
    C. Gains and losses in the patient's weight during the hospitalization
    D. The patient's readiness for self-disclosure
    E. Their own use of language regarding obesity

10. Which of these activities strengthen the nurses' ability to provide culturally competent care to patients who are morbidly obese?
    A. Providing workshops and staff development activities that highlight the etiology, complications, and treatment of obesity
    B. Performing a self-assessment of one's attitudes and biases about obesity
    C. Collaborating with other healthcare professionals when care planning
    D. All of the above

ANSWERS TO NCLEX-TYPE QUESTIONS

1. C   5. A   9. A
2. D   6. D   10. D
3. D   7. D
4. A   8. B

AMERICAN ASSOCIATION OF COLLEGES OF NURSING COMPETENCIES ADDRESSED IN THIS CHAPTER

1. Apply knowledge of social and cultural factors that affect nursing and healthcare across multiple contexts.
2. Use relevant data sources and best evidence in providing culturally competent care.
3. Promote achievement of safe and quality outcomes of care for diverse populations.
4. Advocate for social justice, including commitment to the health of vulnerable populations and the elimination of healthcare disparities.
5. Participate in cultural competence development.

EXERCISE

After reviewing the chapter on Cultural Considerations When Caring for the Patient Who Is Morbidly Obese, please answer the following questions. Discuss your responses with a classmate, colleague, or friend.

A. In reviewing this case example, identify three ways the nurses might have exhibited cultural sensitivity to this patient.
    1.
    2.
    3.

B. Imagine you are the patient in this situation. What would you like to have done for you by the nurses who are caring for you?

C. Among the resources listed on the previous page, which ones would you utilize when caring for this patient? Are there others?

A robust set of instructor resources designed to supplement this text is located at http://connect.springerpub.com/content/book/978-0-8261-8302-6. Qualifying instructors may request access by emailing textbook@springerpub.com.

REFERENCES

Abrams, Z. (2022). The burden of weight stigma. *The American Psychological Association, 53*(2), 52. https://www.apa.org/monitor/2022/03/news-weight-stigma

Adams, M. L. (2022). Accounting for the origins and toll of COVID 19: The key role of overweight in COVID-19. *American Journal of Health Promotion, 36*(2), 385–387. https://journals.sagepub.com/doi/10.1177/08901171211064006

Akkayaoglu, H., & Celik, S. (2020). Eating attitudes, perceptions of body image and patient quality of life before and after bariatric surgery. *Applied Nursing Research, 53*, 151270. https://doi.org/10.1016/j.apnr.2020.151270

Ballard, A. M., Davis, A., Wong, B., Lyn, R., & Thompson, W. R. (2022). The effects of exclusive walking on lipids and lipoproteins in women with overweight and obesity: A systematic review and meta-analysis. *American Journal of Health Promotion, 36*(2), 328–339. https://doi.org/10.1177/08901171211048135

Boutari, C., & Mantzoros, C. S. (2022). A 2022 update on the epidemiology of obesity and a call to action: As its twin COVID-19 pandemic appears to be receding, the obesity and dysmetabolism pandemic continues to rage on. *Metabolism: Clinical and Experimental, 133*, 155217. https://doi.org/10.1016/j.metabol.2022.155217

Brody, J. E. (2017, August). Fat bias starts early and takes a serious toll. *New York Times: Personal Health*. https://www.nytimes.com/2017/08/21/well/live/fat-bias-starts-early-and-takes-a-serious-toll.html

Centers for Disease Control and Prevention. (n.d.-a). *Defining adult overweight & obesity*. Retrieved October 11, 2023, from https://www.cdc.gov/obesity/basics/adult-defining.html

Centers for Disease Control and Prevention. (n.d.-b). *Obesity and overweight*. Retrieved October 11, 2023, from https://www.cdc.gov/nchs/fastats/obesity-overweight.htm

Centers for Disease Control and Prevention. (2022). *Overweight and obesity: Childhood overweight and obesity*. https://www.cdc.gov/obesity/childhood/index.html

Centers for Disease Control and Prevention, National Center for Health Statistics (NHanes). (2021). *National Health Nutrition Examination Survey*. https://www.cdc.gov/nchs/nhanes/participant.htm.

Cuevas, A. G., Cofie, L. E., & Nolte, S. (2022). The association between veteran status and obesity differs across race/ethnicity. *American Journal of Health Promotion, 36*(2), 314–317. https://doi.org/10.1177/08901171211052994

Dao, M. C., Thiron, S., Messer, E., Sergeant, C., Sévigné, A., Huart, C., Rossi, M., Silverman, I., Sakaida, K., Bel Lassen, P., Sarrat, C., Arciniegas, L., Das, S. K., Gausserès, N., Clément, K., & Roberts, S. B. (2020). Cultural influences on the regulation of energy intake and obesity: A qualitative study comparing food customs and attitudes to eating in adults from France and the United States. *Nutrients, 13*(1), 63. https://doi.org/10.3390/nu13010063

Dunagan, P. B., Kimble, L. P., Gunby, S. S., & Andrews, M. M. (2016). Baccalaureate nursing students' attitudes of prejudice: A qualitative inquiry. *Journal of Nursing Education, 55*(6), 345–348. https://doi.org/10.3928/01484834-20160516-08

Epstein, L. (2016). *Why a higher BMI shouldn't raise insurance*. https://www.bartleby.com/essay/BMI-Shouldn-T-Raise-Insurance-Rates-By-86F960752C27620C

Greenberg, J. A. (2013). Obesity and early mortality in the United States. *Obesity, 21*(2), 405–412. https://doi.org/10.1002/oby.20023

Hewitt, E. (2019). Airline passenger of size policies: Will you be forced to buy an extra seat. *Smarter Travel*. https://www.smartertravel.com/airline-passenger-of-size-policies

Hollerbach, B. S., Haddock, C. K., Kukić, F., Poston, W. S. C., Jitnarin, N., Jahnke, S. A., DeBlauw, J. A., & Heinrich, K. M. (2022). Comparisons of baseline obesity prevalence and its association with perceived health and physical performance in military officers. *Biology, 11*(12), 1789. https://doi.org/10.3390/biology11121789

Johnson, S. (2019). What ways are there to measure body fat? *Medical News Today*. https://www.medicalnewstoday.com/articles/326331

Kleinman, A. (1980). *Patients and healers in the context of culture*. University of California Press.

Kubala, J. (2023). *Four ways to measure body fat at home*. Healthline. https://www.healthline.com/health/how-to-measure-body-fat

Lee, K. M., Hunger, J. M., & Tomiyama, A. J. (2021). Weight stigma and health behaviors: Evidence from the eating in America study. *International Journal of Obesity, 45*, 1499–1509. https://doi.org/10.1038/s41366-021-00814-5

National Heart, Lung, and Blood Institute. (n.d.). *Assessing your weight and health risk*. Retrieved October 11, 2023, from https://www.nhlbi.nih.gov/health/educational/lose_wt/risk.htm

National Institutes of Health. (2023). *How does stigma affect patients with overweight, obesity, and diabetes?* National Institute of Diabetes and Digestive and Kidney Diseases. https://www.niddk.nih.gov/health-information/professionals/diabetes-discoveries-practice/how-stigma-affects-patients-with-overweight-obesity-or-diabetes

Obesity Society. (2023). *Country's leading obesity care organizations develop concensus statement on obesity*. https://www.prnewswire.com/news-releases/countrys-leading-obesity-care-organizations-develop-consensus-statement-on-obesity-301734250.html?tc=eml_cleartime

Puhl, R. M., Phelan, S. M., Nudglowski, J., & Kyle, T. K. (2016). Overcoming weight bias in the management of patients with diabetes and obesity. *Clinical Diabetes, 34*(1), 44–50. https://doi.org/10.2337/diaclin.34.1.44

Ryne Paulose-Ram, Jessica E. Graber, David Woodwell, Namanjeet Ahluwalia, "The National Health and Nutrition Examination Survey (NHANES), 2021–2022: Adapting Data Collection in a COVID-19 Environment", American Journal of Public Health 111, no. 12 (December 1, 2021): pp. 2149-2156. https://doi.org/10.2105/AJPH.2021.306517

Southwest Airlines. (2018). *Customers of size policy: Guidelines for customers of size.* https:/www.southwest.com/html/customer-service/extra-seat/index-pol.html

Stierman, B., Afful, J., Carroll, M. D., Chen, T.-C., Davy, O., Fink, S., Fryar, C. D., Gu, Q., Hales, C. M., Hughes, J. P., Ostchega, Y., Storandt, R. J., & Akinbami, L. J. (2021). *National Health and Nutrition Examination Survey 2017–March 2020 prepandemic data files—Development of files and prevalence estimates for selected health outcomes* (National Health Statistics Reports 158). https://www.cdc.gov/nchs/data/nhsr/nhsr158-508.pdf

Van Stiphout, C., Alex, R., Turner, K., Twyman, K., Brown, J., Bowes, B., Charlebois, A., & Quinlan, B. (2022). A quality improvement project to determine the knowledge, attitudes, and beliefs of healthcare providers regarding the treatment of patients with obesity. *Canadian Journal of Cardiovascular Nursing, 32*(2), 11–17. https://cccn.ca/_uploads/63a61347af481.pdf

Wakefield, K., & Feo, R. (2017). Confronting obesity, stigma and weight bias in healthcare with a person centred care approach: A case study . *Australian Nursing and Midwifery Journal, 25*(1), 28–31.

World Health Organization. (2021a). *Fact sheets: Malnutrition.* https://www.who.int/news-room/fact-sheets/detail/malnutrition

World Health Organization. (2021b). *Fact sheets: Obesity and overweight.* https://www.who.int/news-room/fact-sheets/detail/obesity-and-overweight

Yazdani, N., Hosseini, S. V., Amini, M., Sobhani, Z., Sharif, F., & Khazraei, H., (2018). Relationship between body image and psychological well-being in patients with morbid obesity. *International Journal of Community Based Nursing and Midwifery, 6*(2), 175–184. https://doi.org/10.30476/IJCBNM.2018.40825

IMPORTANT WEBSITES

American Obesity Association. Retrieved from www.obesity.org

Implicit Bias Test. Retrieved from implicit.harvard.edu/implicit/selectatest.html

International Obesity Task Force. Retrieved from iotf.org

The American Society for Metabolic and Bariatric Surgery. Retrieved from https://asmbs.org

The Obesity Action Coalition. Retrieved from https://www.obesityaction.org

The Obesity Medicine Association. Retrieved from https://obesitymedicine.org

The Obesity Society. Retrieved from https://www.obesity.org

The Stop Obesity Alliance. Retrieved from https://stop.publichealth.gwu.edu

Weight Loss and Control. Retrieved from www.niddk.nih.gov

Cultural Considerations When Caring for Veterans

Gloria Kersey-Matusiak

The gem cannot be polished without friction, nor man perfected without trials.
—CONFUCIUS

LEARNING OBJECTIVES

After this chapter, the reader will be able to
1. Discuss the healthcare problems experienced by veterans that result from their military service.
2. Describe the social and institutional barriers to veterans making the transition from military service to civilian life.
3. Recall the elements of an appropriate nursing assessment to identify common health concerns experienced by veterans.
4. Apply principles of cultural competency when developing a plan of care for veterans.
5. Identify specific nursing measures to alleviate veterans' health problems and provide support through their transition back to civilian life.

KEY TERMS

Chronic fatigue syndrome

Conscription (draft)

Deployment

Draft

Global War on Terror

Hypervigilance

Improvised explosive device (IED)

Loss of limbs

Medically unexplained illnesses

Military service

Posttraumatic stress disorder (PTSD)

Social reintegration

Suicide

Traumatic brain injury (TBI)

Veterans

INTRODUCTION

Any serious discussion about vulnerable populations in the United States would be incomplete without consideration of the millions of men and women who have either mandatorily or voluntarily placed their lives at risk for the sake of the common good. This chapter provides an overview of U.S. veterans that examines their demographic characteristics, the military culture, physical and psychologic consequences of **military service** during **deployment,** and the impact these consequences have on veterans' future health. The case studies and learning activities in this chapter provide strategies to assist nurses in Veterans Affairs (VA) and non-VA healthcare facilities to better identify and address veterans' healthcare needs during postdeployment and postmilitary transitions.

In this chapter, the term *veterans* refers to all previous members of all branches of the military—the U.S. Army, Navy, Marines, Air Force, and Coast Guard—who have completed their tours of active duty during times of war or peace. The Army continues to be the largest and oldest branch of the military. In 2021, according to a survey by Statista (2022), the Army had 482,416 of all U.S. active-duty personnel, followed by the Navy with 343,223, the Air Force with 328,888, the Marine Corps with 179,378, and the Coast Guard with 44,500 (Data USA, n.d.). The Department of Defense (DoD) issued a press release stating women accounted for "17.3% of active-duty personnel, totaling 231,741 members [in the U.S. military' and 21.4% of the National Guard and reserves at 171,000 members" in 2021 (2022, para. 4). While women were once limited to assigned roles as nurses, cooks, and laundresses, and to lower wages and rank relative to those of men, the role of women in the military has evolved over many decades. In the past, women's participation in the military was limited to 2% of the total number enlisted. For example, "during World War I[,] [w]omen served as nurses, cooks, clerks, and telephone operators. . . . During World War II, [the role of women] expanded to include mechanics, drivers, and even soldiers and pilots" (In the News, 2013, para. 2). In response to the growing outcry by women for equality and the decreasing numbers of men who were enlisting, in January 2013, the Pentagon lifted the ban on women serving in combat roles on the ground, making it possible for them to attain the same military status, rank, and pay as men. All service persons' compensation is determined based on time and grade or rank, and wages are adjusted every 2 years (Defense Finance and Accounting Services, 1949–2018). Promotions are based on a variety of factors. Since 2016, all occupations and positions in the military have been open to women, including combat assignments (Central Intelligence Agency [CIA], 2017). In 2022, the DoD in its report stated, "[t]he over 3 million women who have served in or with the armed forces since the American Revolution have contributed immensely to the strength and resilience of our armed forces" (Patricia Montes Barron as cited in DoD, 2022, para. 6). Barroso (2019) noted that in 2017, nearly one in five commissioned officers in the U.S. military were women.

NURSES IN THE MILITARY

Since the Civil War, nurses have played a special role in the military, voluntarily supporting our troops at home and abroad. During World War II and the Vietnam War, thousands of women and many men supported the U.S. Army and Air Force as nurses; many were wounded and some of them died in the line of duty. During Operations Desert Shield and Desert Storm (1990–1991), 2,214 Army nurses and 972 Air Force nurses were deployed. During the war in Afghanistan, U.S. Army, Navy, and Air Force nurses have provided support for the over 35,000 physically injured U.S. personnel (Scannell-Desch & Doherty, 2012). Since the **Global War on Terror** began, women have had more exposure to combat (Britanica.com, 2017).

Like men, women assigned to combat and noncombat duty in the Persian Gulf often risk being killed or captured. According to the Defense Health Agency (DHA), in 2021 there were 29,645 nurses in the military including 9,598 in the Army, 9,008 in the Reserves/ National Guard, 4,540 in the Navy, 4,036 in the Air Force, 1,352 in the United States Public Health Service, and 1,111 in the DHA (Aker, 2021). According to the American Nurses Association (ANA, n.d.), 35% of active duty nurses in the military are males.

VETERANS BY GENDER, RACE, AND ETHNICITY

According to the U.S. Census Bureau (2023), of the total number of veterans (16.2 million in 2022), women accounted for 1.7 million, or 10.5% of all veterans in the United States, Puerto Rico, and U.S. territories. Non-Hispanic Whites represented 72.3% (11.7 million members) of the veteran population, Black or African Americans represented 12.4% (2 million members), Hispanics of any race represented 8.6% (1.39 million members), Asians represented 2.1% (340,200 members), American Indian and Alaska Natives represented 0.2% (32,400 members), and those listing some other race represented 2.8% (324,000).

VETERANS' NATIONAL ORIGIN AND PLACE OF RESIDENCE

It is important to note that U.S. veterans represent individuals who were born both within and outside of the United States. "According to the U.S. Census, most veterans were born in 1 of the 50 states or in the District of Columbia, while a smaller percentage includes veterans that were born outside the country to American parents and those born in Puerto Rico or other U.S. islands." Since citizenship is not a requirement to join the military, "lawful permanent residents (LPRs) are eligible to enlist. In 2020, 13% (2.3 million) of the U.S. veteran population was born outside the United States or were children of immigrants based on a report by the 2020 U.S. Census Bureau (Buchholz, 2023). The top birth countries from which foreign-born U.S. veterans came were Mexico (68,200), the Philippines (65,200), Cuba, (28,000), Jamaica, (26,000), U.K, (23,100), Panama, (18,800), Germany (16,300), El Salvador (16,200; Buchholz, 2023).

The U.S. state with the highest number of veterans was Texas (1,408,464), followed by Florida (1,356,882), California (1,342,337), Pennsylvania (641,525), and Virginia (641,144; Statista, 2023).

MILITARY CULTURE

According to the Pew Research Center, the individuals we refer to as **veterans** number over 19 million, or 10% of civilians; of these, 11% are women (Schaeffer, 2021).

All branches of the military bring men and women together from diverse generations and racial, ethnic, cultural, religious, geographic, and political backgrounds and place them in unique employment and living situations for sometimes indefinite periods of time. In this setting, a new culture is formed where codes of behavior and patterns of interacting are developed. As part of their military training, members of the armed forces prepare to temporarily relinquish their reliance on family and friends back home in exchange for the camaraderie and support of officers, fellow soldiers, sailors, and Marines. These are the people on whom their daily lives must depend for social, physical, and psychologic support during their tours of duty. In this new environment, servicemen and servicewomen bond with one another around a common cause.

During times of deployment, comrades may share life-altering experiences unmatched by those that occur in their civilian lives. As a result, the brotherhood and sisterhood that develop often creates lasting and cherished relationships that extend beyond the years of active duty. During certain times in U.S. history, military service was not a choice, but a mandatory experience for all males between ages 18 and 35. In 1973, **conscription,** also called the **draft** or mandatory service, ended. Today, military service in the United States is voluntary; however, all men at 18 years of age are required to register with the Selective Service System.

McCaslin and colleagues (2021) examined veterans' perspectives on military culture and on veterans' attitudes, values, beliefs, and behaviors, as well as the role these play after military service. The experiences veterans have while in service in the military are different. The authors believe that overlooking the causes and complexity of veterans' individual reactions to those experiences may result in misdiagnosis by mental health providers. The goal of this research was to identify what aspects of military culture are important for healthcare providers to consider as they care for veterans to inform culturally sensitive mental healthcare for each of them. The authors of this study identified several themes, including military values, beliefs, and behaviors; relationships; occupational habits and practices; acquired skills; communication; affiliation; and psychologic health and well-being. The most frequently noted area within the theme called values, beliefs, and behaviors was related to the "hierarchical command structure" of the military with its clear schedule, objectives, and sense of commitment to working toward a shared, common, and higher purpose. These values instill a selflessness or group spirit different from that found in civilian life. Another cultural attribute is that of the importance of teamwork to accomplish a mission without regard to individual benefit. Participants also discussed the value placed by the military on quick decision-making and getting things done as part of military training. Timeliness or time consciousness was also included, as was striving to be the best, being responsible and dependable, doing what you say, doing your job effectively, not leaving things unfinished, and the importance of being loyal and expecting to have one another's back. Each of these aspects of military life made a lasting impression on veterans' minds. Themes derived from the analysis assist providers to distinguish aspects of cultural transition from psychopathology. The researchers emphasized the importance of training healthcare providers to enhance their sensitivity to military culture when caring for veterans. In a Pew Research Center report of key findings about military veterans, Igielnik (2019) noted that post 9/11 veterans differed from those that served in earlier eras. About one-in-five veterans served on active duty after the terrorist attacks of September 11, 2001. These veterans were more likely to have been deployed and to have served in combat, giving them distinctly different experiences compared to earlier veterans. Most reflect feeling proud for having served (68%) and would endorse military service as a career choice (79%), and most veterans across all eras say the military did a good job preparing them for military life; however, fewer (52%) agree that the military prepared them for the transition to civilian life. About half of post-9/11 veterans say adjusting to civilian life was difficult as compared to the experiences of pre-9/11 veterans (Finnegan et al., 2020; Igielnik, 2019).

Health Challenges

McCaslin and colleagues discussed mental health-related experiences during and following military service within many groups. These experiences included posttraumatic stress disorder (PTSD, 59%), anger (59%), grief (47%), substance use (35%), aggression (29%), and fear (18%). Some of the respondents viewed emotions as liabilities, or weaknesses, and did not want others to know of these feelings for fear that someone would take advantage of them. One stated, "Don't let anyone know you are hurting." The researchers also reported positive reflections by some participants who indicated pride (59% of groups), compassion (29%), and joy (12%). One stated, "I had experiences in the military that inspired me, motivated me, and built me up" (p. 616). More than half of the groups, when discussing coping measures, used substances (59%) or avoidance (42%) as ways of managing stressors.

Some researchers have focused their attention on the mental health issues impacting women veterans. For example, Dyar (2019) described data from the National Center for Veterans Analysis and Statistics (NCVAS) effort to identify nursing care considerations for women veterans. At that time, women represented 9.4% of all veterans. Dyer and colleagues discussed the top five reasons women vets seek services from Veterans Health Administration (VHA): PTSD, major depressive disorders, migraine, lumbo sacral or cervical sprain, and complete removal of the uterus and ovaries representing 33% of all service-connected disabilities. The researchers found that less than 36% of women seek care at the VHA health system. Barriers to accessing care within the system include the belief that the VHA lacked the capacity to meet the needs of women veterans and they had options to receive care elsewhere. Living too far away from a VA facility was another barrier. With the growing number of female veterans seeking help in other systems, the article highlighted healthcare issues specific to female veterans to assist nurses and other health professionals in identifying female veterans' care needs.

Female veterans were found to be at risk for what the author referred to as Gulf War Illness, which the VA (2018) calls chronic multi-symptom illnesses or undiagnosed illnesses. The symptoms are numerous, debilitating, and presumed to be connected to deployment in the Persian Gulf (VA, 2022). In this study, researchers found the chronic symptoms—fatigue, headache, joint pain, indigestion, insomnia, dizziness, respiratory disorders, and memory problems—more prevalent among women (8.4%) compared to men (4.2%). Authors report that women serving in the Gulf War might also have an increased risk for fibromyalgia due to multiple exposures to environmental and psychologic stressors within their time in the service. Data analysis also found a relationship between fibromyalgia and symptoms of depression and PTSD and determined another factor, military sexual trauma (MST), may also be a risk factor for developing fibromyalgia, since 50% of patients reporting sexual trauma in or out of the military also screened positive for fibromyalgia. MST is defined as the psychologic trauma caused by physical assault of a sexual nature while serving in the military, and can include harassment. Women who experience MST seek mental health treatment, but those who report and do not receive it are more likely to attempt suicide. Physical effects of MST are pervasive and include chronic health problems, pain, obesity, higher rates of substance abuse, chronic medical conditions, and mental health. Female veterans may also experience adverse effects on employment in and out of the military, demotions, and decreased rates of employment. In funding year 2022, 199,000 women veterans faced homelessness and were served by VA homeless programs (VA, 2022).

The researchers urged nurses to consider MST if their patient's psychosocial assessments indicated signs of PTSD, but not to assume that all women veterans have experienced MST, and to remember that many women will elect not to report MST. One barrier is lack of knowledge about available services. Collaborative care requires a case manager to aid in assessing VA services. The researchers concluded that most VHA settings focus predominantly on male veterans, so for women, the atmosphere may be unwelcoming, especially if they have encountered MST. Every encounter should offer the most comprehensive, open-minded, nonjudgmental, patient-centeredness care, so that women then feel more comfortable to honestly share their experiences.

Mayfield and colleagues (2021), in an effort to increase psychiatric nurses' awareness of the multiple adversities female veterans face, described the various factors that place female veterans at risk for PTSD, **traumatic brain injury (TBI)**, depressive symptoms, and substance use disorder. The researchers identified multiple traumas that contribute to suicide ideation in female veterans: (a) Women veterans experience higher rates of adverse childhood experiences (ACE), (2) 38% of women report MST, and (3) 33% of women experience intimate partner violence (IPV). These authors encourage the engagement of female veterans as a protective factor in VA clinics, where they are less likely to die by suicide. The authors advocate trauma-informed care (TIC) as a safeguard practiced in the VA settings.

Trauma-Informed Care

Because both male and female military personnel experience multiple traumas, especially during deployments, both groups require and deserve care by health professionals that is trauma informed. Mayfield and colleagues (2021) advocated the use of TIC in responding to female veterans' mental health issues; however, TIC should be used by nurses in the care of any patient for whom trauma is suspected in their history. Using TIC as an approach to care acknowledges the role trauma plays in people's lives and incorporates the four Rs: *realization* of how trauma affects people and families, *recognition* of the signs of trauma, *responds* by applying principles of a trauma-informed approach when giving care, and seeks to *resist retraumatization* of a person by not forcing an individual to re-live or re-encounter previous traumatic experiences. In reviewing the concept of trauma, the Substance Abuse and Mental Health Services Administration's (SAMHSA's) model refers to the three Es: *event, experience,* and *effect.* The model also identifies six key principles: (a) safety; (b) transparency or trustworthiness; (c) peer support; (d) collaboration and mutuality; (e) empowerment, voice, and choice; and (f) cultural, historical, and gender issues.

Principles of a trauma-informed approach include the health professionals' understanding of traumatic stress and how it may impact one's behavior in responding to, or adapting to, that stress. TIC also includes providing patients with a safe, comfortable environment where the patient's dignity, autonomy, and respect is maintained and hope in the possibility of recovery is encouraged through the establishment of an open and trusting relationship between the caregiver and the patient.

Challenges to Reacculturation

Reasons given for the difficult transition back to civilian life included financial, emotional, and professional challenges veterans faced during the transition. These individuals had trouble paying their bills (35%), received unemployment compensation (28%), struggled with alcohol or substance abuse (20%), and had trouble getting medical care for themself or their family (16%; Igielnik, 2019). According to this study, the majority of veterans believe their military service was useful in giving them skills and training that prepared them for a civilian job. This statement was particularly true for commissioned officers (78%) as compared to enlisted service personnel. Despite these positive assertions, the physical and mental health challenges that confront veterans are well documented. For example, in 2021, in the United States about 1.9 million veterans had service-connected disabilities. On the other hand, 11.9 million were without service-related disabilities (Erickson et al., 2024; Vespa, 2020). A study by McCaslin and colleagues (2021) explored veterans' readjustment to civilian life. It found that participants most frequently mentioned mental health concerns across groups affecting their psychologic well-being. These concerns included PTSD (59%), anger (59%), grief (47%), substance use (35%), aggression (29%), and fear (18%). Women in this study reported greater negative experiences of their military service, with some sharing stories of gender and racial discrimination. The authors note that the self-reported negative impact of military service was negatively related to postdeployment support. In previous studies, "social support from military friends and civilian friends and family positively impacts participants' experience of their transition" home and has been predictive of recovery, functioning, and quality of life (McCaslin et al., 2021, 617). Joseph et al. (2022) discussed a need to better understand issues of identity and sense of belonging impacting veterans and encouraged clinicians to focus on the reacculturation process to support them.

Seidenfeld and colleagues (2023) sought to understand how patients experienced nursing care transition interventions (CTI) for clinical and extra medical assistance, as well as how these interventions improve patient outcomes after an ED visit and reduce the need for frequent veteran ED visits. Researchers interviewed 24 participants, 58% male, 50% Black or African American. The authors identified six themes, including experiences during the intervention and elements the patients valued. The participants reported clinical health coaching recommendations covering multiple topics and care coordination activities like appointment scheduling as important. Aspects of transition interventions valued by the participants included interpersonal support, effective communication, connection, and empathy from the interventionalist.

WAR PARTICIPATION AND ITS IMPACT ON VETERANS' HEALTH

Veterans as a group, irrespective of the war in which they may have participated, share several commonalities that distinguish them from their nonveteran counterparts. Those who have been exposed to war at the front lines have encountered experiences unlike any most civilians can fully appreciate, suffering TBIs, PTSD, **loss of limbs**, depressive disorders, anxiety migraines, musculoskeletal injuries, visual and auditory losses, other disabilities, and **suicide** (Ashley & Julaka, 2021).

In addition, individuals serving in the military face the risk of accidental or explosive injury, polytrauma, disability, and psychologic trauma even during noncombat assignments. The VA defined *polytrauma* as two or more injuries occurring in the same incident; affecting multiple body parts or organ systems; and resulting in physical, cognitive, psychologic, or psychosocial impairments and functional disabilities. In addition, according to the VA (2016, 2017), during the Gulf Wars, veterans have been exposed to a variety of environmental and infectious diseases and suffer **medically unexplained illnesses. Chronic fatigue syndrome**, fibromyalgia, functional gastrointestinal (GI) disorders, and undiagnosed illnesses are among this group of unexplained illnesses.

Suicide

Despite the fact that in 2010 the American Psychiatric Association developed guidelines to guide the care of patients demonstrating suicide behaviors (Jacobs et al., 2010), the Association of Behavioral and Cognitive Therapies (ABCT, 2023) reported that suicide among military personnel has been steadily increasing over the last 10 years and death rates by suicide have exceeded those from combat. The increasing prevalence of suicide and suicide attempts is the most serious problem faced by military personnel and veterans. According to the National Veterans Annual Suicide Prevention Report, 399 fewer veterans died by suicide that year; however, there were still 6,261 veterans that died by suicide. The DoD's Report on Suicide in 2021 reported 519 deaths with young, enlisted service personnel at highest risk. In that same year, dependents (202), including 139 spouses, also died by suicide.

Weisenhorn and colleagues (2017) linked high-impact suicide exposure to "psychological health complications, insomnia, **hypervigilance**, and dissociative episodes" with persistent symptoms resulting in PTSD (p. 161). These events pose a devastating problem not just for the victims' immediate family and friends, but for other servicemen and women who are exposed to or hear of the loss of their fellow members of the military, whether in active duty or not.

To address this serious problem, the federal government, through the VA, publishes an Annual Report on Suicide Prevention in which it outlines the annual rates of suicide, comparing both U.S. civilian and military rates, the lethal means used, and suicide prevention next steps. In addition, the American Psychological Association (APA) also publishes its newest research in suicide prevention. As one researcher noted, a key challenge will be making sure people who face barriers to accessing healthcare because of systemic racism or poverty benefit from new innovations. Another researcher, Gregory Simon of the Group Health Research Institute in Seattle, observed that amongthe people who endorsed suicidal ideation on the Patient Health Questionnaire Depression Scale, fewer than 10% engaged in suicidal behavior the next year. On the other hand, half of those who attempt to die by suicide deny ideation beforehand. These behaviors make assessing the risk of suicide difficult. The APA Prevention report also reminds us that suicidal ideation ebbs and flows, so it's hard to determine who is at highest risk and when, since levels of depression may wax and wane.

Wittink and colleagues (2020) conducted eight interviews and focus groups with primary care physicians (PCPs), behavioral health providers (BHPs), and nurses located in six different regions within one VHA's catchment area in the Northeast to determine team members' perceptions of their individual responsibilities and teamwork processes with respect to suicide prevention of veterans. There was consensus across all participants that primary care is a critical venue for suicide prevention. Each group member agreed that a team-based effort utilizing PCPs, nurses, and BHPs leads to shared responsibility. An important theme that emerged from the data was that clinicians have acquired or assumed specified roles. Nurses were recognized as playing a particularly important role in recognizing changes in patients' lives that place them at risk for suicide. BHPs were felt to play a role in further assessing suicide risk and communicating effectively with patients. There was relatively less delineation of the expertise or specific role of PCPs in suicide prevention except as a conduit to the BHPs.

To better understand and prevent suicide, Wolfe-Clark and Bryan (2017) discussed theoretical models that help explain why individuals die in the military by suicide. The authors also identified numerous personal, social, and environmental factors that correlate with suicidal thoughts and behaviors. These factors include family or romantic conflict, legal or disciplinary problems, chronic pain, and MST. Exposure to combat is the military-specific cause most associated with an increased risk of suicidal thoughts. There is a sense that "social isolation has been identified as the strongest predictor of suicidal ideation and attempts" (Wolfe-Clark & Bryan, 2017, p. 480). Another high-risk group consists of patients with serious mental illness, especially those illnesses that interfere with the ability to make sound decisions. Military training and familiarity with firearms also add to a person's capability of inflicting self-harm. Broken relationships, perceiving oneself as being a burden, feeling unloved by others, and social isolation all affect one's self-esteem and may also place someone at higher risk for suicide. Current research is focused on determining who is most at risk and developing appropriate screening tools to assess risk; using wearable devices to measure deviations from physiologic baselines that may indicate higher risk; reassessing current interventions to identify the most crucial elements; and looking for patterns in patients' behavior, not single points in time, since suicidal ideation waxes and wanes. Prevention of suicide and the management of suicide crisis in the military focus on identifying those at risk and assisting them in developing a realistic and effective safety plan to help both the patients and those who are charged with caring for them. Patients contemplating suicide are likely to be among those who are seriously depressed or who have some other mental distress that prohibits them from being able to think clearly during decision-making. Having a written, well-detailed safety plan readily available to them helps minimize the stress of problem-solving. A well-constructed plan will include written strategies for managing feelings of hopelessness and contacting healthcare or other support persons who are available to assist them like the veteran crisis line (veteranscrisisline.net).

The VA has mandated the development and review of a safety plan for every patient at risk for suicide at every VA facility. It is important to note here that patients who are hospitalized in psychiatric facilities following unsuccessful attempts at suicide have been found to be at highest risk immediately after discharge. For this reason, suicide surveillance that includes frequent contact with medical personnel and/or support persons during the initial period following hospitalization is indicated.

To determine what else might be done to engage and treat patients at high risk of suicide, Amato and colleagues (2016) and Beard (2023) explored spirituality and religion as a factor often neglected in suicide prevention. These researchers observed that many empirical studies suggested that certain religious and/or spiritual beliefs, practices, or affiliations may be protective against suicide. The writers argue that several elements of the VA's suicide prevention programs might be strengthened by integrating discussions about religion and spirituality. Further, the researchers propose exploring the role religion and/or spirituality plays during the risk assessment, safety planning, and evidence-based treatment phases of the suicide prevention program. An exploration of patients' spiritual concerns is congruent with principles of patient-centered and culturally competent care.

Whether nurses are caring for veterans in VA facilities or private community hospitals, all nurses are encouraged to keep in mind that during deployment, military personnel are exposed to many physical and psychologic traumas that make veterans more vulnerable to numerous physical and emotional illnesses. Among the most severe, anxiety, serious depression, and PTSD place servicemen and servicewomen and veterans at high risk for suicide. Healthcare literature offers numerous articles about suicide prevention. Hester (2017) discussed the lack of access to mental healthcare as a contributing factor to suicide among servicemen. The American Psychiatric Association has developed criteria for clinicians working with patients at risk for suicide (see Important Websites at the end of this chapter). The VA has also developed a template for safety planning for suicide prevention. Armed with this knowledge and a willingness to integrate patients' religious and/or spiritual considerations into their care planning, all nurses can provide culturally competent, trauma-informed care to veterans. This care is based on veterans' unique cultural needs as former members of the armed forces and offers them the high quality they so deserve.

OTHER HEALTH ISSUES

Loss of Limbs

According to the U.S. Army's Office of Medical History (AMEDD Center of History and Heritage, n.d.), at the end of World War II there was an estimated 1,700 major amputations among veterans compared to 80,000 among civilians who lost one or more limbs during the same period. The Global War on Terror has caused military personnel to sustain more devastating injuries than in past wars. These injuries are referred to as polytrauma or blast injuries. Loss of limbs or musculoskeletal injury are a frequent consequence of exposure to mortar attacks, explosive land mines, suicide bombings, **improvised explosive devices (IEDs)**, or other explosives. Due to advances in medical science, many more of these victims survive, but they suffer visible and invisible disabling injuries for the remainder of their lives. Survivors of these injuries may experience loss of two or more extremities, sometimes accompanied by burns and other soft-tissue injuries as well as damage to major organs. These types of physical injuries result in concomitant psychologic trauma due to changes in body image and the natural grief that accompanies loss of a body part or its function. Veterans who return home with missing body parts must make an adjustment not only to the limitations on their ability to perform activities of daily living (ADL), but to the loss or change in their employment status because of those limitations. These changes in life skills require major adjustments and support by the healthcare personnel who provide care to them. Frequently, the psychologic burden of these injuries often results in alcohol and drug dependence, loss of employment, homelessness, depression, and PTSD. Practitioners must be skilled in providing care that is culturally competent and sensitive to the specific needs of the individual.

TRAUMATIC BRAIN INJURY

More than 450,000 service members were diagnosed with a TBI in the period from 2000 to 2021 (Centers for Disease Control and Prevention [CDC], n.d.). TBI has been described as "a traumatically induced structural injury and/or physiological disruption of brain function as a result of an external force." (O'Neil et al., 2013) Causes of TBIs include blunt injuries, penetrating injuries, acceleration or deceleration injuries as occur in motor vehicle accidents, and explosive blast injuries (most reported). Military TBIs for both sexes are considered mild TBIs (mTBIs, or concussions). This mild type often follows exposure to repeated blasts, causing symptoms that last longer than they do from other causes. The victim may experience confusion or disorientation that lasts less than 24 hours. There may also be concomitant problems that are more easily diagnosed). Identified symptoms of mTBI include headaches, ringing in the ears, difficulty sleeping, irritability, memory losses, mood and anxiety disorders, suicidally, chronic pain, and dizziness or balance problems. Because many of these symptoms mimic other diseases, diagnosis is difficult. Therefore, symptoms could persist long after deployment without diagnosis. The federal government provides a screening tool for nurses and other healthcare personnel, called the brain injury screening tool, to assess military persons postdeployment for symptoms of mTBI. In addition, through its Operation We Are Here, the military provides resources for military veterans to address TBI (www.operationwearehere.com/TBI.html).

POSTTRAUMATIC STRESS DISORDER

PTSD is described as a mental health disorder that is a direct result of exposure to a traumatic event, such as suicide exposure. For many veterans, the memories of their war experiences or other unpleasant encounters during military service are painful and ever-present. For that reason, many seek refuge in the form of antianxiety medication provided by physicians or alternative ways of coping. Sometimes, these alternatives lead veterans to the abuse of legal or illegal substances. These choices are often made in a desperate effort to eliminate horrific images or "flashbacks" that emerge from their psyche and that are often tied to events they witnessed during combat. Friends who may have been killed or seriously injured in front of their eyes become the source of nightmares that keep them from sleeping soundly at night or focusing during the day. Effectively addressing these phenomena requires the assistance of a skillful mental health practitioner. In addition, Lang and colleagues (2016), in a retrospective study of 144 veterans who completed a second-level screening in the polytrauma clinic, found that PTSD and pain severity influenced increased use of healthcare services. They also discovered that 72% of the veterans reported significant PTSD and 87% reported pain symptoms. However, only 45% received adequate mental health treatment. A nurse conducting a veteran's health history can be observant for indications that a referral to a mental health physician for the assessment of PTSD is warranted. Nurses caring for patients with PTSD can maintain a quiet atmosphere, without sudden or harsh noises that might trigger flashbacks or feelings of anxiety. Depression and suicide ideation are among the most serious of the posttraumatic symptoms that veterans experience. These researchers concluded that veterans with high-impact exposure to suicide were twice as likely to experience depression and anxiety as those not exposed to suicide, and 10 times more likely to have PTSD. However, their findings also revealed that veterans who are married are less likely to be highly affected by another person's suicide. The researchers further noted that because return from deployment is a stressful time, continued support from family and friends is needed as a preventive measure to offset PTSD.

MILITARY SEXUAL TRAUMA

Another serious problem affecting both males and females in the military, although less frequently reported by males (10%), is sexual harassment and sexual assault. Considering the current "Me Too" movement, more individuals are being encouraged to report crimes of this nature. Although both women and men in the military experience MST, women are at higher risk of MST and its consequences. Often women are reluctant to disclose the occurrences, fearful of retaliation, especially if victimized by a superior authority in the military. Consequently, in these situations, anxiety, depression, and PTSD may result.

"According to the VA, any sexual activity in which one is involved against his or her will, including sexual harassment, rape, or other sexual assaults while in the military," constitutes sexual trauma (Ganzer, 2016, p. 35). In a more recent report according to Myers (2022), despite the DoD's 17-year efforts in response to their being ordered to set up its Sexual Assault Prevention and Response (SAPR), more "incidents, less reporting, and plummeting confidence in the system to get justice" seems to be the outcome (Myers, 2022). The DoD's 2021 annual report estimated that more than 8% of females and 1.5% of males experienced unwanted sexual contact in 2021, the highest rate since the department began counting in 2004. The estimates that are extrapolated from surveys show that women in the Marine Corps faced the most unwanted sexual incidences; 13.4% of women reported unwanted sexual advances, up from 10.7% in 2018. Men in the Navy were the most affected, with 2.1% of men reporting unwanted sexual adavnces, up from 1% in 2018. Overall, the department counted 7,260 sexual assault reports in 2021 out of an estimated 35,900 incidents for a 20% reporting rate, which marked a significant drop from 2018. Prosecutions are also down; however, the number of perpetrators given non-judicial or administrative punishment like involuntary separation are increasing. Based on this article, the department seems to be focusing its efforts on prevention of these crimes based on 80 recommendations of an independent commission that convened in 2021. Some of the recommendations focused on education and training. Despite these surprisingly large numbers, the military believes that these incidents are underreported. The failure of some men and women to report these crimes is largely due to their fear of retribution or because of offers of benefits in exchange for their silence. Military culture, deployment dynamics, fear of not being believed, stigma, and lack of consequences for perpetrators were identified as factors that contribute to MST underreporting. While much is being done, continued research and additional work still need to be done to combat these terrible crimes (Burns et al., 2014; Myers, 2022).

For many veterans, these experiences leave an indelible mark on their psyche that makes it difficult to resume life as usual when they return home from military duty. Unfortunately, many veterans return home to a society that is unaware of the obstacles they face in transitioning back to civilian life. The time that the individual spends in deployment, the nature of their military experience, and whether the person suffered physical and/or psychologic trauma during their deployment are all factors that influence veterans' ability to transition successfully to civilian life. Moreover, each of the wars in which the U.S. military fought had a different impact on the servicemen, since environmental conditions, length of the war experience, and the type of arms used in battle and other factors varied.

VETERANS IN WORLD WAR II

According to the National WWII Museum (n.d.), over 16 million Americans served in the military in World War II, from 1941 to 1945. At this writing, fewer than 122,000 veterans are still alive from that period, and they are said to be dying at a rate of 230 to 245 a day (National WWII Museum, n.d.). These veterans are in their 90s and older, yet some still remember the darkest moments of those experiences, especially the physical and psychologic trauma they suffered despite having survived the war and reaching home safely. As in all wars, during World War II combat-incurred injuries included TBIs and amputations, usually due to explosions of land mines. Injuries resulted in brain injuries, spontaneous amputations of limbs, soft-tissue damage to other body parts, partial avulsions, and/or vascular damage which, when required, led to physician-determined surgeries to amputate the damaged extremity. Besides the physical consequences of battle, servicemen also sustained invisible injuries that affected aspects of brain functioning.

Long before PTSD was identified as a psychologic consequence of battle trauma, World War II veterans talked of "night terrors, heavy drinking, survivor's guilt, depression, exaggerated startle response, and profound lingering sadness" (Madigan, 2015). These symptoms resulted from witnessing the disfigurement, dismemberment, and/or death of their fellow soldiers during battle. In addition, the anxiety that accompanied the ever-present fear of being injured or killed resulted in some soldiers requiring hospitalization for neuropsychiatric illnesses for 20% of soldiers who fought in World War II. For survivors, injuries from bullets and shrapnel were common, as was the emotional toll the war took on those fortunate enough to survive. Nevertheless, many came home with what was known as shell shock or combat fatigue, what is now called PTSD. An important documentary, *Let There Be Light* (1946), tells the story about therapies and medications, including the use of hypnosis, used to treat the veterans who suffered neuropsychiatric illnesses following this war. Most survivors of World War II went back home to lead productive lives, yet as many veterans of this war continue to age and lose loved ones, residual psychologic problems sometimes recur during their golden years.

VETERANS IN THE KOREAN WAR

During the period from 1950 to 1953, approximately 5.7 million members of the armed forces served in the Korean War. Of that number, 933,000 are alive today with ages ranging from 85 to 89. Veterans of this war were more likely to suffer disabilities related to exposure to a severely cold climate. Some veterans of this war may have also been exposed to ionizing radiation. Soldiers during the Korean War have been depicted in the film and the TV series *M*A*S*H*.

VETERANS IN THE VIETNAM WAR

Veterans of the Vietnam War, who served between 1964 and 1975, are said to be the largest living cohort of United States veterans (U.S. Census Bureau, 2020). The current average age of Vietnam veterans is roughly 71 (Stillwell, 2022). According to Tull (2021) in a study by Congress during the 1980s among Vietnam veterans, approximately 15% of men and 9% of women were found to have PTSD. Those with combat exposure were at a higher risk. In addition, approximately 30% of men and 27% of women had PTSD at some point in their lives following Vietnam. For many Vietnam veterans, the PTSD had become chronic, and for some it was a source of psychologic and social problems with a long-term impact. Many Vietnam veterans are still coping with conditions that go hand and hand with PTSD, including substance abuse, pain, depression, and heart disease, for which PTSD is considered a risk factor.

VETERANS IN THE GLOBAL WAR ON TERROR

The Global War on Terror includes the Gulf Wars in Iraq and Afghanistan. These wars have exposed members of the U.S. military to numerous toxic chemical and environmental hazards. These hazards include infectious diseases, exposures to sand and dust particulates, toxic-embedded fragments, paint, open-air burn pit debris, and combat noises from mortars and missiles (Britannica.com, 2017; VA, 2016). By service period, post-9/11 veterans were the youngest, with a median age of about 37 in 2018.

   The medical problems acquired by veterans during the wars in Iraq and Afghanistan are controversial. Unquestionably, men and women came away from these experiences with a variety of symptoms, collectively named Gulf War illness or syndrome (GWI; GWS). Some veterans associate these symptoms with exposures during their deployment. However, researchers disagree on the extent to which these exposures are directly responsible for the veterans' illnesses.

FACTORS INFLUENCING VETERANS' REINTEGRATION

Veterans are a unique cultural group irrespective of their branch of service, because they share common attributes not always found among civilians. These attributes cross racial and ethnic lines and include characteristics such as loyalty, respect for authority, patriotism, and a willingness to sacrifice their own personal goals for their team members. Unfortunately, too often these courageous men and women return from their roles on the battlefield to a less-than-welcoming environment in society. For many veterans, recollection of their combat or noncombat experiences that may have been traumatic create anxiety, insomnia, and stress that interfere with their routine functioning back at home. For many veterans, it is difficult to discuss their postdeployment feelings and attitudes with civilians who have not shared similar experiences. Moreover, veterans also acquire many skills during their years of service that are not always transferable or applicable to civilian life. Consequently, though highly skilled in some areas, some may find it difficult to find gainful employment in areas where they have expertise. This mismatch between their previous job status in the military and their civilian job status can be a source of anxiety and frustration as they attempt to transition from military service to civilian life. Consequently, these obstacles become barriers to their transition that are difficult to overcome. High rates of postmilitary unemployment, homelessness, relationship problems, an inability to focus on seemingly mundane activities following the excitement of military life, and other issues challenge veterans' **social reintegration** back to civilian life. The postdeployment experience of women is equally complex. While women are still less likely to experience physical injury and disabilities resulting from combat, they are more likely to experience sexual harassment and sexual discrimination and assault. They identify PTSD, major depression, migraines, and lower back pains as theire top four service-connected complaints. All these challenges give rise to depression and, for some, suicide ideation, and the need for mental health intervention. However, many of the numerous VA hospitals around the nation have come under criticism for not adequately addressing veterans' diverse healthcare needs. Many veterans who live far from VA hospitals seek healthcare elsewhere in their communities. Therefore, veterans encounter many nurses who may not be as aware of their specific needs as nurses in military facilities. Consequently, besides the stressful, sometimes life-threatening, experiences veterans may have already endured during deployment, they also find themselves having to battle obstacles to their successful transition back at home without always having effective means of managing these problems. Since veterans seek healthcare services at both VA and nonveteran healthcare facilities, nurses throughout the country have an opportunity to assist them in overcoming obstacles to their transition and to make a positive difference in the attainment of their healthcare goals.

Ashley and colleagues (2021), Davis and colleagues (2023), and Cohen et al., (2018) offered strategies to assist nurses in addressing veterans' healthcare goals. Because veterans are exposed to physical and mental trauma during their military service, they have a higher risk of mental health issues, physical comorbidities, higher rates of unemployment, and increased risk for homelessness and food insecurity. Consequently, the COVID-19 pandemic added an additional strain, worsening these problems (Ashley et al., 2021) These researchers recommend that clinicians screen all adult patients for veteran status. Once established, health professionals should explore the patient's service history and specific health needs. Screening for PTSD, depression, anxiety, and suicidal ideation is also important. The authors warn that because veterans often have access to firearms, they may be at a higher risk for suicide. One key strategy in working with veterans is maintaining patience and a judgment-free setting allowing for open and honest communication where the patient is enabled to express their true feelings (Ashley et al., 2021).

Davis and colleagues (2023) described the formation of a workgroup of VA local recovery coordinators who are mental health clinicians that facilitate systemwide recovery-oriented care within VA medical systems. The goal of the group was to expand critical thought around why antiracism is essential to fully realize mental health recovery. The leaders of this effort were guided by their view of substance abuse and mental health through an antiracist lens. The researchers advocated applying recovery principles to areas affected by racial bias, considering culture without overpathologizing cultural experiences, addressing trauma, acknowledging the impact of racial trauma as a barrier to recovery, and ensuring our mental health systems offer accessible and varied opportunities for healing. The group also identified best practices for incorporating micro and

macro antiracism efforts that address race-based stress and trauma and conduct culturally sensitive outreach through partnerships with communities of color, as well as by
broadening existing diversity, equity, and inclusion (DEI) training. The authors encourage
the education of our workforce at all levels to encourage introspection. They expressed
a desire that these efforts serve as a call to action to place an antiracist lens at recovery
service transformation.

Using Watson's theory of caring, Cohen et al. (2018) sought to understand what is
important to veterans to improve their care. They specifically wanted to learn what caring
meant to veterans. Jean Watson's carative factors provided the framework for this study.
The authors stressed the importance of knowing how veterans experience their care. The
research team interviewed 20 veterans from a variety of service branches: Army (7), Air
Force (2), Navy (5), Coast Guard (1), and Reserves (2). The men ranged in age from 33 to
83 with a mean age of 61. Service included the Korean Conflict, Vietnam Era, Persian Gulf
War, and Operation Iraqi Freedom. The men served between 1950 and 2010 and their tours
of duty lasted from 60 days to 27 years. The veterans had multiple diagnoses, but all discussed anxiety and depression.

The analysis revealed that caring was important to the participants and identified three
themes and subthemes: (a) communicating, which included teaching, explaining, and listening; (b) following up, which included partnering or collaborating; and (c) using specialized knowledge.

The veteran participants interpreted staff members' behaviors in the context of caring.
They provided examples of health professionals' behaviors that exemplified caring behaviors; for example, communicating effectively during follow up to ensure that patients got
what was needed. They also considered behaviors such as calling patients by name, being
professional, being kind, listening, paying attention, explaining in a way that patients
can understand, explaining symptoms, asking if the patient had any questions, expressing concern, giving a patient contact information, making a follow-up call to the patient's
home to ask if the patient was doing alright, and using specialized knowledge; these were
all identified as evidence of caring. "Veterans have disproportionately high rates of mental
illness" (Cohen et al., 2018, p. 165), and many have PTSD, so caring is important to each
of them. All of these strategies offer nurses an opportunity to incorporate best practices
when providing care to veterans and to ensure that the care veterans receive is culturally
competent, trauma-informed, and evidence-based.

IMPORTANT POINTS

- The largest cohort of veterans living today are those who served in the military in Vietnam.
- Veterans share a common culture and identity based on their military experiences including loyalty to the group.
- In 2021, women accounted for 17.3% of active-duty individuals serving in the military.
- Since 2016, all occupations and positions in the military are open to women.
- The race or ethnicity of veterans is linked to age; most older veterans are White, whereas younger veterans are people of color.
- As the U.S. population becomes more racially and ethnically diverse, so does the military.
- According to the U.S. Census, most veterans were born in one of the 50 states.
- The top five states of residence for veterans are Texas, Florida, California, Pennsylvania, and Virginia.
- Citizenship is not a requirement to join the military, and LPRs may and do enlist.

(continued)

IMPORTANT POINTS

(continued)

- Thirteen percent of veterans were born outside of the United States.
- Major problems encountered by servicemen and servicewomen during deployment include polytraumas, TBI, PTSD, sexual trauma, and suicide.
- The numerous physical and psychologic traumas experienced by servicemen and servicewomen during deployment make reintegration back to civilian life challenging.
- Difficulties of veterans during reintegration include feelings of alienation, isolation, and difficulty resuming gender roles.
- Veterans are more likely to experience homelessness than civilians.
- Research shows that veteran women were two to four times more likely than nonveteran women to be homeless. In funding year 2022, 199,000 women veterans were served by VA homeless programs.
- Causes of veterans' homelessness after discharge from the military include MST, PTSD, physical disabilities, and substance abuse.
- Failure by individuals to report unwanted sexual contact is an aspect of military culture due to fear of reprisals, fear of being blamed or not believed, stigma, and lack of consequences for perpetrators.
- Since the Global War on Terror began, the prevalence of suicide among veterans has dramatically increased and surpassed the rate of suicide among civilians.
- Suicide is the leading cause of death in the military, surpassing the rate of death in combat.
- Having feelings of social isolation is the strongest predictor of suicide attempt.
- Persons contemplating suicide are more likely to also be experiencing symptoms of depression and PTSD.

CASE SCENARIO 1

R.J. is a 67-year-old retired veteran who last served in the U.S. Army in Vietnam. During his deployment, R. J. participated in two field operations during which he witnessed several enemy troops being shot and killed. He had been in situations where he had been forced to shoot in his own defense. But the most painful of his war experiences had been witnessing a landmine explosion that severed his army buddy's right leg; R.J. narrowly missed stepping on the land mine himself. After that event, R.J. had continuous nightmares reliving that experience. After 2 years of deployment in Southeast Asia, R.J. was honorably discharged from the Army.

After coming home, R.J.'s nightmares persisted, and he was unable to sleep throughout the night. He sought employment in construction to use the skills he acquired while working with his dad before going to Vietnam. R.J. became frustrated waiting to be called to work. He began drinking heavily, frequently going to his favorite bar on a daily basis. Overeating, drinking, and socializing became his daily routine. R.J. began having severe headaches that were unbearable. A visit to the nearest VA hospital revealed that R.J. was hypertensive and had adult-onset diabetes mellitus. At that time, despite being encouraged to meet with the cardiologist, R.J.'s only concern was his insomnia and nightmares. His physician ordered a tranquilizer to help R.J. sleep and gave him a diuretic to begin treating his moderate hypertension. The physician also encouraged him to come back for follow-up care and advised him to seek counseling for his nightmares, but R.J. did not wish to discuss his nightmares with anyone.

R.J. decided to go to the local hospital near his home instead of the VA hospital, which was several miles away. He wanted to renew his prescription for tranquilizers, since that seemed to be helping his insomnia, and to get medicine for increasing back pain and headaches. The triage nurse in the ED assessed R.J. to be a 67-year-old, 6'3", 278 pounds, White male. The nurse thought R.J. had a rather flat affect; he often stared blankly when questioned. He was pleasant, but seldom smiled, spoke very little, and responded only to specific questions asked by the nurse. He admitted to drinking alcohol daily in large amounts, but also stated he needed the tranquilizers at night to sleep. R.J.'s blood pressure was 186/120, his heart rate was 110, and his respiratory rate was 28 BPM. R.J. was admitted to the medical–surgical unit in a hypertensive crisis.

CASE SCENARIO 2

K.T. is a 40-year-old married, female veteran who was deployed for 12 months in the U.S. Army hospital in Iraq during Operation Enduring Freedom. An RN with a BSN, K.T. is a captain in the Army who served as a nurse in a medical–surgical hospital caring for numerous U.S. and Iraqi soldiers and other Iraqi people impacted by the war. K.T. loved her job and enjoyed working with her fellow soldiers, but missed her husband and 7-year-old daughter, Ariel, who was being cared for by her dad and grandmother at home.

On completing her 12-month tour of duty, K.T. learned that she was finally being sent back to her home base in Philadelphia. One day before her official discharge from deployment, K.T. was assisting a fellow soldier who was transporting a patient by helicopter to another hospital. Suddenly, the squadron was hit by several blasts of mortar fire and many of her fellow soldiers were injured. K.T. was able to crawl to safety and sustained only a few lacerations of her left arm and minor scratches from the debris she encountered while taking cover on the ground. K.T. experienced a slight headache and some ringing in her ears from all the loud combat noise. After her arm was treated, K.T. was given medical clearance to leave for home on her scheduled day of departure.

On returning home, K.T. could not get the images of her last day in Iraq out of her mind. She was unable to sleep at night for more than 4 hours straight and her lingering headache seemed to be getting worse. She became increasingly irritable and depressed and worried about her readiness to resume her old job at the hospital. K.T.'s husband noticed that she had not been "herself" since coming home and encouraged her to seek counseling for her depression at the mental health clinic. Instead, K.T. decided to go to the local community hospital ED to investigate her lingering headache and to get a prescription for her insomnia.

The triage nurse in the ED performed a preliminary assessment and carefully took a nursing history. After hearing of K.T.'s experiences in Iraq, the nurse decided to use a brain injury screening tool to further investigate K.T.'s headaches. The physician ordered a CAT scan that revealed an mTBI. K.T. was admitted to the hospital for further evaluation. The nurse on the receiving unit was somewhat intimidated about caring for a female Army captain, who appeared sad and withdrawn. The nurse introduced herself to K.T., who expressed annoyance and frustration about being admitted. K.T. was certain she would not get any rest now that she was hospitalized.

WHAT NURSES NEED TO KNOW ABOUT THEMSELVES

Application of the Staircase Self-Assessment Model: Self-Reflection Questions

1. Where are you on the Cultural Competency Staircase in working with patients who are veterans? How much do you know about each of these patients' military experiences? How will you progress to the next level?
2. Which case would be the most challenging for you, and why?
3. What attitudes and feelings would you have toward each of these patients? On what are these attitudes based? How might these attitudes influence the care you would give to one of them versus the other?
4. What skills would be useful to nurses when caring for either of these patients?
5. What information or resources would you need to share with these patients to ensure the provision of culturally competent care?
6. During each patient–nurse encounter, what strategies would be useful when addressing specific needs of veterans?

Responses to Self-Reflection Questions

Response: Where are you on the Cultural Competency Staircase in working with patients who are veterans? How much do you know about each of these patients' military experiences? How will you progress to the next level?

In both of the scenarios, the nurse must first consider their comfort level caring for veterans, recognizing the need to have current knowledge of the specific challenges in caring for members of this population. The nurse determines their place on the staircase and advances by following suggestions under Strategies for Progression.

For example, at level 1, the nurse first explores the patient's chart and collects information from the patient, healthcare team, and/or family about recent or previous military experiences impacting the patient's health. Then, the inexperienced nurse would seek assistance or guidance from a more senior nurse or one who is more comfortable caring for veterans. These steps are taken in an effort to establish a positive working relationship between the patient and the nurse in which the patient is able to trust and accept the nurse in the various roles of teacher, advocate, and counselor.

Response: Which case would be the most challenging for you, and why?

The patients' military status, age, gender, and/or race or ethnicity may challenge some nurses, especially those who are inexperienced with diversity. For example, the nurse in Scenario 2 indicates feeling "intimidated" because of the patient's military status. Other nurses may be uncomfortable simply because the patient is also a nurse. Acknowledging these feelings is the first step in preventing them from getting in the way of delivering culturally competent care to the patient.

Having limited knowledge of the circumstances surrounding the patient's hospitalization or about factors contributing to the patient's state of health can also be a barrier to care. In most cases, the patient is the best source of information about their health status. Therefore, nurses must be able to establish a trusting relationship that affords the patient opportunities to share pertinent information in a timely manner. Nurses can overcome any anxiety they may have by focusing their attention on communicating respect for the patient and a sincere desire to learn as much as possible about the patient's perceptions of their clinical situation.

Response: What attitudes and feelings would you have toward each of these patients? On what are these attitudes based? How might these attitudes influence the care you would give to one of them versus the other?

Based on previous experiences with members of the military or other veterans, the nurse may harbor positive or negative biases or hold assumptions about the group based on those experiences. Any assumptions that do not take into account the patient's individuality can interfere with the development of a productive relationship between the patient and the nurse. The culturally competent nurse considers each patient unique with their own personal set of characteristics and clinical expectations.

Together the patient and the nurse work toward the establishment of mutually determined healthcare goals.

Response: What skills would be useful to nurses when caring for either of these patients?

When caring for patients with whom establishing a rapport is potentially challenging, it may be helpful for the nurse to first listen reflectively, making sure to clarify any potentially misunderstood information. Second, it may also be useful to have a communication model in mind or in hand that assists the nurse in communicating effectively. When the patient expresses feelings of anxiety, sadness, mistrust, and depression, the PEARLS communication model, used in medical practice to build relationships between the provider and the patient, may work well in engaging the patient and nurse in the interaction. The mnemonic PEARLS represents *partnership, empathy, acknowledgement, respect, legitimization,* and *support.*

An example of how this mnemonic might be used in Case Scenario 1 is as follows.

P. The nurse explains to R. J. that he wants to work in *partnership* with him in discovering ways to reduce his blood pressure, which if left unchecked is life threatening.
E. The nurse displays *empathy* by acknowledging that the patient appears sad and withdrawn at times, and asks if it would help to talk about it. If comfortable with doing so, the nurses states, "I appreciate how many challenges you've had to face through your work in the military."
A. The nurse commends the patient on taking steps to manage his health problem.
R. The nurse expresses *respect* by stating: "I've never been in the military, but I really admire those who have fought on our country's behalf."
L. The nurse *legitimizes* the patient's situation by saying, "In light of what you've shared with me about your situation, I would probably feel the same way."

Response: What information or resources would you need to share with these patients to ensure the provision of culturally competent care?

The VA provides a variety of services for veterans addressing issues of employment, vocation rehabilitation, homelessness, and the needs of women and minorities. Links to information on these services can be found in the Additional Resources section at the end of this chapter. The nurse in their role of counselor, educator, and advocate can inform the patient of these services or make appropriate referrals.

Response: During each patient–nurse encounter, what strategies would be useful when addressing specific needs of veterans?

The VA has developed a Military Health History Pocket Card available to clinicians for the purpose of obtaining an accurate military health history (VA: Office of Academic Affiliations, 2018). Its website can be found in the Additional Resources section at the end of this chapter. The questions direct the clinician in obtaining information about the nature, location, and type of the veteran's service activity whether or not the service resulted in injury or illness, such as physical or sexual trauma. Questions intended to further explore what the patient was exposed to during deployment, the patient's current living situation, and assistance needs are included in this assessment tool. Nurses can also use the PTSD Assessment Tool Kit by Hanrahan and colleagues (2017).

WHAT INFORMATION DOES THE NURSE NEED TO KNOW ABOUT THE PATIENT?

In addressing both of these scenarios and when caring for all adult patients, the nurse should begin by determining the patient's military status and the nature of those experiences when collecting preliminary data. This information can be sought during the nursing history or cultural assessment phase. After determining the patient's military status, it is critical to also screen for a history of exposures to toxic chemicals, physical traumatic injuries, a history of sexual trauma, depression, PTSD, and suicidal ideation. Having knowledge of the patient's living arrangements and employment status enables the nurse to identify any resources needed to assist the patient. In light of the contributions and sacrifices that servicemen and servicewomen make throughout their lives to ensure the well-being of our society, nurses are compelled to develop strategies that ensure the delivery of culturally competent care when they encounter veterans in their practice.

NCLEX®-TYPE QUESTIONS

1. A health assessment that takes into consideration major healthcare concerns that veterans experience should include screening for:
    A. Physical and sexual trauma, traumatic brain injury (TBI), depression, posttraumatic stress disorder (PTSD)
    B. Loss of hearing and/or vision, insomnia, amputations, paralysis
    C. Chemical or toxic exposures and infectious diseases
    D. Respiratory diseases, loss of limbs, TBI, heart disease
    E. Gunshot wounds, infections, sexually transmitted infections (STIs), toxic syndrome

2. Headaches, tinnitus, insomnia, and memory losses are symptoms that are usually associated with_____ in veterans.
    A. Sexual trauma
    B. posttraumatic stress disorder (PTSD)
    C. Traumatic brain injury (TBI)
    D. Cardiovascular accident (CVA)
    E. Transient ischemic attacks (TIA)

3. The nurse who suspects a patient is experiencing symptoms of posttraumatic stress disorder (PTSD) attempts to prevent an exacerbation by:
    A. Encouraging frequent visitors and patient activities as a distraction
    B. Minimizing stimuli by limiting harsh noises and maintaining a quiet environment
    C. Assisting the patient with activities of daily living (ADLs)
    D. Monitoring the patient carefully and reporting the behavior to a physician
    E. Providing analgesics to promote comfort and minimize pain

4. Failure to report sexual trauma in the military is largely due to:
    A. Fear of reprisals or promises of benefits for silence
    B. Military culture, like loyalty to the group
    C. Fear of not being believed
    D. Lack of consequences for the perpetrator
    E. All of the above

5. The most frequent causes of physical trauma or injury during deployment are:
   A. Explosions from land mines, improvised explosive devices (IEDs), or mortar fire
   B. Accidental injuries due to falls or equipment failure
   C. Motor vehicle accidents
   D. Helicopter crashes
   E. Burns and infections

6. Which statement is true about women and the military?
   A. Women account for about 2% of active-duty enlisted personnel.
   B. Women's roles in the military are limited to nurses, cooks, and secretaries.
   C. All roles, positions, and ranks are now open to women.
   D. Women have never been and are unlikely to be injured or killed in combat.

7. The majority of veterans alive today are those who served in:
   A. World War I
   B. World War II
   C. The Korean War
   D. The Vietnam War
   E. The Persian Gulf

8. Cultural competency skills needed when initially establishing or attempting to establish a rapport with veterans should include:
   A. Reflective listening and use of the PEARLS model
   B. Learning about the veteran's religious and/or spiritual background
   C. Determining the patient's views on time and space
   D. Considering the patient's cultural norms

9. Which of these constitute social barriers to reintegration or transition to civilian life after deployment or service in the military?
   A. Unemployment and homelessness
   B. Depression, alcoholism, and drug abuse
   C. Posttraumatic stress disorder (PTSD)
   D. Feelings of isolation and alienation
   E. All of the above

10. What nursing measures provide the *best* strategy for the nurse to obtain critical information from the patient when caring for veterans who are depressed or withdrawn?
    A. A physical assessment tool to determine injury or disease
    B. A communication tool for facilitating nurse–patient interaction
    C. A cultural assessment tool to explore race, ethnicity, religion, and culture
    D. A nursing health history
    E. Obtaining a partner to assist with care

11. Which of these factors represents the most military-specific cause of posttraumatic stress disorder (PTSD)?
    A. Military culture
    B. Exposure to combat
    C. Lower status and rank
    D. Sexual trauma

12. Servicemen and servicewomen who are contemplating suicide are less likely to reach out for help due to:
    A. Fear of being demoted or released from the military
    B. Stigma and military culture
    C. Upsetting family and friends
    D. Ambivalence about taking their life

13. Military personnel who are exposed to the suicide of friends and colleagues are 10 times more likely to also experience:
    A. Anxiety and depression
    B. Bipolar disease
    C. Behavioral problems
    D. Posttraumatc stress disorder (PTSD)

14. Which of these statements represents the strongest predictor of suicidal ideation?
    A. Pain and sexual trauma
    B. Romantic conflict
    C. Feelings of social isolation
    D. Employment dissatisfaction

15. According to the literature, which of the following represents a high-risk period for reattempts of suicide by persons who are hospitalized?
    A. One day after the initial attempt at suicide
    B. Three months after the initial attempt
    C. One year after hospitalization
    D. The period immediately following discharge

ANSWERS TO NCLEX-TYPE QUESTIONS

1. A	6. C	11. B
2. C	7. D	12. B
3. B	8. A	13. D
4. E	9. E	14. C
5. A	10. B	15. D

AMERICAN ASSOCIATION OF COLLEGES OF NURSING COMPETENCIES ADDRESSED IN THIS CHAPTER

1. Apply knowledge of social and cultural factors that affect nursing and healthcare across multiple contexts.
2. Use relevant data sources and best evidence in providing culturally competent care.
3. Promote achievement of safe and quality outcomes of care for diverse populations.
4. Advocate for social justice, including commitment to the health of vulnerable populations and the elimination of health disparities.
5. Participate in continuous cultural competence development.

SPRINGER PUBLISHING **CONNECT™** | A robust set of instructor resources designed to supplement this text is located at **http://connect.springerpub.com/content/book/978-0-8261-8302-6.** Qualifying instructors may request access by emailing **textbook@springerpub.com.**

REFERENCES

Association of Behavioral and Cognitive Therapies. (2023). *Fact sheet: Military suicide.* https://www.abct.org/fact-sheets/military-suicide/

Aker, J. A. (2021, May 11). *Military nursing highlighted during National Nurses' Week.* https://health.mil/News/Articles/2021/05/11/Military-nursing-highlighted-during-National-Nurses-Week

Amato, J. J., Kayman, D. J., Lombardo, M., & Goldstein, M. F. (2016). Spirituality and religion: Neglected factors in preventing veteran suicide. *Pastoral Psychology, 66,* 191–199. https://doi.org/10.1007/s11089-016-0747-8

AMEDD Center of History and Heritage. (n.d.). *History.* https://achh.army.mil/history/history

American Nurses Association. (n.d.). Male nurse: Why men should consider a career in nursing. Retrieved October 22, 2023, from https://www.nursingworld.org/practice-policy/workforce/male-nursing-careers

Ashley, M., Julaka, S., & Woodward L. (2021). *Nurses in action: Insights into providing care to veterans.* American Psychiatric Nurses' Association. https://www.apna.org/news/providing-mental-health-care-for-veterans/

Barroso, A. (2019). *The changing profile of the U.S. military: Smaller in size, more diverse, more women in leadership.* Pew Research Center. https://www.pewresearch.org/short-reads/2019/09/10/the-changing-profile-of-the-u-s-military

Beard, B. (2023, April 6). Religious identity may impact suicide risk. *Psychology Today*. https://www.psychology-today.com/us/blog/from-lab-to-real-world/202304/religious-identity-may-impact-suicide-risk

Britanica.com. (2017). *Iraq war: 2003–2011*. https://www.britannica.com/event/Iraq-War

Buchholz, K. (2023, November 10). *U.S. fighters from abroad*. Statista. https://www.statista.com/chart/19920/us-veterans-from-another-country/

Burns, B., Grindlay, K., Holt, K., Manski, R., & Grossman, D. (2014). Military sexual trauma among U.S. service-women during deployment: a qualitative study. *American journal of public health, 104*(2), 345–349. https://doi.org/10.2105/AJPH.2013.301576

Centers for Disease Control and Prevention. (n.d.). *Health disparities and TBI*. Retrieved October 22, 2023, from https://www.cdc.gov/traumaticbraininjury/health-disparities-tbi.html

Central Intelligence Agency. (2017). *World fact book*. https://www.cia.gov/the-world-factbook/about/cover-gallery/2017-cover

Cohen, M. Z., Struwe, L., Fletcher, B. S., Kingston, E., Bockman, T., Shimerdla, D., Harrington, R., Robino-West, S., & Ganti, A. K. (2018). The meaning of care for veterans. *International Journal for Human Caring, 22*(4), 159–168. https://doi-org.ezproxy.sju.edu/10.20467/1091-5710.22.4.159

Data USA. (n.d.). (2021). *U.S. coast guard*. https://datausa.io/profile/naics/u-s-coast-guard

Davis, A. G., Davis, B., Williams, Z., Viverito, K., Schwartz, S., Ramos, K., Moreno, J., Jackson, S., Smith, P. A., Gay, J., Aysta, S., & Shiber, N. A. (2023). Antiracism and mental health recovery: Bridging the gap to improve health disparities among veteran populations. *Psychiatric Rehabilitation Journal, 46*(1), 53–54. https://doi.org/10.1037/prj0000535

Defense Finance and Accounting Services. (n.d.). *Military pay charts—1949–2021*. https://www.dfas.mil/MilitaryMembers/payentitlements/Pay-Tables/PayTableArchives

Dyar, K. L. (2019). Nursing care considerations for women veterans. *Med-Surg Matters, 28*(6), 8–10. https://search-ebscohost-com.ezproxy.sju.edu/login.aspx?direct=true&db=ccm&AN=141211814&site=ehost-live

Erickson, W., Lee, C., von Schrader, S. (2024). *2022 disability status report: United States*. /https://www.disability-statistics.org/report/pdf/2022/2000000

Finnegan, A. P., Di Lemma, L., Moorhouse, I., Lambe, R. E., Soutter, E. M., Templeman, J., Ridgway, V., Hynes, C., Simpson, R., & McGhee, S. (2020). Educating nurses to deliver optimum care to military veterans and their families. *Nurse Education in Practice, 42*, 102654. https://doi.org/10.1016/j.nepr.2019.102654

Ganzer C. A. (2016). CE: Veteran women: Mental health-related consequences of military service. *The American Journal of Nursing, 116*(11), 32–39. https://doi.org/10.1097/01.NAJ.0000505583.09590.d4

Hanrahan, N. P., Judge, K., Olamijulo, G., Seng, L., Lee, M., Herbig Wall, P., Leake, S. C., Czekanski, E., Thorne-Odem, S., DeMartinis, E. E., Kelly, U. A., Blair, L., & Longmire. W. (2017). The PTSD toolkit for nurses: Assessment, intervention, and referral of veterans. *The Nurse Practitioner,. 42*(3), 46–55. https://doi.org/10.1097/01.NPR.0000488717.90314.62

Hester, R. D. (2017). Lack of access to mental health services contributing to the high suicide rates among veterans. *International Journal of Mental Health Systems, 11*, 47–50. https://doi.org/10.1186/s13033-017-0154-2

Igielnik, R. (2019, November 7). *Key findings about America's military veterans*. Pew Research Cennter. https://www.pewresearch.org/short-reads/2019/11/07/key-findings-about-americas-military-veterans

In the News. (2013, March). *Women's roles expand in the U.S. military*. https://hmhinthenews.com/womens-expanding-roles-in-the-u-s-military-2

Jacobs, D. G., Baldessarini, R. J., Conwell, Y., Fawcett, J. A., Horton, L., Meltzer, H., Pfeffer, C. R., & Simon, R. I. (2010). *Practice guidelines for the assessment and treatment of patients with suicide behaviors*. American Psychiatric Association. https://psychiatryonline.org/pb/assets/raw/sitewide/practice_guidelines/guidelines/suicide.pdf

Joseph, J. S., Smith-Macdonald, L., Felice, M. C., & Smith, M. (2022). Reculturation: A new perspective on military-civilian transition stress. *Military Psychology, 35*(3), 193–203. https://doi.org/10.1080/08995605.2022.2094175

Lang, K. P., Veazey-Morris, K., Berlin, K. S., & Andrasik, F. (2016). Factors affecting health care utilization in OEF/OIF veterans: The impact of PTSD and pain. *Military Medicine, 181*(1), 50–55. https://doi.org/10.7205/MILMED-D-14-00444

Madigan, T. (2015). Opinion: Their war ended 70 years ago. Their trauma didn't. *The Washington Post*. https://www.washingtonpost.com/opinions/the-greatest-generations-forgotten-trauma/2015/09/11/8978d3b0-46b0-11e5-8ab4-c73967a143d3_story.html

Makaroun, L. K., Halaszynski, J. J., Rosen, T., Haggerty, K. L., Blatnik, J. K., Froberg, R., Elman, A., Geary, C. A., Hagy, D. M., Rodriguez, C., & McQuown, C. M. (2023). Leveraging VA geriatric emergency department accreditation to improve elder abuse detection in older veterans using a standardized tool. *Academic Emergency Medicine, 30*(4), 428–436. https://doi.org/10.1111/acem.14646

Mayfield, B. L., Shaw, R. M., Holland, A., McGuinness, T. M., McCrear, M. D., Patterson, S. G., & Richardson, J. W. (2021). A call to action for women veterans' mental health. *Journal of Psychosocial Nursing & Mental Health Services, 59*(2), 2–4. https://doi.org/10.3928/02793695-20210114-01

McCaslin, S. E., Becket-Davenport, C., Dinh, J. V., Lasher, B., Kim, M., Choucroun, G., & Herbst, E. (2021). Military acculturation and readjustment to the civilian context. *Psychological Trauma: Theory, Research, Practice and Policy, 13*(6), 611–620. https://doi.org/10.1037/tra0000999

Myers, M. (2022). The military's sexual assault problem is only getting worse. *Military Times*. https://www.militarytimes.com/news/your-military/2022/09/01/the-militarys-sexual-assault-problem-is-only-getting-worse/#:~:text=More%20incidents%2C%20less%20reporting%2C%20plummeting,and%20response%20report%2C%20released%20Thursday

National WWII Museum. (n.d.). *WWII veteran statistics*. https://www.nationalww2museum.org/war/wwii-veteran-statistics

O'Neil, M.E., Carlson, K., Storzbach, D., Brenner, L. A., Freeman, M., Quiñones, A., Motu'apuaka, M., Ensley, M., & Kansagara, D. (Eds.). (2013). Definition of MTBI from the VA/DOD clinical practice guideline for management of concussion/mild traumatic brain injury (2009). In *Complications of mild traumatic brain injury in veterans and military personnel: A systematic review*. Department of Veterans Affairs. https://www.ncbi.nlm.nih.gov/books/NBK189784/

Operation We Are Here. (n.d.). *TBI resources for military veterans*. http://www.operationwearehere.com/TBI.html

Pappas, S. (2021, August 25). New research in suicide prevention. *American Psychological Association, 52*(6). https://www.apa.org/monitor/2021/09/news-suicide-prevention

Riordan, J. K., Alexander, S., & Montgomery, I. S. (2019). Use of technology to increase physical activity in female veterans and soldiers aged 19–64 years. *Journal of the American Association of Nurse Practitioners, 31*(10), 575–582. https://doi.org/10.1097/JXX.0000000000000277

Scannell-Desch, & Doherty, M. E. (2012). *Nurses in war: Voices from Iraq and Afghanistan*. Springer Publishing Company.

Schaeffer, K. (2021, April 5). *The changing face of America's veteran population*. Pew Research Center. https://www.pewresearch.org/short-reads/2021/04/05/the-changing-face-of-americas-veteran-population

Seidenfeld, J., Ramos, K., Bruening, R. A., Sperber, N. R., Stechuchak, K. M., & Hastings, S. N. (2023). Patient experiences of a care transition intervention for Veterans to reduce emergency department visits. *Academy of Emergency Medicine, 30*(4), 388–397. https://doi.org/10.1111/acem.14661

Statista. (2022). *Active and reserve United States military forces personnel in 2021 by service branch and reserve component*. https://www.statista.com/statistics/232330/us.-military-force-numbers-by-service-branch-and-reserve-component

Statista. (2023, June 2). *Number of veterans living in the United States in 2021, by state*. https://www.statista.com/statistics/250329/number-of-us-veterans-by-state

Stillwell, B. (2022). *4 important things to know about Vietnam Veterans*. https://www.military.com/history/4-important-things-know-about-vietnam-veterans.html

Tull, M. (2021). The long-term impact of PTSD on Vietnam veterans. *Verywell mind*. verywellmind.com/ptsd-from-the-vietnam-war-2797449?print

U.S. Census Bureau. (2020). *United States Census Bureau releases new report on veterans* (Press Release No. CB20-TPS.30). https://www.census.gov/newsroom/press-releases/2020/veterans-report.html

U.S. Census Bureau. (2023, October 19). *Veterans Day 2023: November 11* (Press Release No. CB23-FF.09). https://www.census.gov/newsroom/facts-for-features/2023/veterans-day.html

U.S. Department of Defense. (2022, December 14). *Press release: Department of Defense releases annual demographics report—Upward trend in number of women serving continues*. https://www.defense.gov/News/Releases/Release/Article/3246268/department-of-defense-releases-annual-demographics-report-upward-trend-in-numbe

U.S. Department of Veterans Affairs. (2016, October). *Fact sheet: Women veterans population*. http://www.va.gov/vetdata

U.S. Department of Veterans Affairs. (2022, December 9). *VA programs to end homelessness among women veterans*. https://www.va.gov/homeless/for_women_veterans.asp

U.S. Department of Veterans Affairs: Office of Academic Affiliations. (2018). *Military health history pocket card for clinicians*. Retrieved from https://www.gov/OAA/pocketcard

U.S. Department of Veterans Affairs: Public Health. (2017, May 16). *Gulf War veterans medically unexplained illnesses*. https://www.publichealth.va.gov/exposures/gulfwar/medically-unexplained-illness.asp

U.S. Government Accountability Office. (2015, July). *Military personnel: DOD is expanding combat service opportunities for women, but should monitor long-term integration progress*. https://www.gao.gov/assets/gao-15-589.pdf

Vespa, J. E. (2020). *Those who served: America's Veterans from World War II to the war on Terror*. https://www.census.gov/content/dam/Census/library/publications/2020/demo/acs-43.pdf

Weisenhorn, D. A., Frey, L. M., van de Venne, J., & Cerel, J. (2017). Suicide exposure and posttraumatic stress disorder: Is marriage a protective factor for veterans? *Journal of Child Family Studies, 26*(1), 161–167. https://doi.org/10.1007/s10826-016-0538-y

Wittink, M. N., Levandowski, B. A., Funderburk, J. S., Chelenza, M., Wood, J. R., & Pigeon, W. R. (2020). Team-based suicide prevention: lessons learned from early adopters of collaborative care. *Journal of Interprofessional Care, 34*(3), 400–406. https://doi.org/10.1080/13561820.2019.1697213

Wolfe-Clark, A.L., & Bryan, C.J. (2017) Integrating two models to understand and prevent military and veteran suicide. *Armed Forces and Society, 43*(3), 478–499. https://doi.org/10.1177/0095327x16646645

IMPORTANT WEBSITES

American Psychiatric Nurses Association (APNA). Retrieved from www.apna.org/
Brain Injury Screening Tool. Retrieved from www.brainline.org/article/tbi-screening-tool
Crisis Chat Line. Retrieved from veteranscrisisline.net
Military Health History Pocket Card. Retrieved from www.va.gov/OAA/pocketcard
Office of Mental Health and Suicide Prevention (2021) National Veterans Suicide Prevention: Annual Report. Retrieved from www.mentalhealth.va.gov/docs/data-sheets/2021/2021-National-Veteran-Suicide-Prevention-Annual-Report-FINAL-9-8-21.pdf
Operation We Are Here. Retrieved from www.operationwearehere.com/TBI.html
Trauma Resilience Initiative. Retrieved from www.traumaresilienceinc.org
U.S. National Suicide Prevention Lifeline. Retrieved from 800 273TALK 8255
Veterans Health Administration. Retrieved from www.va.gov/health
Veterans Suicide Prevention U.S. Department of Veterans Affairs—Suicide Prevention Crisis Line. Retrieved from www.va.gov/health-care/health-needs-conditions/mental-health/suicide-prevention/

Cultural Considerations When Caring for Children of Diverse Backgrounds

Catherine McGeehin Heilferty

There can be no keener revelation of a society's soul than the way in which it treats its children.

—NELSON MANDELA

LEARNING OBJECTIVES

After this chapter, the reader will be able to
1. Identify selected cultural practices related to the care of children at birth, during illness, and at death.
2. Assess the psychologic, sociocultural, spiritual, and/or religious factors influencing the healthcare experiences of children of culturally diverse groups.
3. Analyze the role of the nurse in advocating for culturally diverse children from birth to young adulthood.
4. Discuss cultural and developmental influences on a child's autonomy in medical decision-making.
5. Utilize creative and perceptive cultural assessment and advocacy strategies for children in various healthcare settings.
6. Describe the impact of attitudinal barriers impacting growth and development for children in high-risk settings.

KEY TERMS

Assent

Autonomy

Childhood

Consent

Vulnerability

NURSES' RESPONSIBILITY TO CHILDREN FROM DIVERSE BACKGROUNDS

We investigate cultural considerations in healthcare to discover and mitigate a person's **vulnerability** to maltreatment, inequity in access, and injury. Seen through this lens, children cared for by nurses from a different culture or background than their own are at considerable risk of bias in assessment, care, and follow-up. In this chapter, children are defined as dependents of at least one adult, age newborn to age 18, the legal age of emancipation in

FIGURE 14.1 ■ PERCENTAGE OF CHILDREN AGES 0 TO 17 IN THE UNITED STATES BY RACE AND HISPANIC ORIGIN, 1980 TO 2022 AND PROJECTED 2023 TO 2050

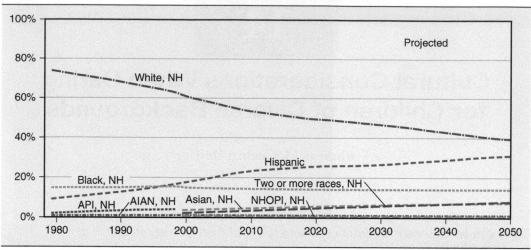

Note: AIAN = American Indian or Alaskan Native; API = Asian or Pacific Islander; NH = non-Hispanic origin; NHOPI = Native Hawaiian or Other Pacific Islander. Each group represents the non-Hispanic population, with the exception of the Hispanic category itself. Race data from 2000 onward are not directly comparable with data from earlier years. Data on race and Hispanic origin are collected separately. Persons of Hispanic origin may be of any race.
Source: Federal Interagency Forum on Child and Family Statistics. (2023). *America's children: Key national indicators of well-being, 2023.* U.S. Government Printing Office. https://www.childstats.gov/pdf/ac2023/ac_23.pdf

most states in the United States. Philosophers and moral theorists define *vulnerability* as susceptibility to harm. It is relational; that is, a person is vulnerable in relation to particular sorts of threats to one's interests. Some persons or groups are especially vulnerable due to a lack of or diminished capacity to protect themselves by virtue of inequalities of power, dependency, capacity, or need (Lulgjuraj & Maneval, 2021; Figure 14.1).

The complexity of the U.S. healthcare system, the differences in access to care from state to state, and issues of sociocultural inequity mean that some U.S. children are born with a disadvantage.

VULNERABILITY AND AUTONOMY

Parents' responsibility to protect and nurture children means that decision-making power within the family structure is inherently imbalanced. No single individual has greater influence on a child's development than the primary caretaker, most often a parent. A parent's responsibility to a child is protection from harm, provision of care and resources, and promotion of development. Parents in different cultures arrive at different conclusions regarding the best balance between teaching children to conform to external expectations and encouraging children to develop internal motivation. Failure to meet children's needs in this area deprives them of the ability to develop self-control and the ability to set and adhere to their own goals (Tiliouine et al., 2022). To that end, as nurses attempt to assess systems, provide care, and teach family members, nurses need to understand the parent–child relationship within the context of culture.

In addition, nurses taking care of children must be aware of the multiple layers of vulnerability that affect a child's well-being. Children are vulnerable due to their dependent relationships with those in authority. To a well child, this is likely a parent, other caregivers, teachers, and so on. When a child is sick, the layers of dependence, and consequently vulnerability, multiply. As a child, the inherent lack of agency, the physical challenge of illness or disability, and the separation from family members during hospitalization or foster care placement, for example, all demand greater attention to the child's vulnerability to emotional, physical, and developmental harm during illness. At every opportunity, nurses must assure a child's capacity for self-care and **assent** to treatment whenever possible.

Nurses should demonstrate proficiency in these efforts in three main care settings: (a) outpatient, which includes primary care, care in long-term care facilities, and care in the family home; (b) emergency and inpatient care; and (c) care in schools. To provide culturally competent care, it is incumbent upon nurses in each of these settings to consider parent beliefs about discipline, safety, nutrition, sleep, and education.

Nurses who care for children are responsible for acquiring and maintaining a sound knowledge base of cultural considerations. Continuing education, like the modules provided by the U.S. Department of Health and Human Services (n.d.) (DHHS), can help nurses maintain a basic level of competency in the ability to provide culturally competent care.

NURSES' RESPONSIBILITY TO CONSIDER CHILDREN IN THE HEALTHCARE SYSTEM AS UNIQUELY VULNERABLE

Decision-making in pediatric healthcare is complex. Children cared for in the healthcare system are uniquely vulnerable to harm because they lack sufficient agency and **autonomy**. Parents or other primary caregivers are looked to for **consent** for providers to treat illness and promote health. Identifying who can give consent should be the first step in any discussion about treatment options. Parents with very conservative backgrounds may consider children as without voice in medical decision-making. Children unaccustomed to being asked to participate in any kind of decision-making may hesitate to make their own healthcare choices.

In some cultures, assessing authority in family relationships can be quite complex. Responsibility for "parental consent" can be complicated by informal relationships of responsibility. Biological parents may have responsibility for some day-to-day supervision of the child, but an extended family membera grandmother, for example—may have legal medical decision-making responsibility. It is important for nurses to assess and respect the formal and informal roles that each family member plays in the health of the child. This can be particularly challenging in emergency situations. In the absence of a person with clear legal responsibility for decision-making on behalf of the child, nurses should consult with social workers and members of the institution's ethics committee.

At every opportunity, children in the healthcare system should be included in information sharing and decision-making to the developmental degree that they are able. In the seminal policy statement titled *Informed Consent in Decision-Making in Pediatric Practice*, the American Academy of Pediatrics (AAP's) Committee on Bioethics outlined the complexity of the issue, provided a framework for decision-making, and made recommendations for practitioners. The themes threaded through each of the nine recommendations are (a) the importance of inclusion of the child in decision-making to the highest ability possible; (b) limiting the harm and promoting the benefits of care in each interaction; and (c) that children, especially adolescents, living with a complex chronic disease should be considered to have advanced, personal, and experiential knowledge of their illness that informs their decision-making in unique ways (Katz et al., 2016).

WHAT PARENTS SAY THEY NEED FROM HEALTHCARE PROVIDERS

Owing to their unique and heightened sense of responsibility for a child's well-being, most parents enter healthcare relationships with high expectations of caregivers. Most parents expect to be informed and to participate actively in decision-making and will hold caregivers accountable for outcomes. As important as these elements are, what most parents want is to be heard and understood.

A qualitative study of Muslim parents of children with life-limiting conditions aimed to assess participants' experiences with the American healthcare system. Thematic analysis of in-depth interviews resulted in new knowledge about the value parents place on open, honest communication, the varied concerns about how providers will react to their religious affiliation, and the importance of leaning heavily into faith and accepting God's plan during times of serious illness (Kolmar et al., 2023).

A 3-year prospective grounded theory study in three pediatric settings aimed to conceptualize "best practice health care [pediatric] providers" (BPHCPs). In all, 34 parents and 80 practitioners were observed in 80 encounters. Researchers found that BPHCPs were those that shared a broad worldview; valued equity, family-centered care, and integrity; and demonstrated a commitment to authentic engagement. BPHCPs had both extensive disciplinary knowledge and knowledge about a wide variety of general topics, such as cultural practices, spiritual issues, farming, music, and local sports teams. BPHCPs valued social justice, so they provided equitable care to all, regardless of how different parents were from themselves. BPHCPs also recognized that persons are part of larger wholes (families, cultures) and that everyone is both affected by and affects these larger wholes (Davies et al., 2017).

WHERE DO CHILDREN ENCOUNTER THE HEALTHCARE SYSTEM?

Cultural Considerations for the Pediatric Nurse in Outpatient, Medical Home, and Home Care Settings

Nurses caring for children in outpatient settings must provide comprehensive care in condensed visits. Assessing the cultural influences on healthcare and establishing a trusting relationship in brief encounters can be exceptionally challenging. The assessment models in Chapter 2 and at the end of this chapter can help nurses arrive at an understanding of parent and child health beliefs and values quickly and effectively.

In a synthesis of 24 qualitative studies of parenting practices of African immigrants in destination countries, Salami and colleagues (2017) suggested that clinicians be aware of and sensitive to the specific practices, values, and needs of this growing group. The authors found common features of parenting for African immigrants in destination countries: (a) changes in discipline practices across transnational borders and the use of physical discipline; (b) respect as a deeply embedded value of parenting; (c) integration of cultural values into parenting; and (d) integration of religious practices into parenting. Challenges faced by this population noted by the authors included lack of informal/community support, access to services and lack of formal support; cultural conflict in parenting; fear related to social services; and language barriers.

Sixteen million children in the United States—21% of children—live in food-insecure homes. The AAP recommends a two-item screening tool that can be used in pediatric outpatient settings across the country. The child or caregiver answers these statements, yes or no:

1. Within the past 12 months, we worried whether our food would run out before we got money to buy more.
2. Within the past 12 months, the food we bought just didn't last, and we didn't have money to get more (Gitterman et al., 2015).

In 2021, the AAP published a toolkit for helping families living with food insecurity that includes screening, interventions, and advocacy resources for those working with children and families. Multilanguage support materials and the use of interpreters were advised, as well as tailoring food available onsite to family preferences (AAP, n.d.).

One frequent subject of discussion during well-child visits is parent–child bed sharing, or co-sleeping, a practice common across cultures. Each year in the United States, approximately 3,500 infants die of sleep-related incidences, including sudden unexpected infant death (SUID) and accidental suffocation and strangulation in bed. Parents should be advised that safe sleeping for infants includes supine positioning; use of a firm, flat sleep surface; room sharing without bed sharing; and avoidance of soft bedding and overheating (Moon et al., 2022).

Interestingly, studies about bed sharing have suffered from design limitations and a lack of convincing evidence to date. In addition, claims that there are psychosocial, developmental, or other benefits to be gained from the practice are as yet unconvincing in the literature as well. Much more study is necessary, as is sensitivity when discussing the practice (Mileva-Seitz et al., 2017). Nurses should review all of the evidence regarding risks and benefits of bed sharing with parents without judgment.

Many barriers to mental health exist for minority children. Nurses must identify these barriers and work to overcome them. Black and Latino children receive outpatient mental healthcare at far lower rates that White children, despite reports of equal incidence across race and culture. Use of emergency care for mental health crises were the same regardless of background, indicating that while the incidence may be the same, ongoing adequate outpatient mental healthcare is lacking for minority children (Marrast et al., 2016). Akobirshoev and colleagues (2020) demonstrated that racial/ethnic minority children with disabilities experience additional disparities in healthcare access outcomes that are greater than the sum of the effects from either characteristic alone. In addition, the researchers demonstrated that disparities persist across all selected geographies even for children living in states or metropolitan cities with the best healthcare systems in the United States.

For children whose family members speak a language other than English, limits to health education in the outpatient setting can be disruptive and may affect health outcomes. The Latino Consortium of the AAP Center for Child Health Research identified language problems as significant when considering health outcomes of Latino children. The report by the consortium noted that Latino parents in one primary care clinic cited language barriers as the single greatest barrier to healthcare access. Parents identified the lack of Spanish-speaking healthcare staff and inadequate interpreter services as the principal problems. Studies were cited that found that medical interpreters were frequently not called when needed, were inadequately trained, or were not available at all. The authors cited another study that demonstrated an increased risk of medical errors when interpreters were poorly trained or unavailable (Flores et al., 2002). This recognition across healthcare settings has led to a transition in thinking beyond an individual nurse's responsibility for self-assessed culturally competent care to include institutional accountability for adequately addressing language barriers as a safety issue (Truong et al., 2014). Despite expanded use of professional interpretation since the early 2000s, language barriers continue to pose challenges in parents and children's perceptions of being heard and understood. The use of family members to translate complex medical terminology created feelings of dependency, isolation, and powerlessness, negatively affecting their relationships with their child or spouse (whoever was translating for them; Tulli et al., 2020).

Nurses in clinics, primary care settings, and working in homecare must either speak the language of the family or have access to adequate interpretation services. In hospitals or schools, where the need for interpretation services is great, institutions often sometimes financially support in-person assistance with language differences. In the United States, while agencies are federally obliged to provide equal access to care, which includes language assistance, just 13 states mandate third-party reimbursement for medical interpretation services (Gunzel, 2012). In clinics and at home, however, in-person interpretation often is not feasible. Ideally, agencies that provide outpatient services invest time and energy into hiring nurses from diverse backgrounds who can speak the family's preferred language. Language-line services that use telephone interpretation can be useful in these situations.

Health outcomes for children in the community setting can be improved through outreach by healthcare providers. Outreach is successful when meaningful and personal connections are made between healthcare providers and community members. Including community leaders and healers when offering health teaching and trying to improve access to the healthcare system is effective in disease prevention and management. In one pilot study of differences between care in the community and in large institutions, some pediatrician offices reported advertising job openings in small, ethnic-specific newspapers in order to increase the diversity of the office workforce. Since every culture values the health of children, culturally competent pediatric care can serve as a template for improving access for adults as well (Dent et al., 2021).

Cultural Considerations for the Pediatric Nurse in Emergency Care and Inpatient Hospital Settings

Accurate and culturally competent communication is essential when children are hospitalized. Under even the best of circumstances, the environment can be intimidating to parents and children. It is difficult to know who can answer questions about the child's care. Events and family–provider interactions happen quickly, often separated by prolonged periods of anticipatory waiting. These challenges are more complicated if English fluency is lacking. When communication is a key factor in successful health outcomes and in ensuring a child's safety, nurses can decrease risk by facilitating accurate communication.

Family members and pediatric oncologists completed a survey of perceptions of prognosis communication. Of the 281 parents of various races and ethnicities who participated in the study of disparities in prognosis communication among parents of children with cancer, 205 (79%) were White, 23 (6%) were Black, 29 (8%) were Hispanic, and 24 (7%) were Asian/other. Furthermore, 87% of parents wanted as much detail as possible about their child's prognosis, with no significant differences by race/ethnicity. However, physician beliefs about parental preferences for prognosis communication varied based on parent race/ethnicity, with physicians considering Black and Hispanic parents less interested in details about prognosis than Whites (Ilowite et al., 2017).

Cultural Considerations for the School Nurse

For children underserved and underinsured in the U.S. healthcare system, the school nurse can be an important link to health promotion services (Schroeder et al., 2018). School nurse services vary widely in the United States and are regulated by state boards of nursing and education. Many states have no specific guidelines for baseline school nurse education beyond licensure; some require a school nurse certification in addition to licensure (Steed et al., 2022). No standard exists for the appropriate nurse staffing for schools. The National Association of School Nurses (NASN) recommends a ratio of 225 nurses to one student.

At a time when much of disease management for children is occurring in outpatient and primary care settings, school nurses in K–12 schools are being asked to monitor and treat both chronic and acute health issues. Health experts have long recognized the benefits for students with health problems and developmental delays to attend school. It is not uncommon for school nurses to care for students with medical problems such as type 1 diabetes and seizure disorders; students with mental health and emotional issues such as depression, anxiety, and attention deficit disorders; and students with complex medication and feeding issues requiring feeding tube management and central line access.

In addition to attending to more complex illness issues, school nurses are taking on greater responsibility for students' primary care screening. Well-child baseline assessment of weight, vision, and hearing, the hallmark of early school nursing, has expanded to include assessments of health issues related to poverty, culture, nutrition, sleep, and safety. School nurses have teamed with other healthcare professionals to anticipate and meet these needs. Progressive school districts have invested in adequate nurse staffing and in partnerships with academic health centers to create school-based health centers (SBHC) that can address disparities in health and education outcomes. SBHCs provide comprehensive child and adolescent health screening, treatment, and teaching as well as referral to advanced care as indicated (School Based Health Alliance [SBHA], 2022).

SBHCs represent an opportunity for nurses to engage in truly interdisciplinary, comprehensive preventative care for children. If the aspirations of comprehensive school-based care are to be realized, nurses must embrace culturally competent care in practical ways. The majority of children using SBHCs are impoverished, underinsured, and members of minority communities (Kjolhede, 2021; SBHA, 2022). The NASN (2016) suggested specific strategies for meeting the needs of students from diverse backgrounds. The Cultural Competency Assessment Checklist, developed by the NASN, provides succinct prompts for nurses to use in interactions with students and caregivers to facilitate communication, improve understanding, and demonstrate respect (Appendix 14.A).

Dr. Susan B. Hassmiller, the senior advisor for nursing for the Robert Wood Johnson Foundation, recently reflected on her observation of the work of Melissa Kunz, a school nurse at a Wilmington, Delaware, high school:

> Kunz not only knew what the students needed, but understood that their family situations and where they lived affected their health. Watching Kunz in action, I realized that the competencies for school nursing are similar to those needed in intensive care units and emergency rooms, but are just being executed in a much different environment. . . . [S]chool nurses . . . need a [similar] vigilant and experienced ear to understand what kids aren't saying, including the internal hurts, bullying, depression, anxiety over relationships and tests, family stress and trauma, and hunger. School nurses need to be ready at a moment's notice for whatever may walk through the door and make accurate assessments for conditions that may not be readily apparent. (Hassmiller, 2016, para. 9)

School nurses may be the first healthcare contact for family members with questions or concerns about a student's gender identity. School nurses are uniquely positioned to provide support, advocate, and provide health education for lesbian, gay, bisexual, transgender, queer, and intersex (LGBTQ)[1] students. The school-age years are a time of development in many facets of identity, not the least of which is gender. School nurses can make referrals and collaborate with other school services. They can role-model acceptance and encourage LGBTQ students to form groups for personal support or political change. They can be an agent of peace and understanding to prevent bullying and other alienating behaviors (NASN, 2016). A recent systematic review of the literature on bullying of LGBTQ students reported that in schools where policies prohibiting bullying included language that explicitly protect students based on gender identity and sexual identity, lower rates of victimization and higher rates of interventions by educators were found (Hall, 2017).

MEMBERS OF THE PEDIATRIC HEALTHCARE TEAM

Pediatric nurses are often responsible for making referrals to and coordinating services among social workers, physicians, early intervention therapists, school therapists, social service agencies, medical interpreters, and many others. In every instance, nurses must incorporate an understanding of the family's culture and the family members' ability to

---

1   This is the official designation used by the Human Rights Campaign, the largest U.S. civil rights organization.

participate in the plan of care. Professional interpretation during conversations with each specialist should be provided for non-English speakers.

In outpatient, hospital, and school settings, social workers provide and organize child protective services; arrange supplemental insurance and other financial supports; and provide psychologic counseling for families under stress. The federal government of the United States recognizes the particular vulnerability of children who are ill or injured by providing financial support in the form of Supplemental Security Income (SSI) benefits; the Children's Health Insurance Program (CHIP), managed by the states using Medicaid funding; and Supplemental Nutrition Assistance Program (SNAP) and Women, Infants, and Children (WIC) support. All of these programs are subject to the winds of American politics and federal budgeting.

Nurses working with children collaborate with physicians and advanced practice nurses in the hospital to accomplish specific health goals. In the outpatient and school settings, nurses emphasize the importance of consistent, regular primary care. In each instance, nurses must consider the values, abilities, and beliefs of families from many cultures. One of the most comprehensive services offered to children in the United States with or at risk for physical, speech, and other developmental delays is the Early Intervention program. Through Early Intervention, children receive regular physical, occupational, and speech therapy, coordinated to maximize their development.

Children with chronic illness or developmental delays are vulnerable in the school setting to bullying, academic setbacks, and family separations, and may require more time to accomplish objectives. School nurses work together with family members, social workers, and educational specialists to develop individualized educational plans (IEPs). All members of the school team should plan care and teaching within the context of the child's cultural background.

SOCIAL DETERMINANTS OF CHILDHOOD HEALTH: NURSES CARING FOR MARGINALIZED CHILDREN

Children Living in Poverty

Almost half of young children in the United States live in poverty or near poverty. Poverty and related social determinants of health can lead to adverse health outcomes in **childhood** and across the life course, negatively affecting physical health, socioemotional development, and educational achievement. With an awareness and understanding of the effects of poverty on children, pediatric health practitioners in many settings can assess the financial stability of families, link families to resources, and coordinate care with community agencies (AAP, 2016).

Children with limited resources are at increased risk for low birth weight, chronic diseases like asthma, obesity, high blood pressure, increased accidental injuries, toxic stress, lack of school readiness, and adverse childhood events such as neglect, physical and emotional abuse, and parental incarceration (AAP, 2016). Child poverty is greater in the United States than in most countries with comparable resources. In a 2012 report from the United Nations Children's Fund (UNICEF), of 35 member nations of the Organisation for Economic Cooperation and Development (OECD), the United States ranked 34th in child poverty. A 2014 report from the same organization ranked the United States 35th of 40 member nations, above only Chile, Mexico, Romania, Turkey, and Israel. In the policy statement and report titled *Poverty and Child Health in the United States*, the AAP Council on Community Pediatrics (Gitterman et al., 2016) identified specific programs that have helped ameliorate the effects of poverty on children's health (Table 14.1). Research in recent years supports the assertion that these safety net programs have had a positive effect on health outcomes for children in the United States.

TABLE 14.1 ■ PUBLIC- AND PRIVATELY FUNDED PROJECTS AIMED AT IMPROVING CHILD HEALTH BY MITIGATING THE EFFECTS OF POVERTY

PROGRAM	HEALTH BENEFIT	RISK
U.S. Tax Policy Earned Income Tax Credit and Child Tax Credit	Decreased incidence of low-birth-weight infants; fewer preterm births; increased use of prenatal care	Subject to federal tax policy created and approved by Congress
Direct Aid TANF—formerly "welfare"	Decreased food and housing insecurity	Block grant to states, so subject to state policies and regulations; tethered to work requirements that may mean need for child care so a single parent can work
Access to Comprehensive Healthcare CHIP Patient Protection and ACA or "Obamacare"	Increased coverage for millions of Americans; increased use of preventative care; dependent children covered through age 26; coverage for preexisting conditions; coverage for dental, mental health, and substance abuse services in addition to medical/surgical care	Federal law, but has been challenged in Congress and the Supreme Court. Most effective when universal coverage is achieved
Early Childhood Education Early Head Start Head Start	Access to educational, nutritional, health, and social services	Subject to federal funding
SNAP; WIC; School Lunch Program	Funding for nutritional support	Subject to federal funding
Home Visiting Nurse–Family Partnership	Benefit of the ACA: first-time, low-income mothers receive weekly visits at home by a nurse beginning in the second trimester	
Family and Parenting Support in the Medical Home	Comprehensive healthcare and education in primary care settings	
Interventions for Adolescents and Parents of Young Children	Job training combined with child care benefit	

ACA, Affordable Care Act; CHIP, Child Health Insurance Programs; SNAP, Supplemental Nutrition Assistance Program; TANF, Temporary Assistance to Needy Families; WIC, Women, Infants, and Children.
Source: Gitterman, B. A., Flanagan, P. J., Cotton, W. H., Dilley, K. J., Duffee, J. H., Green, A. E., Keane, V. A., Krugman, S. D., Linton, J. M., McKelvey, C. D., & Nelson, J. L. (2016). Poverty and child health in the United States. *Pediatrics, 137*(4), e20160339. https://doi.org/10.1542/peds.2016-0339

LGBTQ Children

The NASN developed a comprehensive, specific, and supportive policy statement on caring for LGBTQ school children. LGBTQ students need school nurses to

- Recognize that the health risks are disproportionately higher for LGBTQ students and provide culturally competent care in a safe, private, and confidential setting.
- Make referrals for evidence-based care to healthcare professionals knowledgeable about the healthcare needs of LGBTQ youth.
- Provide support and resources for families about local and national organizations that are available to help them to support their children.
- Advocate for the creation and enforcement of inclusive zero-tolerance bullying policies; attend and promote professional development programs for school leadership and personnel to understand and meet the needs of LGBTQ students; promote inclusive health education and curriculum for all students; and encourage a welcoming, inclusive environment with safe spaces in the school, that is, health office, counselor's office, and classrooms.

- Promote student-led gay–straight alliances and other clubs supported by faculty and administrators to improve the school climate for all students, regardless of their sexual orientation, gender identity, or gender expression.
- Provide support for students by advocating for practices and policies that promote the physical, psychologic, and social safety of all students regardless of their sexual orientation, gender identity, or gender expression.

Encourage the use of gender-neutral school forms, dress codes, changing space, and bathrooms; use students' preferred names and pronouns; and protect confidentiality when contacting others if the student is not "out/open" to family or to others at school (NASN, 2016).

IMPORTANT POINTS

- In 2021, 22% (73.6 million children) of the population of the United States were between 0 and 18 years old.
- Twenty-five percent of all U.S. children are native-born children of at least one foreign parent.
- Three percent of all U.S. children (2.26 million) are foreign born of foreign-born parents.
- The percentage of English language learners (ELLs) varies by location; 12.2% in cities, 8.9% in suburbs, and 3.5% in rural areas (U.S. Census Bureau, 2023).
- No single individual has greater influence on a child's development than the primary caretaker, usually the parents.
- The nurse's responsibility to children of diverse backgrounds includes self-awareness, awareness of multiple layers of vulnerability of sick children, respect for and acceptance of difference, dedication to equal access to safe quality care, and continuing education.
- Nurses need to understand the parent-and-child relationship within the context of culture.
- In each care setting, the nurse must consider the parents' beliefs about discipline, safety, nutrition, sleep, and education.
- In the absence of a person with clear legal responsibility for decision-making on a child's behalf, nurses should consult with social workers and members of their institution's ethics committee.
- At every opportunity, children in the healthcare system should be included in information and decision-making as they are developmentally able.

WHAT NURSES NEED TO KNOW ABOUT THE PATIENT

Selecting a Cultural Assessment Model

CASE SCENARIO PART 1

Carmen brings her 9-year-old daughter, Ariana, to the ED of the local children's hospital on a Tuesday after school for another asthma exacerbation. This is the third ED visit in the last 3 months. When the triage nurse realizes Carmen's primary language is Spanish, she uses the basic words she knows for a brief physical and family assessment. The nurse directs questions to Ariana, who speaks English for her mother. She asks the assistant to arrange for a professional interpreter to visit as soon as possible.

IMPORTANT POINTS

- Sixteen million children live in food-insecure houses.
- Studies reveal a high risk for obesity in minority children.
- Cultural factors may contribute to children's obesity.
- Culturally appropriate care should include nutritional counseling.
- Bed sharing, a common practice across cultures, is associated with high rates of SUID.
- Black and Hispanic infants are bed sharing at increasing rates.
- Infants should not share the same bed surface with parents until the baby turns 1 year old.
- Many barriers to mental health exist for minority children; however, Black and Latino children receive care at lower rates.
- Although language is the single greatest barrier to healthcare access for Latino children, just 13 states provide third-party reimbursement for medical interpretation services.
- When English fluency is lacking, nurses can ensure a child's safety and decrease health risks by facilitating accurate communication.
- Nurses must have an acceptance of cultural differences in perception and management of pain.
- Family-centered care must be personalized.
- No standard exists for appropriate school nurse staffing; the Association of School Nurses recommends 225 students to one nurse.
- School nurses take on responsibility for well-child screening and assessments and for medical issues like diabetes mellitus (DM), seizure disorders, and mental health problems.

CASE SCENARIO PART 2

Through Ariana, Carmen tells the nurse that Ariana has had a cold for a week. Today, she says her chest feels tight. This morning she started "wheezing like the last time when it was so bad." Carmen says she thinks Ariana needs to be in the hospital again. The interpreter is meeting with another family and will arrive in an hour. The nurse assesses Ariana's vital signs and respiratory system. Her vital signs are concerning, she is short of breath, and she is only able to answer questions with difficulty. Carmen and Ariana both look confused and fearful.

IMPORTANT POINTS

- Progressive school districts partner with academic health centers to form SBHCs.
- School nurses are uniquely positioned to provide support and advocacy for LGBTQ children.
- Almost half of young children live in poverty or near poverty; child poverty is greater in the United States than in most countries with comparable resources.
- Children with limited resources are at risk for low birth weight; chronic diseases like asthma, obesity, and high blood pressure; increased accidental injuries; toxic stress; lack of school readiness; neglect; physical abuse; and parental incarceration.
- After investigation by Child Protective Services (CPS), 650,000 children are substantiated as victims of maltreatment; over 1,500 child deaths are attributed to abuse or neglect annually, and 80% of child maltreatment occurs in those younger than 4 years.
- The trauma of child abuse has lifelong physical, emotional, and mental consequences.

(continued)

IMPORTANT POINTS

(continued)

- Nurses and nurse practitioners (NPs) are in a unique position to recognize and protect children against abuse through collaboration with CPS, social workers, and other members of the healthcare team for prompt reporting of suspected abuse.
- The likelihood of child maltreatment, primarily neglect, increases as high as 42% during a parent's military deployment.
- Immigrant children are most likely to be uninsured, receive inconsistent routine care, receive inadequate screening and immunizations, live below the poverty level, have less access to quality early education programs, and live with a parent who faces the threat of deportation.

CASE SCENARIO PART 3

Ariana is admitted to the hospital. The interpreter visits to say hello, explains the next steps, and invites Carmen and Ariana to ask questions. The interpreter learns that Carmen's husband, Bayardo, works 12 hours a day, 6 days a week at a dairy farm in the suburbs. Carmen, Bayardo, and Ariana were born in Guatemala, and are living in the United States without documentation. Ariana's younger sister was born in the United States. Carmen tells the nurse through the interpreter that she was unable to purchase the refills of Ariana's prescriptions for her daily medicine. Educational, financial, and social support will be needed in the coming days.

IMPORTANT POINTS

- Undocumented children face unique health challenges.
- The Dream Act, passed by Congress in 2002, was expanded by President Obama with the Deferred Action Childhood Arrivals (DACA) program to cover older undocumented children.
- In 2017, President Trump attempted to discontinue the DACA program, which would exacerbate inadequate access to healthcare; however, the outcome of this effort is still being decided in the courts.

WHAT NURSES NEED TO KNOW ABOUT THEMSELVES

Application of the Staircase Self-Assessment Model: Self-Reflection Questions

1. Where are you on the Cultural Competency Staircase regarding delivering care to children from diverse backgrounds?
2. What encounters have you had with children diagnosed with asthma? How is care for children with asthma different than care for children with other childhood illnesses?
3. How might the nurses in this case scenario feel about caring for Ariana? How would you feel, and why?
4. What skills are needed to care for a child from another culture competently who is living with asthma?

5. What factors influence the nurse's motivation to provide culturally competent care to children with chronic illnesses?
6. What do the nurses need to know about this patient in order to provide this patient with culturally competent care?
7. What services will be consulted for help in supporting Ariana and her family educationally, financially, and socially?

Responses to Self-Reflection Questions 1, 2, 3, 4, 5, and 6

Response: Where are you on the Cultural Competency Staircase regarding delivering care to children from diverse backgrounds?

Refer to Chapter 1 when considering your answer.

Response: What encounters have you had with children diagnosed with asthma? How is care for children with asthma different than care for children with other childhood illnesses?

Care for children with chronic illness is complex under ideal circumstances. Financial, cultural, and social barriers to seeking care multiply the challenges that families face. Insufficient support for chronic health concerns often results in repeated exacerbations of the illness. In some cases, this can become life-threatening.

Response: How might the nurses in this case scenario feel about caring for Ariana? How would you feel, and why?

Although not ideal, the ED nurse's use of Ariana as an interpreter until a professional was available may have been a sign of respect for Carmen's fear and done out of a sense of urgency to offer information. Nurses feel a host of emotions when caring for children with chronic illness in childhood. Frustration and sympathy are common. Some nurses may feel resentment toward a family using the ED as a substitute for primary care or may feel angry at a healthcare system poorly designed to help people from diverse backgrounds. It is also possible that nurses feel pride and satisfaction in being able to compassionately guide families through a complex health system at a time of stress and fear.

Response: What skills are needed to care for a child from another culture competently who is living with asthma?

Nurses caring for children with chronic illnesses rely on all of the scientific and artistic skills of nursing: vigilant assessments, careful actions, anticipatory critical thinking and compassion, patience, and caring behaviors. Culturally competent nurses caring for children and family members are careful in communication: They listen reflectively, use professional interpretation, and are both physically and mindfully present during interactions. Pediatric nurses need to be proficient in cultural assessment skills and willing to model culturally competent care for newer nurses.

Response: What factors influence the nurse's motivation to provide culturally competent care to children with chronic illnesses?

Nurses must be mindful of the possibility that personal and previous professional experiences with chronic illness can influence their thinking and actions. This family may have lacked adequate access to care. Presumptions about the cultural values, beliefs, and practices of each family should be set aside to allow for open-minded, respectful care. Nurses should reflect on prior successes and on positive role modeling in working with families from any culture. When working with persons without citizenship documentation, nurses need to treat family members with respect in a nonjudgmental way.

Response: What do the nurses need to know about this patient in order to provide this patient with culturally competent care?

Nurses should be assessing the values and routines of daily life. Consider these questions: Is it important that all family members be present at times of significant decision-making? Is it important to them that someone stay with Ariana at all times? Where does she sleep at home? Are there special objects that will provide comfort for her? What is the family's faith practice? Is connection to community members essential during hospitalization? How does the family manage transportation needs?

NCLEX®-TYPE QUESTIONS

1. Potential complications of poor maternal nutrition during pregnancy include which of the following? *Select all that apply.*
   A. Low-birth-weight infants
   B. Prematurity
   C. Inhibited growth and development
   D. Genetic anomalies

2. What are examples of the layers of vulnerability that children are subject to in the healthcare system? *Select all that apply.*
   A. Autonomy
   B. Dependency
   C. Lack of agency
   D. Physical and emotional immaturity

3. During a family interaction on a pediatric inpatient unit, a nurse recognizes that the parents of the sick child speak Spanish in the home. When should a professional medical interpreter be consulted?
   A. After trying to have a sibling provide interpretation
   B. During physician rounds only
   C. If the Spanish-speaking housekeeping staff are unavailable
   D. Immediately and at any time essential health information is being communicated during the hospitalization

ANSWERS TO NCLEX-TYPE QUESTIONS

1. A, B, and C
2. B, C, and D
3. D

AMERICAN ASSOCIATION OF COLLEGES OF NURSING COMPETENCIES ADDRESSED IN THIS CHAPTER

1. Apply knowledge of social and cultural factors that affect nursing and healthcare across multiple contexts.
2. Use relevant data sources and best evidence in providing culturally competent care.
3. Promote achievement of safe and quality outcomes of care for diverse populations.
4. Advocate for social justice, including commitment to the health of vulnerable populations and the elimination of healthcare disparities.
5. Participate in continuous cultural competence development.

A robust set of instructor resources designed to supplement this text is located at http://connect.springerpub.com/content/book/978-0-8261-8302-6. Qualifying instructors may request access by emailing textbook@springerpub.com.

REFERENCES

Akobirshoev, I., Mitra, M., Li, F., Dembo, R., Dooley, D., Mehta, A., & Batra, N. (2020). The compounding effect of race/ethnicity and disability status on children's health and health care by geography in the United States. *Medical Care, 58*(12), 1059–1068. https://doi.org/10.1097/MLR.0000000000001428

American Academy of Pediatrics. (n.d.). *Screen and intervene: A toolkit for pediatricians to address food insecurity.* https://frac.org/aaptoolkit

American Academy of Pediatrics. (2016, March 9). *Poverty and child health.* https://www.healthychildren.org/English/family-life/Community/Pages/Poverty-and-Child-Health.aspx

Davies, B., Steele, R., Krueger, G., Albersheim, S., Baird, J., Bifirie, M., Cadell, S., Doane, G., Garga, D., Siden, H., Strahlendorf, C., & Zhao, Y. (2017). Best practice in provider/parent interaction. *Qualitative Health Research, 27*(3), 406–420. https://doi.org/10.1177/1049732316664712

Dent, R. B., Vichare, A., & Casimir, J. (2021). Addressing structural racism in the health workforce. *Medical care, 59*(Suppl. 5), S409–S412. https://doi.org/10.1097/MLR.0000000000001604

Flores, G., Fuentes-Afflick, E., Barbot, O., Carter-Pokras, O., Claudio, L., Lara, M., McLaurin, J. A., Pachter, L., Ramos-Gomez, F. J., Mendoza, F., Valdez, R. B., Villarruel, A. M., Zambrana, R. E., Greenberg, R., & Weitzman, M. (2002). The health of Latino children: urgent priorities, unanswered questions, and a research agenda. *JAMA, 288*(1), 82–90. https://doi.org/10.1001/jama.288.1.82

Gitterman, B. A., Chilton, L. A., Cotton, W. H., Duffee, J. H., Flanagan, P., Keane, V. A., Krugman, S. D., Kuo, A. A., Linton, J. M., McKelvey, C. D., Paz-Soldan, G. J., Daniels, S. R., Abrams, S. A., Corkins, M. R., de Ferranti, S. D., Golden, N. H., Magge, S. N., & Schwarzenberg, S. J. (2015). Promoting food security for all children. *Pediatrics, 136*(5), e1431–e1438. https://doi.org/10.1542/peds.2015-3301

Gitterman, B. A., Flanagan, P. J., Cotton, W. H., Dilley, K. J., Duffee, J. H., Green, A. E., Keane, V. A., Krugman, S. D., Linton, J. M., McKelvey, C. D., & Nelson, J. L. (2016). Poverty and child health in the United States. *Pediatrics, 137*(4), e20160339. https://doi.org/10.1542/PEDS.2016-0339

Gunzel, J. G. (2012). A right to a medical interpreter, but not a guarantee. *Public Insight Network.* https://www.publicinsightnetwork.org/2012/07/11/medical-interpreter/

Hall, W. (2017). The effectiveness of policy interventions for school bullying: A systematic review. *Journal of the Society for Social Work and Research, 8*(1), 45–69. https://doi.org/10.1086/690565

Hassmiller, S. (2016, May 11). Why school nurses are the ticket to healthier communities. *Robert Wood Johnson Foundation.* https://www.rwjf.org/en/culture-of-health/2016/05/why_school_nursesar.html

Ilowite, M. F., Cronin, A. M., Kang, T. I., & Mack, J. W. (2017). Disparities in prognosis communication among parents of children with cancer: The impact of race and ethnicity. *Cancer, 123*(20), 3995–4003. https://doi.org/10.1002/cncr.30960

Katz, A. L., Webb, S. A., Macauley, R. C., Mercurio, M. R., Moon, M. R., Okun, A. L., Opel, D. J., & Statter, M. B. (2016). Informed consent in decision-making in pediatric practice. *Pediatrics, 138*(2), e20161485. https://doi.org/10.1542/PEDS.2016-1485

Kjolhede, C., Lee, A. C., De Pinto, C. D., O'Leary, S. C., Baum, M., Beers, N. S., Bode, S. M., Gibson, E. J., Gorski, P., Jacob, V., Larkin, M., Christopher, R., Schumacher, H., & Council on School Health. (2021). School-based health centers and pediatric practice. *Pediatrics, 148*(4), e2021053758. https://doi.org/10.1542/peds.2021-053758

Kolmar, A., Kamal, A., & Steinhauser, K. (2023). "Between wings of hope and fear": Muslim parents' experiences with the American Health Care System. *Journal of Palliative Medicine, 26*(1), 73–78. https://doi.org/10.1089/jpm.2022.0154

Lulgjuraj, D., & Maneval, R. E. (2021). Unaccompanied hospitalized children: An integrative review. *Journal of Pediatric Nursing, 56*, 38–46. https://doi.org/10.1016/j.pedn.2020.10.015

Marrast, L., Himmelstein, D. U., & Woolhandler, S. (2016). Racial and ethnic disparities in mental health care for children and young adults. *International Journal of Health Services, 46*(4), 810–824. https://doi.org/10.1177/0020731416662736

Mileva-Seitz, V. R., Bakermans-Kranenburg, M. J., Battaini, C., & Luijk, M. P. C. M. (2017). Parent–child bed-sharing: The good, the bad, and the burden of evidence. *Sleep Medicine Reviews, 32*, 4–27. https://doi.org/10.1016/j.smrv.2016.03.003

Moon, R. Y., Carlin, R. F., Hand, I., & The Task Force on Sudden Infant Death Syndrome and the Committee on Fetus and Newborn. (2022). Evidence base for 2022 updated recommendations for a safe infant sleeping environment to reduce the risk of sleep-related infant deaths. *Pediatrics, 150*(1), e2022057991. https://doi.org/10.1542/peds.2022-057991

National Association of School Nurses. (2016). *LGBTQ students: The role of the school nurse.* Author.

Salami, B., Hirani, S., Meharali, S., Amadu, O., & Chambers, T. (2017). Parenting practices of African immigrants in destination countries: A qualitative research synthesis. *Journal of Pediatric Nursing, 36*, 20–30. https://doi.org/10.1016/j.pedn.2017.04.016

School Based Health Alliance. (2022). *SBHA and National Association of School Nurses joint statement.* https://www.sbh4all.org/sbha-and-national-association-of-school-nurses-joint-statement

Schroeder, K., Malone, S. K., McCabe, E., & Lipman, T. (2018). Addressing the social determinants of health: A call to action for school nurses. *Journal of School Nursing, 34*(3), 182–191. https://doi.org/10.1177/1059840517750733

Steed, H., O'Toole, D., Lao, K., Nuñez, B., Surani, K., & Stuart-Cassel, V. (2022, December 14). *State laws on school nursing outline copious responsibilities for nurses.* Child Trends. https://doi.org/10.56417/2161j1674h

Tiliouine, H., Benatuil, D., & Lau, M. (2022). *Handbook of children's risk, vulnerability and quality of life.* Springer.

Truong, M., Paradies, Y., & Priest, N. (2014) Interventions to improve cultural competency in healthcare: a systematic review of reviews. *BMC Health Services Research, 14*(9), 99. https://doi.org/10.1186/1472-6963-14-99

Tulli, M., Bukola Salami, B., Begashaw, L., Meherali, S., Yohani, S., & Hegadoren, K. (2020). Immigrant mothers' perspectives of barriers and facilitators in accessing mental health care for their children. *Journal of Transcultural Nursing, 31*(6), 598–605. https://doi-org.udel.idm.oclc.org/10.1177/1043659620902812

U.S. Census Bureau. (2023, December 18). *Explore census data.* https://data.census.gov/

U.S. Department of Health and Human Services. (n.d.). *Culturally competent nursing care: A cornerstone of caring.* https://ccnm.thinkculturalhealth.hhs.gov

IMPORTANT WEBSITES

Agency for Healthcare Research and Quality. Retrieved from www.ahrq.gov

Assuring Cultural Competence in Health Care: Recommendations for National Standards and an Outcomes-Focused Research Agenda (CLAS Standards). Retrieved from www.researchgate.net/publication/237467036_Assuring_Cultural_Competence_in_Health_Care_Recommendations_for_national_standards_for_culturally_and_linguistically_appropriate_services_in_health_care_CLAS

The California Endowment. Retrieved from www.calendow.org

The Commonwealth Fund. Retrieved from www.cmwf.org

Cross Cultural Health Care Program. Retrieved from www.xculture.org

Hablamos Juntos. Retrieved from www.ncbi.nlm.nih.gov/pmc/articles/PMC2988148

Health Resources and Services Administration. Retrieved from www.hrsa.gov

Joint Commission on Accreditation of Hospital Organizations. Retrieved from www.jointcommission.org

National Business Group on Health. Retrieved from www.businessgrouphealth.org

National Center for Cultural Competence. Retrieved from https://nccc.georgetown.edu

National Center on Minority Health and Health Disparities, National Institutes of Health. Retrieved from www.nimhd.nih.gov

National Health Law Program. Retrieved from www.healthlaw.org

The Network for Multicultural Health. Retrieved from futurehealth.ucsf.edu/TheNetwork/Default.aspx?tbid=.html

Office of Minority Health. Retrieved from www.minorityhealth.hhs.gov

Toward Culturally Competent Care: A Toolbox for Teaching Communication Strategies. Retrieved from https://archive.org/details/towardculturally00muth

Transcultural Nursing Society. Retrieved from www.tcns.org

Resources for Small Practice Settings to Provide Interpreter Services

Addressing Language Access Issues in Your Practice: A Toolkit for Physicians and Their Staff Members: California Academy of Family Physicians and CAFP Foundation. Retrieved from www.aafp.org/pubs/fpm/issues/2014/0300/p16.html

Providing Language Services in Small Health Care Provider Settings: Examples From the Field: The Commonwealth Fund. Retrieved from https://collections.nlm.nih.gov/catalog/nlm:nlmuid-101254934-pdf

Resources for Translated Health Education Materials and Forms

Cultural Responsiveness and Equity. Retrieved from https://www.nasn.org/nasn-resources/resources-by-topic/cultural-responsiveness-equity

Healthy Roads Media. Retrieved from https://www.migrantclinician.org/resource/healthy-roads-media.html

Immunization Action Coalition. Retrieved from https://www.immunize.org/

Improving Cultural Competency in Children's Health care: Retrieved from https://nichq.org/resource/expanding-perspectives-improving-cultural-competency-childrens-health-care

Multicultural Health Communication Service. Retrieved from www.mhcs.health.nsw.gov.au

APPENDIX 14.A

NATIONAL ASSOCIATION OF SCHOOL NURSES

Cultural Competency Assessment Checklist

As you conduct an assessment for the children you serve, remember to assess for cultural needs. Following is a checklist of what to assess. Remember not to assume and to be sensitive to how you ask questions so as not to offend. The best way of doing this is by saying, "Tell me about …."

Before you assess a student and the student's family, be aware of your own biases and how they may influence how you interpret results. "Bracket" them or put them to the side as much as possible so you can be open to the needs of your families.

This list can be used when ensuring you have addressed cultural needs in the care plan. "Tell me about":

- Language
- Cultural identification
- Religious identification
- Will this impact health practices?
- View of health
- Cause of sickness (i.e., germ theory, "curse")
- Health practices
- Medication
- Traditional healing
- Food
- Support network
- Social determinants
- Education/literacy level
- Environmental concerns
- Socioeconomic status
- Comprehension
- Are you and the student/family on the same page?
- Do you understand them?
- Do they understand what you have said?

Source: Reprinted with permission, National Association of School Nurses. (2016). *LGBTQ students: The role of the school nurse.* Author.

Cultural Considerations for Advanced Practice Registered Nurses

Janet Roman

Far and away the best prize that life offers is the chance to work hard at work worth doing.

—THEODORE ROOSEVELT

LEARNING OBJECTIVES

After this chapter, the reader will be able to
1. Explore the role of the advanced practice registered nurse (APRN).
2. Examine cultural factors influencing the practice of APRNs.
3. Examine factors influencing the provision of culturally competent care by APRNs to clients of diverse backgrounds.
4. Investigate cultural variations and barriers to care provided by APRNs.
5. Illustrate strategies for improving access to care, communication, and patient outcomes by APRNs.
6. Discuss APRN practice with unique populations and situations.

KEY TERMS

APRN

Certified nurse anesthetist (CRNA)

Certified nurse-midwife (CNM)

CLAS Standards

Clinical nurse specialist (CNS)

DEFINING THE ADVANCED PRACTICE REGISTERED NURSE

APRNs are an integral part of the healthcare system, with their roots dating back to the 1890s (Hibbert et al., 2017). RNs who attain complex decision-making skills and advanced clinical competence through graduate education with a master or doctoral degree are considered to be APRNs. The umbrella of APRN includes the roles of **clinical nurse specialist (CNS)**, nurse practitioner (NP), **certified nurse anesthetist (CRNA)**, and **certified nurse-midwife (CNM;** Hibbert et al., 2017). In the 1950s the CNS role developed to meet the needs of the chronically ill and was the first nursing specialty to be formally recognized (Hibbert et al., 2017). The NP role was developed in the 1960s to fill the gap in primary care due to a lack of physicians serving rural and underserved populations (Hibbert et al., 2017; Woo et al., 2017). Each state regulates the scope of practice and the criteria for entry into advanced practice. APRN graduates must be eligible for national certification, which is used for state licensure (American Nurses Association, 2023). APRNs are educated in one or more of six populations: family (across the life span), adult-gerontology, pediatrics, neonatal, women's health, or psych-mental health (APRN Consensus Group, 2008).

As the use of APRNs continues to grow to meet the needs of our population which is living longer, the diversity in our nation is also growing. Frey (2021) reports the 2020 U.S. Census revealed minorities make up over 40% of the population. However, the APRN workforce is not reflective of the national diversity make-up where only 29% are minorities (National Healthcare Quality and Disparities Report, 2021). By 2050, the United States will consist of individuals from racial or ethnic minority backgrounds comprising over half of the population, according to Barksdale and colleagues (2017). Although nurses need to develop the ability to communicate and interact with people from various backgrounds, the diversity of the nursing workforce should be closer to those of the population at large to foster better interaction and communication according to the Institute of Medicine (2011). Steps should be taken to recruit, retain, and foster the success of diverse individuals. One way to accomplish this is to increase the diversity of the nursing student body according to the Institute of Medicine (2011). Let's explore the cultural considerations for the APRN.

CULTURAL CONSIDERATIONS FOR THE ADVANCED PRACTICE REGISTERED NURSE

Cultural competence has been proven to be an important component of healthcare delivery, and APRNs need to be sensitive and respectful of culturally rooted ideas and practices in order to provide culturally competent care (Lau & Rodgers, 2021). Cultural safety skills encompass cultural awareness, knowledge, and skills (Lau & Rodgers, 2021). To build cultural competence, APRNs must be motivated to learn about culturally diverse individuals. Cultural awareness involves self-reflection of one's own attitudes and bias toward the similarities and differences in others (Lau & Rodgers, 2021). Cultural knowledge is an understanding derived from cultural health beliefs and values. The APRN should be ready for cultural humility, which Lau and Rodgers (2021) describe as a combination of self-reflection, action to redress power imbalances, and collaboration. The cultural skills of awareness, knowledge, sensitivity, and competence can be enhanced with diversity training (Lau & Rodgers, 2021).

CULTURAL FACTORS INFLUENCING THE PRACTICE OF ADVANCED PRACTICE REGISTERED NURSES

During clinical health assessments of patients from culturally or linguistically diverse backgrounds, APRNs frequently rely on the use of family or friends as interpreters to minimize the effects of the patients' poor language skills, according to Pirhofer and colleagues (2022). Sometimes APRNs do not discuss the cultural aspects of health for fear of offending patients (Pirhofer et al., 2022). The National Institutes of Health (NIH) developed standards to improve culturally and linguistically appropriate services (CLAS) that could be adapted to improve equity and eliminate health disparities. The use of CLAS can benefit those at greatest risk of disparities, including racial and ethnic minorities, patients with limited English proficiency, and those with low health literacy, according to Ng and colleagues (2017). The **CLAS Standards** provide the framework for APRNs to meet the needs of diverse patients and addresses three overarching areas: leadership, communication and language, and continuous improvement and accountability (Ng et al., 2017).

CULTURAL VARIATIONS AND BARRIERS TO CARE PROVIDED BY ADVANCED PRACTICE REGISTERED NURSES

Cultural safety deals with the balance of power between APRNs and patients, whereby APRNs must acknowledge and prioritize patients' dignity and right to self-determination, according to Pirhofer and colleagues (2022). Cultural safety requires APRNs to reduce bias and achieve equity within the healthcare environment (Pirhofer et al., 2022). The change in healthcare environment is challenging as APRNs must translate the learned educational material into clinical practice and assess for areas of improvement (Pirhofer et al., 2022). Cultural safety was previously difficult to achieve because APRNs had varying definitions and because it is a continual process with no endpoint. Continuous training was highlighted by APRNs because some expressed the basic education received in nursing school and APRN job onboarding was not enough (Pirhofer et al., 2022). Barriers to cultural safety were reported by APRNs as prejudices or stereotypes transformed from various aspects of a culture; difficulty communicating, and visitation by many relatives, made their jobs more difficult. Patients at times did not receive the care they were entitled to, and APRNs sometimes rejected patients by refusing to care for them (Pirhofer et al., 2022). Religion, dietary requirements, and the time required to adapt to cultural nuances presented additional barriers for providing cultural safety by APRNs.

STRATEGIES FOR IMPROVING ACCESS TO CARE, COMMUNICATION, AND PATIENT OUTCOMES BY ADVANCED PRACTICE REGISTERED NURSES

The presence of a culturally safe environment requires a multifaceted approach to include healthcare providers and organizations to facilitate access to healthcare and achieve equity within the workforce (Pirhofer et al., 2022). The healthcare culture should be one where patients and APRNs create suitable healthcare solutions together by making communication paramount, thus building relationships while receiving information (Pirhofer et al., 2022). Self-reflection, sensitivity, understanding, and empathy are important for APRNs to continuously improve cultural safety (Pirhofer et al., 2022). Quality control can be garnered from the patient's feedback after encounters with APRNs (Pirhofer et al., 2022).

Communication has been identified by APRNs as one of the largest barriers to care, hindering access to care, and possibly contributing to unmet patient needs (Pirhofer et al., 2022). One thought by Pirhofer and colleagues (2022) was that work might be more rewarding if APRNs acknowledged individuality within their colleagues. This acknowledgement could foster curiosity about other cultures, which would increase the APRNs' knowledge and understanding of not only their patients but their colleagues, too (Pirhofer et al., 2022). Healthcare teams could identify colleagues that relate with a diverse culture and potentially have that colleague lead or facilitate the plan of care, giving APRNs easier access to patients (Pirhofer et al., 2022). Organizations should invest in interpreter services to cover the vast languages encountered and include various media and applications (Pirhofer et al., 2022). With the advances of modern technology and cell phones, translation can occur immediately and seamlessly (Pirhofer et al., 2022). Pirhofer and colleagues (2022) identified suggestions by APRNs such as holding language classes, building prayer rooms, expanding chaplaincy, holding cultural festivals, and even introducing a qualified care expert as a contact person.

Building a multicultural care team has benefits for the patients and the organization as a whole. Teams with a higher degree of diversity had diverse resources from language skills to religious and cultural understanding with an increased openness toward diverse cultures, according to Pirhofer and colleagues (2022). Healthcare teams of culturally diverse employees are better prepared to grasp the importance of cultural safety. The philosophy of cultural safety must be embedded in the mission of the organizations and displayed by all healthcare team members. Other helpful services disseminated through the organization could be cultural safety rounds or briefings that included reflection rounds. Cultural safety can be accomplished through continuing education where cultural safety specifically is taught in addition to cultural issues (Pirhofer et al., 2022). Educational attainment by APRNs was a significant predictor of cultural awareness, cultural sensitivity, and cultural competency, leading to cultural safety (Pirhofer et al., 2022). Additionally, an assessment for the presence of prejudice, discrimination, and even racism in the healthcare organization and culture must be conducted along with the development and implementation of remedial strategies using diversity management and leadership, according to Pirhofer and colleagues (2022).

DIFFERENTIATING ADVANCED NURSING FROM NURSING PRACTICE

Advanced health assessment, advanced diagnostic and reasoning, and advanced care planning are integral parts of advanced practice nursing. Addressing diversity, equity, and inclusion is crucial in all aspects of advanced practice nursing. APRNs must have a cultural awareness and knowledge of the beliefs, values, and practices of the patient population being served (Rhodes & Petersen, 2018). During an advanced health assessment, detailed information must be gathered to the extent a differential diagnosis can be pondered. A relationship with the patient at the onset of the assessment sets the tone for the encounter and provides the initial opportunity for providing culturally competent care. Mutual trust is a vital aspect in the relationship. Rhodes and Petersen (2018) reveal that patients must feel involved in their healthcare. After establishing a relationship with the patient, APRNs should elicit the chief complaint or reason for the visit. All associated history and symptoms of the present illness should be obtained including any treatments, noting their success or failure to relieve symptoms. Obtaining thorough family, social, past medical, and surgical histories are paramount. Patient interview and history taking includes a head-to-toe review of systems, both physical and psychologic. The information-gathering process is concluded with a thorough physical examination. APRNs must understand that equal care cannot be defined as the same care in a culturally diverse population because this care will not be considered equally good by all patients, according to Rhodes and Petersen (2018; Box 15.1).

The APRN reviews all data collected, taking into consideration the patient's beliefs, cultural norms, religious practices, and family/support relationships. A list of differential diagnoses is compiled starting with the most likely and severe illness. Each diagnosis requires consideration for any further diagnostic testing that may be needed to confirm or rule out the diagnosis. Close attention must be given to cultural and religious preferences at every juncture of the process. The APRN must be cognizant of religious and cultural norms regarding blood draws, blood products, and animal-based products. Once all testing has been completed and a diagnosis confirmed, the APRN creates a treatment plan. The patient should be involved in devising the treatment plan as well as their support system if appropriate.

BOX 15.1   Helpful Cultural Assessment Tips

What culture does the patient identify?

How strictly does the patient adhere to cultural norms associated with that culture?

What are the patient's social, ethnic, and religious affiliations and beliefs?

What is the patient's perception of health, illness, and healthcare providers?

Are there any religious practices that APRNs need to be aware of when creating care plans?

What type of support system is available to the patient?

Would the patient be more comfortable being assessed by someone of the same gender?

Source: Rhodes, J., & Petersen, S. W. (2018). *Advanced health assessment and diagnostic reasoning* (3rd ed.). Jones & Bartlett Learning.

UNDERSTANDING AUTONOMOUS PRACTICE FOR ADVANCED PRACTICE REGISTERED NURSES

Historically, APRNs must have a collaborative practice agreement with a physician in order to practice in most states. Autonomous practice or full practice authority (FPA) eliminates the requirement of a practice agreement and allows APRNs to practice to the full extent of their education and training. Each state has individual rules and regulations for the licensure of autonomous practice APRNs, but most require some practice hours as an APRN and most limit the practice scope to primary and family care. Additionally, autonomous practice is generally granted to NPs in general practice and is not designated for specialty NPs, CRNAs, and, in some cases, midwives. As of April 2022, 26 states, the District of Columbia, and two U.S. territories have FPA for NPs, according to Kapu (2022). In states with FPA, underserved minority patients have increased access to care, with streamlined care and lower costs (Kapu, 2022).

To put APRN practice limitations into perspective, there were many tasks and care options that APRNs were not able to provide or were limited in some states. In addition to the requirement of physician supervision, APRNs cannot order certain medications or treatments like rehabilitation services, coordinate involuntary psychiatric hospital admissions during mental health crisis, certify hospice illnesses, sign death certificates, or even order diabetic shoes. These are just a few examples of limitations imposed on APRN practice in varying states. Now, with autonomous practice, studies have shown that states with FPA are ranked among those with the best access to care (Kapu, 2022). Kapu (2022) reports that 19 of the highest ranked states for access to care have FPA laws in place. Conversely, nine of the 10 lowest ranked states for overall health do not have FPA laws (Kapu, 2022). This data shows the impact of allowing APRNs to practice autonomously.

TELEHEALTH AND THE COVID-19 PANDEMIC

The COVID-19 pandemic caused the healthcare system to pivot abruptly! During a very narrow window of time, healthcare as we knew it was forced from face-to-face office and hospital visits to remote, no contact patient interactions. Many states had bans on indoor gatherings, which included healthcare visits. Most non-urgent care was initially cancelled until a manner of patient care could be devised that limited or eliminated contact. Telehealth patient visits were quickly embraced by the healthcare industry and payor sources like the Centers for Medicare and Medicaid Services (CMS) to mitigate risks for transmission of the COVID-19 virus, increase access to care, expedite patient triage, and conserve use of personal protective equipment, which was in short supply at the beginning of the pandemic (Demeke et al., 2021). In March 2020, CMS granted pay parity between in-person and telehealth visits, as reported by White-Williams and colleagues (2023).

Telehealth includes a range of virtual communications: telephone calls, remote monitoring, and videoconferencing, according to White-Williams and colleagues (2023). Though telehealth reduced geographical barriers and improved access to care, health inequities persisted. White-Williams and colleagues (2023) report that low-income communities had a lack of resources and technological support to maintain telehealth use. Early studies of telehealth use among minorities showed that Hispanics and Black people were less likely to use telehealth services than White people. This research showed that audio visits were utilized more than video visits, especially in Black patients, and Hispanic patients missed more telehealth visits than their Black and White counterparts (White-Williams et al., 2023).

As telehealth use broadens, it is important to consider health equity as disparity in minority groups persists (White-Williams et al., 2023). Studies show that telehealth use increased during the pandemic. However, people with limited English proficiency utilized telehealth services less than those proficient in English. Health equity could continue to mount for people who have a lack of access to healthcare services (White-Williams et al., 2023). In addition to racial and ethnic trends noticed during the COVID-19 pandemic with telehealth use, trends were identified in regions of the nation and between rural and urban areas. Healthcare centers in the Northeast and West showed significantly higher use of telehealth than in Southern regions. Similar trends were identified in urban healthcare centers where their telehealth use surpassed that of rural health centers. Health centers in the South and in rural areas report challenges with the logistics of implementing telehealth and limited broadband access, according to Demeke and colleagues (2021).

MIGRANTS, REFUGEES, AND ASYLUM SEEKERS

Migrants are people who go to other countries on their own volition to live for any reason. Sometimes this includes people who are displaced because of natural disasters or poor economic opportunities, according to Shaffer and colleagues (2019). Refugees are persons outside their country seeking asylum due to a serious threat to their lives, war, violence, fear of persecution, or serious public conflict or disorder, according to Shaffer and colleagues (2019). Both migrants and refugees experience challenges addressing their healthcare needs and require culturally competent care for improved outcomes (Lau & Rodgers, 2021). Healthcare workers are often the first people migrants meet during their resettlement, and APRNs play a vital role. The goal for resettlement is self-sufficiency through employment and acculturation into their new environment. Health is a part of the resettlement process and refugees generally receive a health assessment early in the process, most often performed by APRNs in some locations (Balcom et al., 2017).

Migrants and refugees are vulnerable and often have similar shared experiences regarding trauma, violence, harassment, separation from family members, torture, social isolation, discrimination, financial insecurities, and human trafficking, to name a few (Lau & Rodgers, 2021; Shaffer et al., 2019). APRNs providing care to migrants and refugees should begin with self-reflection and awareness of their own biases, beliefs, culture, and identity. APRNs must put the plight of migrants and refugees into context, recognizing their unique experiences and journey. There is an imbalance of power in this vulnerable population, making open communication and respectful listening by APRNs paramount to creating a safe environment, as well as building trust and rapport (Lau & Rodgers, 2021). Lau and Rodgers (2021) reflect on the importance of APRNs displaying sensitivity to difficult topics and recognizing the "whole person," including biopsychosocial and spiritual needs. APRNs should devise comprehensive plans of care addressing the social determinants of health, prevention, and health promotion. This inclusive approach can improve outcomes in the migrant and refugee population.

DIVERSITY IN ADVANCED PRACTICE NURSING EDUCATION

The American Association of Colleges of Nursing (AACN) provides the foundation for nursing education in the United States with a primary focus on competency-based learning, according to Spies and Feutz (2023). Competency is the application of knowledge learned, with a blending of knowledge, skills, and attitudes toward the provision of care, as stated by Spies and Feutz (2023). The AACN Essentials focus on competencies across nursing programs, differentiating entry level or undergraduate from advanced or graduate levels (Spies & Feutz, 2023). The AACN Essentials are composed of 10 domains, each consisting of competencies with subcompetencies that reflect the educational level of the students (Spies & Feutz, 2023). The AACN Essentials should be aligned with the institution program outcomes, then cross walked through the curriculum (Spies & Feutz, 2023). Regarding diversity, equity, and inclusion, the AACN Essentials identify specific competencies and subcompetencies that should be reflected in the nursing curriculum. A prime example is Domain 3: Population Health of the AACN Essentials. The competency 3.1 is to manage population health. The entry-level subcompetency 3.1i identifies ethical principles to protect the health and safety of diverse populations (AACN, 2021). Competency 6.4, which is to work with other professionals to maintain a climate of mutual learning, respect, and shared values, calls for APRNs to practice self-assessment to mitigate implicit biases toward team members and to integrate diversity, equity, and inclusion into team practices, according to the AACN (2021). Faculty can use a step-by-step approach to incorporate the AACN New Essentials into the curriculum for APRNs.

IMPORTANT POINTS

1. The term APRN includes clinical nurse specialists (CNS), nurse practitioners (NPs), certified nurse anesthetists (CRNA), and certified nurse-midwives (CNMs).
2. The APRN workforce consists of 29% minorities, which is not reflective of the national diversity.
3. Over 40% of the U.S. population is a minority group member.
4. Advanced health assessment, advanced diagnostic reasoning, and advanced care planning are integral parts of advanced practice nursing.
5. Cultural awareness involves self-reflection of one's own attitudes and biases toward similarities and differences in others.
6. The National Institutes of Health (NIH) developed CLAS Standards that provide a framework for APRNs to meet the needs of diverse patients.
7. Promoting cultural safety requires APRNs to reduce bias and achieve equity within the healthcare environment.
8. Between APRNs and their clients, communication is the biggest barrier to the provision of culturally competent care.
9. Suggested strategies for APRNs to enhance care include holding language classes, holding cultural festivals, and building multicultural care teams.
10. APRNs recognized that equal care is not the same care in working with culturally diverse populations.
11. The APRN reviews all data and considers the patient's beliefs, cultural norms, religious practices, and family /support relationships.
12. The APRN can use the helpful Cultural Assessment Tips by Rhodes and Petersen (2018) to assess culturally diverse patients' care needs.

CASE SCENARIO

Abigail is a 32-year-old female who is currently cancer free after being treated with chemotherapy for cancer. Abigail has been diagnosed with chemo-induced cardiomyopathy that led to heart failure with a reduced ejection fraction (HFrEF). She has been hospitalized multiple times over the past year for heart failure (HF) exacerbations. She is the daughter of migrant workers and now works on a farm picking blueberries. The farm is far from her home; however, workers receive free bus transportation provided by the company. The rural community where Abigail lives does not contain a supermarket with 25 miles. There is one pharmacy locally, which is always crowded, and limited public transportation. Abigail does not own a car and cannot afford taxi or ride share services. Abigail has health insurance from her employer, but the out-of-pocket deductibles and copays are high on her limited income. After paying rent and expenses, Abigail has little money left to purchase groceries, so she utilizes the local church food pantry for groceries. The food pantry provides nonperishable foods which most often are canned or processed.

She is following up as an outpatient with the HF APRN after the latest hospital discharge. The APRN reviews the hospital records and notes Abigail's abnormal lab values indicative of excessive fluid accumulation. The APRN reviewed pharmacy records and noted Abigail's diuretics had not been refilled as ordered.

During the history and physical, the APRN asks Abigail about her diuretic or water pill use, or lack thereof. Abigail says she takes the water pill when she can. The APRN asks what a typical day of meals entails. Abigail replies that she skips breakfast; eats chips, pretzels, or peanuts available free in the company breakroom; and has a regular dinner at home. A regular dinner consists of canned vegetables, canned meats, and canned starches. The APRN counsels Abigail on the importance of taking her diuretics as ordered and eating fresh or frozen vegetables, meats, and starches, then scheduled a follow-up appointment for 1 month. One month later at the follow-up appointment, the APRN notes that Abigail had been seen in the ED twice for HF exacerbation with elevation in the same lab values, indicating excessive fluid accumulation as in previous hospitalizations. The APRN counsels Abigail again on the importance of taking her diuretics as ordered and eating fresh or frozen vegetables, meats, and starches, then schedules a 1-month follow-up appointment. This time Abigail had been seen once in the ED for HF exacerbation with excessive fluid accumulation. The APRN becomes frustrated with Abigail, documenting that she is noncompliant with the treatment plan.

However, the APRN does not know that Abigail has a 2-hour commute each way on a bus that does not have a bathroom, making it difficult to take diuretics on workdays. She tried taking the water pills once at work but was reprimanded for leaving her workstation often. Abigail tried taking the water pills after returning home from work in the evening, but then reports being up all night using the bathroom. After days of interrupted sleep, her body was weak and tired, making it challenging to perform her duties on the farm.

WHAT NURSES NEED TO KNOW ABOUT THEMSELVES

Application of the Staircase Self-Assessment Model: Self-Reflection Questions

When considering Abigail's case, ask yourself the following questions. If you are the APRN caring for Abigail:

1. Where am I on the Cultural Competency Staircase? What actions have I taken to progress to the next level?
2. How many encounters have I had with migrant workers? People from rural areas?
3. What do I know about the community I serve regarding access to food, medication, public transportation, and so on?
4. How many encounters have I had with people with financial or food insecurity? What are my beliefs or attitudes toward people with financial or food insecurity?
5. What assumptions, stereotypes, or generalizations underlie my beliefs about Abigail or people with her socioeconomic status?
6. What do I know about Abigail's health beliefs, attitudes, and values and how do these differ from my own? Did I truly try to get to the root of Abigail's issues before labeling her "noncompliant"?
7. What resources have I familiarized myself with that could benefit Abigail or anyone in her situation?

Responses to Reflection Questions 1, 2, 3, 4, 5, and 6

Response: Where am I on the Cultural Competency Staircase? What actions have I taken to progress to the next level?

You have heard consistently throughout this text the steps and questions for nurses to ask themselves to determine their level on the staircase. This is a crucial process to becoming culturally aware of your patients' needs. Understanding your patient's cultural background will facilitate improved healthcare outcomes. Starting at step one, how much do you value becoming culturally competent? How much do you know about your own culture? How much do you know about other cultural groups? In this case scenario, Abigail is the daughter of migrant workers, lives in a rural community, and is socioeconomically disadvantaged.

Response: How many encounters have I had with migrant workers? People from rural areas?

Migrant workers are people who cross borders to live in other countries, usually because of unfavorable conditions resulting from poor economic opportunities (Shaffer et al., 2019). Though Abigail is not a migrant worker, she is a child of migrants and therefore may experience some challenges. Migrants often leave behind their families and friends. They have to adapt to new surroundings and may experience language and cultural barriers.

Response: What do I know about the community I serve regarding access to food, medication, public transportation, and so on?

Rural areas generally lack grocery stores, which is compounded by a lack of public and individual transportation, according to Bardenhagen and colleagues (2017). The grocery stores or convenience stores sell prepacked foods that lack nutrients. Fresh fruits and vegetables are scarce, possibly due to poor infrastructure. Undeveloped or poorly maintained roads and storage present access barriers (Bardenhagen et al., 2017). This description of rural areas describes Abigail's situation. Her neighborhood lacks a grocery store within 25 miles, she does not have personal transportation and she relies on public transportation that is limited.

Response: How many encounters have I had with people with financial or food insecurity? What are my beliefs or attitudes toward people with financal or food insecurity?

Financial insecurity defines itself. Many times, migrant workers do not receive wages high enough to cover basic life necessities of food, shelter, and clothing. This financial insecurity leads to food insecurity. People without sufficient wages often have to choose between how their limited income will be utilized on shelter, food, clothing, and so on. Abigail relies on the local food pantry for food. She is at the mercy of the church for her daily meal plans. Although her APRN suggested a meal plan lower in sodium with fresh or frozen meats, vegetables, and starches, Abigail does not have access to the foods on the list.

Response: What assumptions, stereotypes, or generalizations underlie my beliefs about Abigail or people with her socioeconomic status?

APRNs should familiarize themselves with resources in the communities they serve. Collaboration with social workers and community nurses can aid in gathering this vital data.

Response: What do I know about Abigail's health beliefs, attitudes, and values, and how do these differ from my own? Did I truly try to get to the root of Abigail's issues before labeling her "noncompliant"?

In the case scenario regarding Abigail, how much time was devoted by the APRN to get a good understanding of Abigail's health attitudes, beliefs, or values? The APRN did not address these matters with Abigail. The APRN thought that her job was done by counseling Abigail on more than one occasion on her diet and healthcare needs. However, did the APRN delve further into why Abigail was unsuccessful? Did the APRN assess Abigail's resources for foods or medications? It is important for the APRN to ensure patients have the means to obtain medications ordered and also have access to the foods in the treatment plan.

NCLEX®-TYPE QUESTIONS

1. The umbrella term APRN refers to which of these groups of nurses? *Select all that apply.*
   A. Nurses with 10 years or more of experience
   B. Nurses who are clinical nurses specialists (CNS)
   C. Nurses who are certified nurse-midwives (CNM)
   D. Nurses who are certified nurse anesthetists (CRNA)
   E. Nurses who are nurse practitioners (NP)

2. According to the U.S. Census Bureau 2020, which statement about the APRN workforce is true? *Select all that apply.*
   A. 40% of all APRNs are minority group members.
   B. The APRN workforce does not reflect the national diversity make-up.
   C. 29% of APRNs are minority group members.
   D. The APRN workforce closely matches the national diversity make-up.

3. The National Institutes of Health's (NIH's) CLAS Standards were intended to address which of the following goals? *Select all that apply.*
   A. Assist patients in need of financial support.
   B. Assist patients with low literacy.
   C. Improve culturally and linguistically appropriate services
   D. Provide nutritional support

4. Which of the following statements reflect barriers to the promotion of cultural safety by APRNs? *Select all that apply.*
   A. Prejudice or stereotypes
   B. Difficulties communicating
   C. Visitation by relatives
   D. Time required to attend to cultural nuances

5. The largest barrier to APRNs and hindering access to care, resulting in unmet care needs, is:
   A. A lack of patient motivation
   B. Communication problems
   C. Limited resources
   D. Adequate time to care for patients

6. Effective strategies for addressing problems APRNs face when working with cultural diverse clients include which of the following? *Select all that apply.*
   A. Identifying colleagues that can facilitate care planning for diverse groups
   B. Investing in interpreters
   C. Utilizing families to translate or interpret the patient's needs
   D. Holding language classes for staff members

7. In the care of culturally diverse patients by APRNs, which statement is accurate?
   A. Equal care means giving the same care to all.
   B. Equal care may mean giving differential treatment based on an individual's needs.
   C. To ensure fairness, care should be identical.
   D. Care should be based on the cultural group with whom an APRN is working.

8. When should the APRN pay attention to the cultural and religious preferences of their clients?
   A. During the history-taking interview or first encounter
   B. During special religious holidays
   C. When a client indicates a religious preference
   D. At every juncture of the nursing process

9. The APRN's treatment plan should be developed between:
   A. The client and the APRN
   B. The APRN and the physician
   C. The family and the APRN
   D. The family, the APRN, and the physician

10. In most states, APRNs practice:
    A. Autonomously
    B. With a collaborative practice agreement with a physician
    C. To the fullest extent of their training and education
    D. With a limited scope of practice

11. Autonomous practice is generally granted to nurse practitioners (NPs) who are:
    A. Specialty care nurses
    B. In general family practice
    C. Certified nurse anesthetists (CRNAs)
    D. Working in urban areas

12. What statement about APRNs, migrants, and refugees is accurate? *Select all that apply.*
    A. During migrant and refugee's resettlement, health assessments are often performed by APRNs.
    B. Before providing care to migrants, the APRN should begin with a self-reflection.
    C. APRNs should treat all migrants the same because of their shared experiences.
    D. APRNs must place the plight of the migrant in context, recognizing each client's unique experiences.

ANSWERS TO NCLEX QUESTIONS

1. B, C, D, and E
2. B and C
3. B, C, and D
4. A, B, C, and D

5. B
6. A, B, C, and D
7. B
8. D

9. A
10. B
11. B
12. A, B, and D

AMERICAN ASSOCIATION OF COLLEGES OF NURSING COMPETENCIES ADDRESSED IN THIS CHAPTER

1. Apply knowledge of social and cultural factors that affect nursing and healthcare across multiple contexts.
2. Use relevant data sources and best evidence in providing culturally competent care.
3. Promote achievement of safe and quality outcomes of care for diverse populations.
4. Advocate for social justice, including commitment to the health of vulnerable populations and the elimination of healthcare disparities.
5. Participate in continuous cultural competence development.

ESSENTIAL CORE COMPETENCIES FOR GRADUATE EDUCATION THIS CONTENT ADDRESSES

American Association of Colleges of Nursing Advanced: Nursing Education

2.1. **Engage with the individual in establishing a caring relationship.**
  2.1d. **Promote caring relationships to effect positive outcomes.**
  2.1e. **Foster caring relationships.**
2.2. **Communicate effectively with individuals.**
  2.2g. **Demonstrate advanced communication skills and techniques using a variety of modalities with diverse audiences.**

2.3. Integrate assessment skills in practice.

2.3h. Demonstrate that one's practice is informed by a comprehensive assessment appropriate to the functional area of the advanced nursing practice.

3.2. Engage in effective partnerships.

3.2e. Challenge biases and barriers that impact population health outcomes.

 A robust set of instructor resources designed to supplement this text is located at http://connect.springerpub.com/content/book/978-0-8261-8302-6. Qualifying instructors may request access by emailing textbook@springerpub.com.

REFERENCES

American Association of Colleges of Nursing. (2021). *The essentials: Competencies for professional nursing education.* https://www.aacnnursing.org/Portals/0/PDFs/Publications/Essentials-2021.pdf

American Nurses Association (2023). *Types of nurse practitioner specialties.* https://www.nursingworld.org/practice-policy/workforce/what-is-nursing/types-of-nurse-practitioner-specialties/

Balcom, D., Carrico, R. M., Goss, J., Smith, M., Van Helden, S., Ford, R. A., Mutsch, K., & Bosson, R. S. (2017). The role of the nurse in the care of refugees: Experiences from the University of Louisville global health program. *Kentucky Nurse, 65*(1), 6–7.

Bardenhagen, C. J., Pinard, C. A., Pirog, R., & Yaroch, A. L. (2017). Characterizing rural food access in remote areas. *Journal of Community Health, 42*, 1008–1019. https://doi.org/10.1007/s10900-017-0348-1

Barksdale, C. L., Rodick 3rd, W. H., Hopson, R., Kenyon, J., Green, K., & Jacobs, C. G. (2017). Literature review of the national CLAS Standards: Policy and practical implications in reducing health disparities. *Journal of Racial and Ethnic Health Disparities, 4*(4), 632–647. https://doi.org/10.1007/s40615-016-0267-3

Demeke, H. B., Merali, S., Marks, S., Pao, L. Z., Romero, L., Sandhu, P., Clark, H., Clara, A., McDow, K. B., Tindall, E., Campbell, S., Bolton, J., Le, X., Skapik, J. L., Nwaise, I., Rose, M. A., Strona, F. V., Nelson, C., & Siza, C. (2021). Trends in use of telehealth among health centers during the COVID-19 pandemic—United States, June 26–November 6, 2020. *MMWR. Morbidity and Mortality Weekly Report, 70*(7), 240–244. https://doi.org/10.15585/mmwr.mm7007a3

Frey, W. H. (2021, August 13). New 2020 census results show increased diversity countering decade-long declines in America's White and youth populations. *Brookings Metro.* https://www.brookings.edu/articles/new-2020-census-results-show-increased-diversity-countering-decade-long-declines-in-americas-white-and-youth-populations

Hibbert, D., Aboshaiqah, A. E., Sienko, K. A., Forestell, D., Harb, A. W., Yousuf, S. A., Kelley, P. W., Brennan, P. F., Serrant, L., & Leary, A. (2017). Advancing nursing practice: The emergence of the role of advanced practice nurse in Saudi Arabia. *Annals of Saudi Medicine, 37*(1), 72–78. https://doi.org/10.5144/0256-4947.2017.72

Institute of Medicine. (2011). *The future of nursing: Leading change, advancing health.* National Academies Press. https://www.ncbi.nlm.nih.gov/books/NBK209871

Kapu, A. N. (2022, July 29). *States with full practice authority ensure access to nurse practitioners.* https://www.nurse.com/blog/states-with-full-practice-authority-ensure-access-nurse-practitioners

Lau, L. S., & Rodgers, G. (2021). Cultural competence in refugee service settings: A scoping review. *Health Equity, 5*(1), 124–133. https://doi.org/10.1089/heq.2020.0094

National Healthcare Quality and Disparities Report. (2021). *Advanced practice registered nurses by race (left) and U.S. population racial and ethnic distribution (right), 2019.* Agency for Healthcare Research and Quality (U.S.). https://www.ncbi.nlm.nih.gov/books/NBK578535/figure/ch2.fig20

Ng, J. H., Tirodkar, M. A., French, J. B., Spalt, H. E., Ward, L. M., Haffer, S. C., Hewitt, N., Rey, D., & Scholle, S. H. (2017). Health quality measures addressing disparities in culturally and linguistically appropriate services: What are current gaps? *Journal of Health Care for the Poor and Underserved, 28*(3), 1012–1029. https://doi.org/10.1353/hpu.2017.0093

Pirhofer, J., Bükki, J., Vaismoradi, M., Glarcher, M., & Paal, P. (2022). A qualitative exploration of cultural safety in nursing from the perspectives of advanced practice nurses: Meaning, barriers, and prospects. *BMC Nursing, 21*(1), 1–14. https://doi.org/10.1186/s12912022-00960-9

Rhodes, J., & Petersen, S. W. (2018). *Advanced health assessment and diagnostic reasoning* (3rd ed.). Jones & Bartlett Learning.

Shaffer, F., Bakhshi, M., Farrell, N., & Alvarez, T. (2019). The role of nurses in advancing the objectives of the global compacts for migration and on refugees. *Nursing Administration Quarterly, 43*(1), 10–18. https://doi.org/10.1097/NAQ.0000000000000328

Spies, L. A., & Feutz, K. (2023). Developing and implementing entrustable professional activities to prepare global nurses. *Journal of Transcultural Nursing, 34*(1), 100–105. https://doi.org/10.1177/10436596221125896

White-Williams, C., Liu, X., Shang, D., & Santiago, J. (2023). Use of telehealth among racial and ethnic minority groups in the United States before and during the COVID-19 pandemic. *Public Health Reports (Washington, D.C.: 1974)*, 138(1), 149–156. https://doi.org/10.1177/00333549221123575

Woo, B., Lee, J., & Tam, W. (2017). The impact of the advanced practice nursing role on quality of care, clinical outcomes, patient satisfaction, and cost in the emergency and critical care settings: A systematic review. *Human Resources for Health*, 15(1), 63. https://doi.org/10.1186/s12960-017-0237-9

IMPORTANT WEBSITES

American Association of Nurse Anesthesiology. Retrieved from www.aana.com

American Association of Nurse Practitioners. Retrieved from www.aanp.org

American College of Nurse-Midwives. Retrieved from www.midwife.org

American Psychiatric Nurses Association. Retrieved from www.apna.org

Gerontological Advanced Practice Nurses Association. Retrieved from www.gapna.org

National Association of Pediatric Nurse Practitioners. Retrieved from www.napnap.org

16

Delivering Culturally Competent Care to Victims of Human Trafficking

Gloria Kersey-Matusiak

The inspiration you seek is already in you. Be silent and listen.

—RUMI

LEARNING OBJECTIVES

After this chapter, the reader will be able to

1. Discuss the problem of human trafficking as a global and national concern.
2. State the incidence of human trafficking and its impact in the United States.
3. Explain the mechanisms that facilitate the acquisition of human beings for trafficking.
4. Identify states with the highest prevalence of human trafficking.
5. Recall the profiles of victims and perpetrators of human trafficking.
6. Identify national and state efforts to combat human trafficking.
7. Discuss medical problems that may result from human trafficking.
8. Develop strategies for individuals to combat human trafficking in the United States.
9. Describe the culturally competent nurses' role in providing ethical and trauma-informed care to victims of human trafficking.

KEY TERMS

Autonomy

Beneficience

Commercial sexual exploitation of children (CSEC)

Domestic servitude

Effects

Ethics of Care Model

Event

Experienced

Forced labor

Justice

National Action Plan (NAP)

Nonmaleficence

Red flags

Sexual exploitation

Trafficking warning signs

Trauma-informed care

INTRODUCTION

The problem of human trafficking is a global concern that happens on every continent and "almost every country around the world, including the United States" (Youth.gov, n.d., para. 1). It is the "buying and selling of people" (UNICEF, 2016 para. 1,), a form of slavery that according to the International Labor Organization thrives in a $150 billion-dollar industry that makes its profits through the exploitation of an estimated 20.9 million people around the world. The business of trafficking human beings involves all races, ethnicities, ages, gender identities, social classes, and nationalities who are forced to work in inhumane conditions for little or no pay, or to engage in criminal activities like prostitution for the benefit of perpetrators who often escape punishment for their crimes. Traffickers force individuals who are held captive to work as prostitutes, or in restaurants, factories, farms, and private homes, for a profit (Paton, 2020). Human trafficking is a violation of human rights, and a serious crime against federal, state, and international law (King, 2009). For nurses and other health professionals, human trafficking is also a public health emergency (Paton, 2020) for which preventive measures and interventions for its elimination are urgently needed.

TYPES OF HUMAN TRAFFICKING

There are several types or forms of human trafficking; these include forced **sexual exploitation**, **forced labor**, and **domestic servitude** (Morris, 2023; Paton, 2020). Within the United States, the most common form is sex trafficking; however, labor trafficking is more common among foreign nationals (Association of Women's Health, Obstetric and Neonatal Nurses, 2016). The United States is ranked as one of the worst countries globally for human trafficking, and an estimated 199,000 incidents occur in the country every year (World Population Review, 2023). In 2017, law enforcement agencies reported more than 1,200 cases of human trafficking, but that figure was much lower than the actual number of trafficking victims that year. In 2020, the United States had 8,839 human trafficking cases reported, with most cases involving sex trafficking in massage/spa businesses and pornography. According to Amy Farrell, a researcher at Northeastern University who studies human trafficking, it is hard to estimate the magnitude of the problem because state and regional law enforcement records reflect less than 10% of trafficking victims in the area. In addition, "state and local police often don't have the specialized training necessary to identify human trafficking when they see it. [It is also] difficult to persuade a victim of human trafficking to [cooperate] with . . . police" (Callahan, 2019, paras. 2–3). However, these are but a few of the reasons human trafficking in all its forms is able to thrive in the United States and elsewhere.

OTHER MECHANISMS AND FACTORS CONTRIBUTING TO TRAFFICKING

There are many contributing factors that facilitate the ongoing trafficking in persons, yet three factors play a major role in sustaining its proliferation. According to UNICEF (2016), first, perpetrators enjoy a high reward for very little risk of being caught. Human trafficking is the second most profitable illegal industry, second only to the drug trade. Second, human trafficking, like other industries, relies on the economic principles of supply and demand. The high demand drives the market to provide a high volume of people to meet that demand. As consumers demand cheap goods, corporations demand cheap labor, forcing those at the bottom of the supply chain to exploit workers. Third, systemic inequalities and disparities (e.g., geographical displacement, extreme poverty, women who are uneducated) make certain groups more vulnerable to exploitation (UNICEF, 2016). Traffickers seek the most vulnerable and underserved individuals, those who are desperate to find work, housing, or to escape domestic violence, or those who face the threat of persecution by gangs or other bad actors in their homeland. However, not all victims are immigrants; American citizens are victimized too by trafficking.

Among other factors contributing to these crimes, according to Amy Farrell, director and associate professor of criminal law at Northeastern University, sometimes sex crimes are classified in broader categories such as a general sex offense or another catchall phrase into which sex trafficking becomes harder to determine. Also, "state and local police often lack the specialized training necessary to identify human trafficking when they see it" (Callahan, 2019), and when they do, it is difficult to convince victims of trafficking to collaborate with police for reasons of safety and survival.

MYTHS AS BARRIERS TO VICTIM IDENTIFICATION

Citizens of the United States hold many misconceptions and myths about human trafficking. The U.S. Department of Homeland Security (DHS) published a list that indicates widespread misinformation about the facts related to human trafficking. These misconceptions make it difficult for victims of trafficking to be recognized and for citizens to act when they witness someone who is being victimized. For example, many Americans believe that human trafficking only happens in other countries. In the United States, trafficking occurs in cities, suburbs, and rural towns (Office on Trafficking in Persons, 2019). Some citizens believe that human smuggling and human trafficking are the same. In actuality, human smuggling involves moving a person across a country's border with that person's consent. However, trafficking is based on exploitation by force, fraud, or coercion to hold a person against their will for forced labor or sexual exploitation. Another myth is that labor trafficking only occurs in developing countries; it actually happens in the United States, too, but it is reported less often. Others believe that victims of trafficking can reach out for help when they are in public. Victims of trafficking both fear and depend on perpetrators. They depend on them for sustenance, especially if they are minors while they are being held hostage. Victims may be fearful of the perpetrator's retribution toward them or their families. Survivors of trafficking sometimes fear having contact with police, since many trafficking persons have been criminalized for crimes they were forced to commit by the perpetrator. These misconceptions serve as barriers to combatting trafficking crimes.

PROFILE OF TRAFFICKING VICTIMS

Anyone can become a victim of human trafficking. In the United States, both citizens and foreign nationals have been victimized. Women and girls of color are disproportionately vulnerable to sex trafficking, as roughly 66% are people of color (Human Trafficking Collaborative, 2019). Although 94% of sex trafficking victims are female (Human Trafficking Collaborative, 2019), researchers for an ECPAT-USA paper that examined the **commercial sexual exploitation of children (CSEC)**, entitled "And Boys Too" (Friedman, 2013), found that the voices of male victims have often gone unheard. This study revealed various factors that accounted for the underreporting of men and boys involved in sexual trafficking. These factors included the unwillingness of boys to self-identify as having been exploited due to shame, stigma about being gay, or being perceived as gay by their family and community, as well as a lack of screening by law enforcement or social service officers who disbelieved boys can be victims of CSEC. Findings revealed "vast underreporting of boys who were victims of trafficking and that much needs to be done to protect children" (Friedman, 2013).

Human trafficking is facilitated online and through social media. Some traffickers use love and affection as a way of coercing individuals who are vulnerable, such as people who lack education, those looking for jobs, runaways, people trying to escape violence or sexual or physical abuse in their homes, and persons who are LGBTQ. In addition, 47% of people living in extreme poverty are among those who were victims of trafficking. Thus,

TABLE 16.1 ■ SIGNS THAT MIGHT INDICATE SOMEONE IS A VICTIM OF TRAFFICKING

SIGNS THAT YOUTH IS BEING TRAFFICKED	ADDITIONAL SIGNS OF SEX TRAFFICKING	SIGNS TO OBSERVE DURING TRAVEL
• Misses school regularly • Frequently runs away from home • Frequent travel to other cities or towns • Exhibits bruises or other signs of physical trauma, withdrawn behavior, depression, anxiety, or fear • Lacks control over their schedule • Is hungry, malnourished, or inappropriately dressed based on weather; shows signs of drug addiction • Has coached or rehearsed responses to questions	• Demonstrates a sudden change in attire, behavior, or material possessions (has expensive items) • Is uncharacteristically promiscuous • Has a boyfriend or girlfriend that is noticeably older • Attempts to conceal recent scars • Shows a sudden change in attention to hygiene	• Has a travel companion who controls ticket, documents, and movement • Avoids eye contact with travel companion • Lacks knowledge of travel plans and destination

Source: Youth.gov. (n.d.). *Human trafficking: The problem*. Retrieved January 8, 2024, from https://youth.gov/youth-topics/trafficking-of-youth/the-problem

being poor, living in abusive domestic situations, being homeless, or being a member of the LGBTQ community places individuals at greater risk of trafficking.

Youth.gov identified potential indications that a young person is being trafficked. See Table 16.1. These indicators include someone who misses school on a regular basis, or frequently runs away from home; frequently travels to other cities or towns; exhibits bruises or other signs of physical trauma; displays withdrawn behavior, depression, anxiety, or fear; lacks control over their schedule, identification, or travel documents; is hungry or malnourished; is inappropriately dressed for the weather; shows signs of drug addiction; and/or has coached/rehearsed responses to questions. Victims are often lured with false promises of love, money, or simply a better life (Paton, 2020; Youth.gov, n.d.). It is important to note that minors under age 18 are considered victims by law enforcement when trafficked, even if they have been forced or coerced to participate in illegal activities. There is mandatory reporting of suspected child abuse (Paton, 2020), so suspected trafficking of a minor is reportable to the DHS or Child Protective Services in one's state.

PROFILE OF PERPETRATORS

Perpetrators of human trafficking represent every social, ethnic, and racial group. These individuals exploit others by taking control of their lives by threatening physical and emotional abuse and keeping victims "dependent and in bondage" (Paton, 2020, para. 2). Perpetrators can come from large national gangs, criminal organizations, local street and motorcycle gangs, and individuals with no affiliation with any group or organization. They can be either men or women. The Bureau of Justice Statistics reported that the number of persons prosecuted for human trafficking in 2020 was 1,343, an 84% increase from 2011. However, only 658 persons were convicted of a federal human trafficking offense. Of the 1,169 defendants charged in U.S. district court, 92% were male, 63% were White, 18% were Black, 17% were Hispanic, 95% were U.S. citizens, and 66% had no prior convictions. At the end of the year, among 47 states that reported data, 1,564 persons were in the custody of a state prison for human trafficking (Lauger et al., 2022).

STATES WITH THE HIGHEST PREVALENCE OF HUMAN TRAFFICKING

Table 16.2 features a list of the top 10 U.S. states with the highest rates of trafficking. According to World Population Review, California consistently has the highest number of human trafficking cases in the United States. For example, California had 1,334 cases reported in 2020, followed by Texas with 987 cases, Florida with 738, and New York with 414 cases. Perhaps

TABLE 16.2 ■ STATES IN THE UNITED STATES WITH THE HIGHEST RATES OF TRAFFICKING PER 100,000 PEOPLE

STATE	PER 100,000 PEOPLE
1. Mississippi	6.38
2. District of Columbia	6.08
3. Nevada	5.80
4. Missouri	4.32
5. Nebraska	3.65
6. California	3.43
7. Oregon	3.29
8. Florida	3.26
9. Texas	3.24
10. Arkansas	3.23

Source: World Population Review. (2023). *Human trafficking statistics by state.* https://worldpopulationreview.com/state-rankings/human-trafficking-statistics-by-state

not coincidentally, these states are the most populated in the United States and have very high immigrant rates. In contrast, Rhode Island had the lowest number of cases and the lowest rate of trafficking, based on its population (World Population Review, 2023).

CURRENT EFFORTS TO COMBAT TRAFFICKING

According to the White House National Action Plan, "human trafficking disproportionately impacts the most vulnerable and underserved members of our society" (The White House, 2021). The White House's **National Action Plan (NAP)** reflects the U.S anti-trafficking goal, but also broader efforts to address inequities for marginalized groups and the U.S. government's commitment to gender and racial equity. The plan integrates recommendations from survivors' lived experiences about how to prevent human trafficking, provide resources, and protect and respond to the global needs of trafficking survivors. A central focus of U.S. and global anti-trafficking efforts includes prevention, protection, prosecution, and partnerships. (See National Action Plan in Important Websites.)

Laws impacting immigrants who are victims of trafficking include the Victims of Trafficking and Violence Protection Act of 2000. It consists of two divisions: the Trafficking Victims Protection Act (TVPA) and the Violence Against Women Act (VAWA). The U.S. government also created T and U visas that are intended to encourage victims of serious crimes like trafficking to cooperate with law enforcement to assist in the prosecution of traffickers. T visas are for noncitizens who are living in the United States due to being trafficked into the country (U.S. Department of Labor, 2015). An applicant for a U visa may have traveled to the United States and then became a victim of trafficking and/or other serious crimes. Both visas, if awarded, give survivors legal status to live in the United States

MEDICAL PROBLEMS RESULTING FROM HUMAN TRAFFICKING

At some point in time, most victims of trafficking will connect with healthcare services because of the conditions in which they are forced to live. Yet, one survey of trafficking survivors found that while still held captive, 87.8% went unidentified despite having interacted with healthcare providers; 67% of these survivors were seen in the ED, although victims of trafficking might also be seen in any other area offering healthcare services (Paton, 2020). Unfortunately, victims of trafficking usually delay seeking help until their health needs are serious.

According to the U.S. Department of State, most trafficking victims, although not all, are women. Consequently, women are at high risk for gynecologic and obstetric problems, such as sexually transmitted infections, unintended pregnancies, repetitive abortions or miscarriages, trauma to the rectum or vagina, and infertility. Women who are trafficked seldom use primary care and therefore may have many untreated illnesses about which they are unaware (Association of Women's Health, Obstetric and Neonatal Nurses, 2016). In addition, victims of trafficking often experience both physical and psychologic abuse. Physical injuries from abuse and torture can be evidenced by burns, lacerations, missing or broken teeth, malnutrition, dehydration, substance use disorders, depression, anxiety, and posttraumatic distress syndrome (Association of Women's Health, Obstetric and Neonatal Nurses, 2016). In addition the Drug Enforcement Administration (DEA, 2022) warned the public of an emerging trend to target young Americans with brightly colored fentanyl pills in 26 states. Other **red flags** (see Table 16.3) that someone has been victimized by trafficking include if the patient appears withdrawn, nervous, fearful, and avoids eye contact; displays distrusting or disruptive behavior; is unwilling or hesitant to answer questions about the injury or illness; offers an inconsistent history or explanation of the chief complaint; and shows signs of physical abuse, self-inflicted injuries, or suicide attempts (Paton, 2020).

TRAFFICKING AND THE ROLE OF THE NURSE

Nurses are uniquely positioned as health professionals to mitigate harmful effects of trauma because they have opportunities for intimate encounters with patients. These encounters afford the nurse time to recognize **trafficking warning signs** (see Table 16.4), consider any possible risk factors, and conduct an appropriate assessment to confirm any suspicions the nurse might have. The culturally competent nurse locates a quiet, private space when possible, establishes a trusting relationship with the patient, and observes the patient for any indications of physical or psychologic trauma or abuse. The nurse engages the patient and seeks honest and open nonjudgmental discussion about the patient's life situation, while demonstrating "acceptance and compassion" (Paton, 2020, "What To Do"). When speaking with the patient, the nurse listens actively and attempts to establish a rapport with the patient that promotes a sense of physical and psychologic safety.

However, even when suffering harsh treatment at the hands of perpetrators, victims who are being trafficked are usually reluctant to share information about their situation out of fear for their own safety or that of family members (Association of Women's Health, Obstetric and Neonatal Nurses, 2016). Perpetrators can manipulate their victims to

TABLE 16.3 ■ PATIENT'S TRAFFICKING RED FLAGS

• Inconsistent history or explanation about the injury or illness	• Is unwilling or hesitant to answer questions about the injury or illness
• Nervousness, fearfulness	• Shows signs of physical abuse, or self-inflicted injuries
• Avoids eye contact; appears withdrawn.	• Makes suicide attempts
• Displays distrusting or disruptive behavior	

Sources: Data from Paton, F. (2020, September 25). *Human trafficking in the health care setting: Red flags nurses need to know.* NurseLabs. https://nurseslabs.com/human-trafficking-health-care-setting-red-flags-nurses-need-know; U.S. Department of Homeland Security. (2020). *Human trafficking 101 information sheet.* https://www.dhs.gov/blue-campaign/materials/human-trafficking-101

TABLE 16.4 ■ WARNING SIGNS OF TRAFFICKING

• No identification
• Inability to keep appointments
• Tattoos or branding
• Accompanied by a person who does not allow the patient to speak or be alone with healthcare staff
• Conflicting stories or misinformation
• May not speak English
• Lacks documentation of age, immunization, and healthcare encounters

Sources: Data from Paton, F. (2020, September 25). *Human trafficking in the health care setting: Red flags nurses need to know.* NurseLabs. https://nurseslabs.com/human-trafficking-health-care-setting-red-flags-nurses-need-know; U.S. Department of Homeland Security. (2020). *Human trafficking 101 information sheet.* https://www.dhs.gov/blue-campaign/materials/human-trafficking-101

believe they are caring for them at the same time they are abusing them. They might also threaten victims about revealing their identity or discussing the situation with authorities. Therefore, nurses must be strategic in maintaining the patient's confidentiality while seeking the appropriate resources and referrals to assist and protect the patient who has experienced or who is currently experiencing trafficking. It is critical that the nurse remembers that this is a potentially life-threatening situation, and the focus should be on protecting the victim against further harm or being retraumatized. Like other victims of prolonged high-stress situations, patients who are determined to be victims of trafficking require **trauma-informed care**.

TRAUMA-INFORMED CARE

In 2014, the Substance Abuse and Mental Health Services Administration (SAMHSA) developed a framework (see Important Websites at the end of the chapter) that could be used among health practitioners, researchers, and trauma survivors to support them in their work to reduce the effects of severe trauma on survivors. Their research resulted in the development of the following concepts relating to trauma: an **event** or series of events or set of circumstances that is **experienced** by an individual as physically or emotionally harmful or life threatening and that has lasting adverse **effects** on that individual's functioning and well-being. The events may have occurred as a single event or a series over time (SAMHSA, 2014). Similar experiences may impact individuals differently; therefore, situations considered traumatic to one person may not be to another. So, it is an individual's unique interpretation of the experience that matters. Adverse effects from a traumatic event may happen immediately or have a delayed response with a lasting impact on that person's ability to cope with the normal stressors of life: to trust relationships; to manage cognitive processes, like memory, attention, and thinking; to regulate behavior; or to control the expression of emotions. Culturally competent nurses incorporate the six principles of SAMHSA's trauma-informed model in their practice: (a) Safety; (b) Trustworthiness and Transparency; (c) Peer Support; (d) Collaboration and Mutuality; (e) Empowerment, Voice, and Choice; and (f) Cultural, Historical, and Gender Issues.

WHAT NURSES CAN DO

The nurse who suspects a patient is a victim of trafficking obtains a history, performs a thorough physical assessment, and utilizes available resources to assist the patient. The nurse should follow the hospital's action plan for trafficking situations if one exists. While ensuring the patient's safety, nurses can offer help and assure the patient that confidentiality will be maintained. The nurse should take care to not force or insist that the patient disclose information they do not wish to disclose as it may cause that person to be retraumatized by reliving their past or current trafficking experiences, posing an internal conflict and creating fear of the perpetrator's retaliation.

Macias-Konstantopoulos (2017) discussed the ethical challenges nurses face when interviewing, assessing, and providing care for patients who have been victims of trafficking. The author discussed the **Ethics of Care Model**, which includes the ethical principles that guide nursing practice in its Code of Ethics: respect for **autonomy, nonmaleficence, beneficence,** and **justice.** Guided by these principles, the culturally competent nurse realizes that regardless of the circumstances or context in which the nurse meets the patient who is a victim of trafficking, every patient deserves dignified and respectful healthcare. This means that the nurse ensures privacy, confidentiality, and an interpreter, if needed. Despite the common use of the term *victim* of trafficking, patients retain their rights of self-determination and decision-making and decide if and when, to disclose their experiences, and what events they reveal. Nonmaleficence obligates healthcare professionals to first do no harm and to act in the patient's best interest (beneficence). It makes sense then that a nurse would seek to remove the trafficked persons from their captors; however, forcibly doing so might place the patient in even greater harm or risk, or cause undue stress, anxiety, or fear. Equally harmful would be "probing for details," by asking personal, embarrassing, and unnecessary questions that can only cause more harm by compelling the patient to relive a difficult and stressful situation. However, when the patient is a child, mandatory reporting laws in all 50 states obligate nurses to report child abuse (Macias-Konstantopoulos, 2017).

When we consider justice or fairness as it relates to survivors of trafficking, they have limited access to healthcare for all the reasons discussed earlier in this chapter. Trafficking victims' focus is largely on surviving, so the crime of trafficking mostly remains concealed. The victims of trafficking appear in minute clinics, urgent care centers, and EDs only when they are in desperate need of services. As the author states, "the unique circumstances surrounding the care of trafficked persons appears to challenge . . . the fair [or just] distribution of resources" (Macias-Konstantopoulos, 2017, p. 83).

Healthcare professionals are at a disadvantage because many have not received the training needed to recognize signs and symptoms of trafficking, or to assess or respond to these patients' needs. Professionals are also faced with weighing the benefits and potential risks of treatment options when the likelihood of nonadherence to the treatment plan and/or medication regime is great, given the inconsistent access to care the trafficked patient may have. In the case of sexually transmitted infections (STIs) and in the treatment of conditions and/or injuries where follow-up care is needed, health professionals must decide on the most practical and effective approach for the patient. They must also consider public health concerns and the potential spread of communicable diseases. The author of this article also advocated implementation into policies and practices plans that include trauma-informed ethics of care, which integrate knowledge of the widespread impact of trauma, the signs and symptoms of trauma, and responses that actively resist retraumatization of victims (Macias-Konstantopoulos, 2017).

Kusterbeck (2023) reviewed 2,780 ED visits and concluded that "[m]ost ED visits for intentional, interpersonal violence-related injuries to youth 10–15 years resulted from family violence" (para. 1). In this study, 19.2% were peer violence-related injuries, but 54.7% involved family violence. The author also notes that more than half of violence-related injuries happen at home. The article reminds us that social-work consults may be needed to evaluate the safety of a child's home and that ED screening for prevention of future violence is critical. Researchers suggest using a standardized tool to screen for factors that identify youth at risk and the appropriate interventions. Under the federal Child Abuse Prevention and Treatment Act, ED and healthcare professionals are mandatory reporters and have a legal requirement to report suspected child abuse to relevant authorities in a timely fashion. When teens present with violent injuries, they should also be screened for trafficking and sex work as well as other forms of trafficking. Since state laws vary regarding the process, it is the responsibility of health professionals to know the specific responsibilities where they practice. Failure to make a timely report of suspected child abuse or neglect can result in criminal, civil, or licensure actions. All states provide reporters with immunity when the report of abuse is made in good faith; that is, the evidence clearly indicates abuse or negligence and the facts of the case are clearly and objectively documented. Quotes with statements from caregivers are an example of objectively documenting the facts. Detailed observations of the child's injuries and behavior are equally important. An assessment of whether the suspected perpetrator will remain in the home after a child's discharge is another important fact to include in the documentation. Any agreed-upon safety measures to protect the child should also be documented in the medical record (Kusterbeck, 2023). In addition, Child Protective Services' (CPS's) planned response with the time frame should be documented as well. If the patient is medically ready for discharge, CPS will determine if the child can safely return home.

SUMMARY

The culturally competent nursing care of trafficked persons is complex and must be evidence based. Healthcare literature offers much information about the scope and impact of human trafficking in the United States on all its citizens and noncitizens. To effectively provide comprehensive care to patients who are recipients of trafficking crimes, nurses must first be educated about the health-related issues affecting the men, women, and children who are victimized. Vigilance is critical in interviewing and assessing patients who present with risk factors, warning signs, or obvious red flags that suggest a need for more careful observation, history taking, or collaboration with health professionals with more experience working with members of this population (Scannel et al., 2018). Teens presenting with violent injuries should be screened for sex trafficking as well. The focus during a nurse's interaction with a suspected victim of trafficking is primarily on maintaining the patient's safety and the provision of optimum care. Regardless of the patient's circumstances, the nurse acts in the patient's best interest. Using an ethical and trauma- informed approach, the nurse respects the patient's right to autonomy and to make the choice to accept offered help or to seek it later. However, in the case of minors (i.e., those under 18 years of age), nurses and other healthcare professionals are mandatory reporters.

IMPORTANT POINTS

- Human trafficking is a violation of human rights, as well as federal, state, and international law, that occurs in almost every country in the world, including the United States.
- Trafficking in persons means making a profit from the sale of individuals who are forced to work as prostitutes or as forced labor in restaurants, factories, farms, or private homes.
- The International Labor Organization estimates that trafficking is a $150-billion industry.
- Types of human trafficking include: sexual exploitation, forced labor, and domestic servitude.
- The three factors that facilitate trafficking are (a) high reward, low risk of being caught; (b) high demand drives the market for greater supply; and (c) systemic inequities and disparities make certain groups more vulnerable to exploitation.
- Myths and misconceptions create barriers to combatting trafficking.
- While women and girls of color are disproportionately vulnerable to sex trafficking, men and boys are also victims of sex trafficking.
- Risk factors for human trafficking include poverty, lack of education, homelessness, unemployment, being a victim of domestic violence or other physical or psychologic abuse, and/or being a member of the LGBTQ community.
- Some indicators of a young person being a victim of trafficking include frequently missing school; running away from home; displaying withdrawn behavior, depression, anxiety, or fear; and/or exhibiting signs of trauma.
- Of 1,169 defendants charged in district court, 92% were male, 63% were White, 18% were Black, 17% were Hispanic, and 95% were U.S. citizens.
- The top four states with the highest numbers of trafficking cases were California, Texas, Florida, and New York. Rhode Island had the lowest rate of trafficking.
- Medical problems associated with trafficking include gynecologic problems, STIs, trauma to the rectum and vagina, multiple abortions, infertility, evidence of abuse like broken teeth, malnutrition, dehydration, substance abuse, and posttraumatic stress disorder (PTSD).
- When caring for trafficking survivors, nurses are encouraged to integrate ethical principles and trauma-informed care in their practice.
- Teens presenting with violent injuries should be screened for sex trafficking as well.
- Nurses must consider trafficking of minors reportable offenses and document all facts objectively.

CASE SCENARIO

Ifekerenma, or Karenma as she is called, was born in a little town in the south-eastern part of Nigeria where she lived with her mother, father, and five siblings. Karenma was the youngest child. The family was very poor, and it had always been her dream to come to the United States. At age 14, one of her father's cousins who lived in America offered to bring her to come to live with him and his American wife. Kerenma was ecstatic; she would go to school in the city in America where her cousin lived and one day become a nurse. Her cousin promised that he would also get her a part-time job working with one of his friends so she would have pocket money. The couple would also acquire citizenship for her, as he and his wife were already American citizens.

In exchange for her good fortune, Karenma agreed to work part-time for her cousin's friend and help with housework in their three-bedroom house. Karenma was happy to have her own small bedroom. Soon after her arrival, Karenma learned that she was being held responsible for all the cooking and cleaning in her cousin's house. She was also driven each morning to a factory that her cousin's friend owned. There, Karenma met several girls her age who worked on an assembly line packaging fruits, vegetables, and dry goods. Karenma was scheduled to work there for 6 days a week from 6 a.m. until 6 p.m. during the entire summer months. In the fall, they would revise her work schedule so she could attend school. Gradually she was also asked to cook for the couple and was rarely allowed out of the house. She was only permitted to go to work, come home, and do her chores.

Soon after her arrival, both her aunt and uncle became verbally and physically abusive, beating and punishing her for not cleaning the house to their satisfaction or sometimes not wanting to go to work. They accused her of being ungrateful for all they were doing for her and sending money to her family as well. Karenma wished she could return to her parents and siblings, but still believed one day she would achieve her dream and did not want to disappoint her family. She would one day make enough money to send for them. One day her uncle's wife beat Karenma so badly with an electric cord that while trying to escape the blows, Karenma tripped and fell down a flight of stairs.

In the ED, the couple told the staff that Karenma had an accident and fell down the steps at home. Karenma never made eye contact with the staff and allowed her uncle to respond to the nurse's questions. The patient was holding her left arm at the elbow and the nurse asked Karenma if her arm hurt. Karenma responded by slowly nodding her head, while looking at her cousins. The nurse asked if Karenma spoke English and they said yes, but she is very shy and not used to being in the United States. The nurse asked the couple to wait in the waiting room while she completed the physical assessment. When offering Karenma the patient gown she noticed how the patient was reluctant to get undressed, but needed help in putting the gown on. The nurse was appalled on seeing the large fresh lacerations and old scars on Karenma's back and legs.

WHAT NURSES NEED TO KNOW ABOUT THEMSELVES

Application of the Staircase Self-Assessment Model: Self Reflection Questions

1. Where are you on the Cultural Comptency Staircase regarding your knowledge of patients who come from this cultural, ethnic, and socioeconomic background? How will you progress to the next level?

2. How comfortable are you about exploring the possibility that the patient is a recent immigrant who is being victimized by trafficking?
3. What about this situation is the most challenging for you?
4. What resources will you need to plan safe, ethical, trauma-informed care for this patient?
5. What barriers to this patient's care have you identified?

Responses to Self-Reflection Questions 4 and 5

Response: What resources will you need to plan safe, ethical, trauma-informed care for this patient?

After performing the physical assessment of this patient, the nurse suspects that there are indications of abuse. After questioning the patient about the source of the lacerations, the nurse should follow any hospital plans that exist for the treatment of patients who are suspected of being abused. An example of such a plan may be found at the Mayo Clinic website: www.mayoclinic.org/diseases-conditions/child-abuse/diagnosis-treatment/drc-20370867.

Because the patient is a minor at age 14, the Mayo Clinic recommends a thorough assessment that includes physical examination, lab tests, x-rays, information about the child's medical history, observation of the child's behavior, observations of interactions between the parents or caregivers and the child, discussions with caregivers, and discussion with the child.

Response: What barriers to this patient's care have you identified?

One major barrier is the limited communication by Karenma, who is reluctant to speak about what happened to her. The nurse establishes a rapport with the patient and attempts to provide an environment of safety

WHAT THE NURSE NEEDS TO KNOW ABOUT THE PATIENT

1. After reviewing the scenario, what facts do you have about the patient?
2. What are the patient's immediate needs?
3. What resources and/or strategies are available to address this patient's healthcare needs?
4. How will you ensure the patient receives optimal trauma-informed culturally competent care?

Responses to Patient Assessment Questions

Response: After reviewing the scenario, what facts do you have about the patient?

Besides knowing that this patient is a minor, the nurse further determines that the couple accompanying the patient are not her parents, but relatives with whom she is now living. In observing the interactions between the child and her caregivers, the nurse considers that the relationship seems strained. The adults speak on Karenma's behalf, not allowing her to respond. Since she is English-speaking and 14 years of age, this behavior is inappropriate. The fact that Karenma does not make eye contact with anyone and appears sad or intimidated is a warning sign or red flag, as are the fresh lacerations and old scars on her back. The account that the caregivers offer about Karenma's injuries does not explain the other old and new injuries.

Response: What are the patient's immediate needs?

An x-ray of the patient's arm is needed to help determine the full extent of this patient's physical injuries. Considering the mounting physical evidence, Karenma's immediate needs include being protected from further abuse by the caregivers and to not provoke any retaliation by them toward Karenma.

Response: What resources and/or strategies are available to address this patient's healthcare needs?

A team approach will be helpful ultimately in addressing the needs of this patient. Ideally, such a team might include nurses, a pediatrician, a social service representative, and a psychotherapist.

Because Karenma is only 14 years of age, this case will need to be reported to the local CPS. The nurse must document all of the facts of the case including conversations with the adults accompanying the patient, Kerenma's own statements, the nurse's observations about the patient's behavior, and the results of the physical assessment. The CPS officials will need to further investigate the situation to determine whether this is a case of child abuse and/or human trafficking and if it is safe for Karenma to return to her cousin's home.

Response: How will you ensure the patient receives optimal trauma-informed culturally competent care?

The nurse in this situation establishes a respectful rapport with all parties in this situation to determine the best approach to provide safe, patient-centered care to Karenma. Recognizing that the patient is in a precarious living situation, the nurse interviews the patient privately and attempts to gain her trust by assuring confidentiality while explaining the patient's rights and her entitlement to be free of physical and emotional abuse. The nurse must also share her obligation to contact CPS, given the teen's age. The follow-up and disposition of the child when medically stable will be determined by hospital policy, the results of the investigation, and the decisions by CPS.

NCLEX®-TYPE QUESTIONS

1. Which statements are true about the problem of human trafficking? *Select all that apply.*
   A. The problem of human trafficking occurs in almost every country around the world.
   B. The United States is one of a few countries not faced with human trafficking.
   C. Human trafficking is a violation of federal, state, and international law.
   D. International labor industries estimate human trafficking to be a $150-billion industry.
   E. The victims and perpetrators of human trafficking are largely foreign nationals.

2. What rationale explains why human trafficking is called a public health emergency? *Select all that apply.*
   A. Victims of trafficking are at high risk for traumatic physical injuries.
   B. Many victims of trafficking acquire communicable diseases.
   C. Victims of trafficking have limited access to healthcare treatment facilities.
   D. Mental health issues including suicide occur among trafficking victims.
   E. Many victims of trafficking are children.

3. Which statement is accurate about perpetrators of human trafficking? *Select all that apply.*
   A. The majority of those engaged in human trafficking are caught and prosecuted.
   B. Most human traffickers are foreign nationals or immigrants living in the United States.
   C. Most defendants charged in district courts were U.S. citizens.
   D. Most human traffickers represent racial minority members.
   E. Traffickers are mostly affluent individuals with connections to foreign government.

4. Which state has consistently had the highest human trafficking rates in the United States?
   A. Rhode Island
   B. New York
   C. Texas
   D. California

5. Which groups of individuals are the most likely targets of human trafficking? *Select all that apply.*
   A. Runaway children
   B. Victims of domestic violence
   C. Victims of child abuse
   D. Individuals living in poverty.
   E. Legal permanent residents of the United States

6. The nurse interviews and examines a patient and considers which of these a "red flag" suggesting human trafficking? *Select all that apply.*
   A. The patient does not make eye contact and seems nervous and anxious.
   B. The nurse notices burn injuries to the patient's back.
   C. The man accompanying the patient responds to the nurse for the patient.
   D. The patient who is female and Asian Indian requests a female nurse.
   E. The patient asks the nurse to explain a medical term.

7. Which statement is true about the incidence of males who are victims of trafficking? *Select all that apply.*
   A. Human trafficking of men is extremely rare.
   B. Males are victims of human trafficking, but it is underreported.
   C. Men can more easily cope with trafficking.
   D. Boys and men are reluctant to reveal incidents of trafficking due to shame and fear of being perceived as gay.
   E. Men and boys who are LGBTQ are vulnerable targets of trafficking.

8. Which of the following are the most likely reasons survivors reluctantly discuss their trafficking situations with health professionals? *Select all that apply.*
   A. Most have bonded or are in love with their captors.
   B. Most victims are untrusting and fear retaliation against them or family members.
   C. Some survivors do not realize they are victims of deceit or manipulation.
   D. Most victims are focused on survival over escape.
   E. Most victims eventually escape without assistance from officials.

9. When determining the probability of a patient being victimized by trafficking, which response by the nurse is appropriate? *Select all that apply.*
   A. Convince the patient to reveal the name and location of their captor to promote safety.
   B. In the case of a child who is a suspected victim of trafficking, the nurse should report the suspicion to immediate supervisors and the Department of Health and Human Services (DHHS) or Child Protective Services (CPS).
   C. Seek a private location to interview the patient suspected of being a victim of trafficking.
   D. Give a reluctant patient information about how to follow-up later to obtain help.
   E. Report injuries that look suspicious to the police with or without the patient's permission.

10. Which is a strategy nurses can use to plan care for trafficking persons? *Select all that apply.*
    A. Follow the hospital's action plan for working with trafficked persons.
    B. Seek programs that provide training in caring for trafficked persons.
    C. Consider the ethical principles in the nurses' Code of Ethics as a guide to inform care.
    D. Observe for warning signs and red flags.
    E. Integrate trauma-informed care in caring for trafficked patients.

ANSWERS TO NCLEX QUESTIONS

1. A, C, and D
2. A, B, C, D, and E
3. C
4. D

5. A, B, C, and D
6. A, B, and C
7. B, D, and E
8. B, C, and D

9. B, C, D, and E
10. A, B, C, D, and E

AMERICAN ASSOCIATION OF COLLEGES OF NURSING COMPETENCIES ADDRESSED IN THIS CHAPTER

1. Apply knowledge of social and cultural factors that affect nursing and healthcare across multiple contexts.
2. Use relevant data sources and best evidence in providing culturally competent care.
3. Advocate for social justice, including commitment to the health of vulnerable populations and elimination of healthcare disparities.

 SPRINGER PUBLISHING CONNECT™ | A robust set of instructor resources designed to supplement this text is located at http://connect.springerpub.com/content/book/978-0-8261-8302-6. Qualifying instructors may request access by emailing textbook@springerpub.com.

REFERENCES

Association of Women's Health, Obstetric and Neonatal Nurses. (2016). Human trafficking. *Journal of Obstetric, Gynecologic & Neonatal Nursing*, 51(6), E1–E3. https://doi.org/10.1016/j.jogn.2016.04.001

Callahan, M. (2019, August 16). Human trafficking, the problem is much bigger than we think. *Northeastern Global News*. https://news.northeastern.edu/2019/08/16/human-trafficking-in-the-us-is-a-much-bigger-problem-than-we-think

Drug Enforcement Administration. (2022). *DEA warns of brightly-colored fentanyl used to target young Americans*. https://www.dea.gov/press-releases/2022/08/30/dea-warns-brightly-colored-fentanyl-used-target-young-americans

Friedman, S. A. (2013). *And boys too*. ECPAT USA. https://static1.squarespace.com/static/594970e91b631b3571be12e2/t/5977b2dacd0f688b2b89e6f0/1501016795183/ECPAT-USA_AndBoysToo.pdf

Human Trafficking Collaborative: University of Michigan. (2019). *Who are the victims*? https://humantrafficking.umich.edu/about-human-trafficking/who-are-the-victims/

King, L. (2009, January 30). *International law and human trafficking*. United Nations Office on Drugs and Crimes. https://sherloc.unodc.org/cld/uploads/res/bibliography/international_law_and_human_trafficking_html/InternationalLaw.pdf

Kusterbeck, S. (2023). Family violence implicated in injury-related ED visits. *Relias Media*. https://www.reliasmedia.com/articles/149042-family-violence-implicated-in-injury-related-ed-visits

Lauger, A. D., Kaeble, D., & Motivans, M. (2022, October). *Human trafficking data collection activities, 2022*. U.S. Department of Justice, Office of Justice Programs, Bureau of Justice Statistics. https://bjs.ojp.gov/sites/g/files/xyckuh236/files/media/document/htdca22.pdf

Macias-Konstantopoulos, W. L. (2017). Caring for the trafficked patient: Ethical challenges and recommendations for health care professionals. *AMA Journal of Ethics*, 19(1), 80–90. https://doi.org/10.1001/journalofethics.2017.19.1.msoc2-1701

Morris, G. (2023). How nurses can recognize and report human trafficking. *Nurse Journal*. https://nursejournal.org/articles/how-nurses-recognize-and-report-human-trafficking

Office on Trafficking in Persons. (2019, February 20). *Myths and facts about human trafficking*. https://www.acf.hhs.gov/otip/about/myths-facts-human-trafficking

Paton, F. (2020, September 25). *Human trafficking in the health care setting: Red flags nurses need to know*. NurseLabs. https://nurseslabs.com/human-trafficking-health-care-setting-red-flags-nurses-need-know

Scannell, M., MacDonald, A. E., Berger, A., & Boyer, N. (2018). Human trafficking: How nurses can make a difference. *Journal of Forensic Nursing*, 14(2), 117–121. https://doi.org/10.1097/JFN.0000000000000203

Substance Abuse and Mental Health Services Administration. (2014). *SAMHSA's concept of trauma and guidance for a trauma-informed approach*. https://ncsacw.acf.hhs.gov/userfiles/files/SAMHSA_Trauma.pdf

UNICEF. (2016, January 6) *How trafficking exists today*. UNICEF USA. https://www.unicefusa.org/stories/how-trafficking-exists-today

U.S. Department of Labor. (2015). *Fact sheet: The department of labor expands its support of victims of human trafficking and other crimes*. https://www.dol.gov/general/immigration/20150402u%26tfactsheet

The White House. (2021, December 4). *Fact sheet: The national action plan to combat human trafficking (NAP)*. https://www.whitehouse.gov/briefing-room/statements-releases/2021/12/03/fact-sheet-the-national-action-plan-to-combat-human-trafficking-nap

World Population Review. (2023). *Human trafficking statistics by state*. https://worldpopulationreview.com/state-rankings/human-trafficking-statistics-by-state

Youth.gov. (n.d.). *Human trafficking: The problem*. Retrieved January 8, 2024, from https://youth.gov/youth-topics/trafficking-of-youth/the-problem

IMPORTANT WEBSITES

Mayo Clinic Diagnosis and Treatment Plan for Suspected Child Abuse. Retrieved from https://www.mayoclinic.org/diseases-conditions/child-abuse/diagnosis-treatment/drc-20370867

The National Action Plan and The White House Action Plan. Retrieved from www.whitehouse.gov/wp-content/uploads/2021/12/National-Action-Plan-to-Combat-Human-Trafficking.pdf

National Human Trafficking Hotline. Retrieved from https://humantraffickinghotline.org/en

National Human Trafficking Resource Center. Retrieved from www.eeoc.gov/national-human-trafficking-resource-center

Substance Abuse and Mental Health Services Administration Guidance for a Trauma-Informed Approach. Retrieved from https://store.samhsa.gov/product/SAMHSA-s-Concept-of-Trauma-and-Guidance-for-a-Trauma-Informed-Approach/SMA14-4884

U.S. Department of Health and Human Services. Retrieved from www.hhs.gov

Index